THIRD

The Phlebotomy Textbook

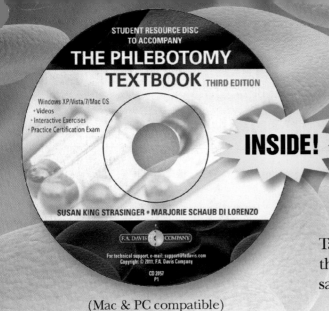 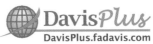
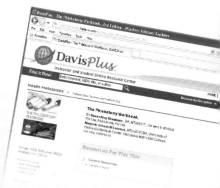
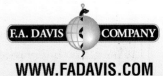

THIRD EDITION

The Phlebotomy Textbook

Susan King Strasinger, DA, MLS(ASCP)
Faculty Associate
Clinical Laboratory Science Program
The University of West Florida
Pensacola, Florida

Marjorie Schaub Di Lorenzo, MLS(ASCP)SH
Phlebotomy Technician Program Coordinator
Nebraska Methodist College
Omaha, Nebraska

Adjunct Instructor
Clinical Laboratory Science Program
University of Nebraska Medical Center
Omaha, Nebraska

F.A. Davis Company • Philadelphia

F. A. Davis Company
1915 Arch Street
Philadelphia, PA 19103
www.fadavis.com

Printed in the United States of America

Last digit indicates print number: 10 9 8 7 6 5

Senior Acquisitions Editor: Christa Fratantoro
Manager of Content Development: George W. Lang
Developmental Editor: Karen Carter
Art and Design Manager: Carolyn O'Brien

As new scientific information becomes available through basic and clinical research, recommended treatments and drug therapies undergo changes. The author(s) and publisher have done everything possible to make this book accurate, up to date, and in accord with accepted standards at the time of publication. The author(s), editors, and publisher are not responsible for errors or omissions or for consequences from application of the book, and make no warranty, expressed or implied, in regard to the contents of the book. Any practice described in this book should be applied by the reader in accordance with professional standards of care used in regard to the unique circumstances that may apply in each situation. The reader is advised always to check product information (package inserts) for changes and new information regarding dose and contraindications before administering any drug. Caution is especially urged when using new or infrequently ordered drugs.

Library of Congress Cataloging-in-Publication Data

Strasinger, Susan King.
   The phlebotomy textbook / Susan King Strasinger, Marjorie Schaub Di Lorenzo. – 3rd ed.
      p. ; cm.
   Rev. ed. of: The phlebotomy workbook / Susan King Strasinger, Marjorie Schaub Di Lorenzo. 2nd ed. c2003.
   Includes bibliographical references and index.
   ISBN 978-0-8036-2057-5
   1. Phlebotomy–Practice. I. Di Lorenzo, Marjorie Schaub, 1953- II. Title.
   [DNLM: 1. Phlebotomy–methods. 2. Blood Specimen Collection–methods. 3. Clinical Laboratory Techniques. QY 25]
   RB45.15S774 2011
   616.07'561–dc22

                                                            2010040771

To Harry, you will always be my editor-in-chief.
SKS

To my husband, Scott, and my children,
Michael, Christopher, and Lauren, and daughter-in-law Kathy,
for their encouragement, patience, and support.
MSD

Preface

Significant updates and formatting changes have been made to *The Phlebotomy Textbook*, 3rd edition. The title of this 3rd edition has been changed to reflect the technical advances that offer student and instructor interaction by computer rather than the previous written format using perforated workbook pages. *The Phlebotomy Textbook*, 3rd edition, remains comprehensive, integrating theory and procedures with particular attention to preexamination variables and safety procedures. Detailed procedure explanations are accompanied by the visual reinforcement of boxes, tables, highlighted technical and safety tips, and preanalytical considerations. Recognizing the expanding role of the phlebotomist, this textbook includes additional information on point-of-care testing, arterial puncture, and central venous access devices, as well as specimen processing and other special collection procedures such as bone marrow and other body fluid collections.

New additions to the third edition include key points to highlight important information at the end of each chapter, full-color step-by-step instruction for all procedures, review questions in a multiple-choice format to prepare for certification examinations, clinical situations to emulate actual patient scenarios and promote critical thinking and evaluation, and a student CD-ROM. Included at the back of the text, the student CD-ROM contains interactive exercises, video clips of venipuncture and dermal procedures, and a mock certification exam with 100 questions.

Additional student resources can be found on the DavisPlus website. These resources include student quizzes and animations that demonstrate concepts such as reasons for failure to obtain blood collection, hemolysis, blood flow through the heart, and carbon dioxide/oxygen transport.

For educators who adopt this text for their course, an Instructor's Resource CD-ROM is available. This valuable CD-ROM contains the following educator ancillaries:

- Instructor's Guide with Internet resources, lecture outlines, additional clinical situations, critical thinking review questions, answers to study questions and clinical situation exercises, procedure evaluation forms, and sample course schedules.
- ExamView Pro test generator with more than 1200 questions.
- PowerPoint presentation with lecture points and illustrations.
- Image ancillary including over 300 figures from the text.

These instructor ancillaries are also available via the instructor-only, password-protected area on our DavisPlus website.

As with previous editions, this edition is designed to provide up-to-date and accurate information that can be used as an instructional text for phlebotomy technician programs, medical laboratory technician and medical laboratory science programs, medical assisting programs, and cross-training of nurses and other allied health personnel. It is an excellent reference for health-care professionals currently practicing phlebotomy, for in-house training programs, or for independent study for national certification examinations and employee continuing education.

The format of this book has been changed to arrange the chapters in a logical organization that can be used as a syllabus for teaching the course. Each chapter builds on information from previous chapters. The book is divided into four sections.

Section 1, Phlebotomy and the Health-Care Field, describes the role of the phlebotomist in the health-care delivery system. Major topics include ethical, legal, and regulatory issues; clinical laboratory personnel and laboratory tests and their clinical correlations; interpersonal and communications skills; and the latest safety and infection control requirements.

Section 2, Body Systems, presents the anatomy and physiology of the body systems and includes the disorders and diagnostic tests for each system. Emphasis is placed on the circulatory system, including the composition of blood, and the structure and function of the vascular and cardiac system. A chapter on medical terminology is included to facilitate understanding and communication in the health-care setting.

Section 3, Phlebotomy Techniques, describes the various types of phlebotomy equipment and phlebotomy theory and procedures. Venipuncture complications, preexamination variables, special collection techniques, and dermal puncture are covered. A chapter on quality phlebotomy and management that addresses quality assessment is included.

Section 4, Additional Techniques, presents information on arterial blood collection, point-of-care testing, and the collection and processing of nonblood specimens, such as bone marrow and other body fluids. Computer applications and the phlebotomist's role using a LIS is an important part of this unit.

The Phlebotomy Textbook, 3rd edition, is written to comply with the guidelines established by national certifying organizations and the essentials published by the National Accrediting Agency for Clinical Laboratory Science (NAACLS). All procedures are written in accordance with the standards developed by the Clinical and Laboratory Standards Institute (CLSI) and the Occupational Safety and Health Administration (OSHA), thus enabling this text to be used as a current reference in any health-care setting.

Highlighted features of this 3rd edition include:

- Key terms and objectives at the beginning of each chapter to emphasize important concepts.
- Increased numbers of colored illustrations, photographs, diagrams, charts, and tables to easily visualize important information.
- **Full-color step-by-step procedures with instructions to visualize the technique.**
- Special collection procedures, including venous access devices, arterial blood collection, bone marrow collection, and point-of-care testing.
- Color-highlighted Technical Tips to emphasize important points and to help avoid complications.
- **Color-highlighted Safety Tips to protect health-care workers and patients.**
- **Color-highlighted Preexamination Considerations to avoid erroneous laboratory test results.**
- Numerous clinical situation exercises to facilitate critical thinking.
- An expanded legal chapter including the prevention of medical errors, confidentiality, malpractice, incident reporting, informed consent, and HIV consent.
- Correlation of laboratory tests, diagnostic procedures, diseases, and disorders for each body system.
- **Key Points at the end of each chapter to summarize important information.**
- **Multiple-choice study questions to simulate certification examination questions.**
- Cross-reference icons that draw attention to related content in other chapters.
- Appendices listing collection requirements for frequently ordered laboratory tests, answers to study questions and clinical situations, and abbreviations.
- A complete color tube guide listing the different types of collection tubes, the additives, the number of inversions required, and the laboratory uses of the tubes.

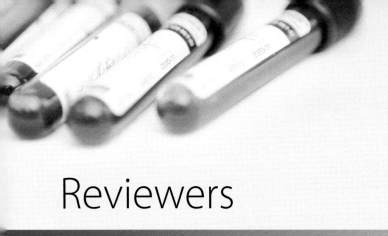

Reviewers

Wayne Aguiar, MS, MT(ASCP)SM
Director, Phlebotomy and Clinical Laboratory Education Programs
Hartford Hospital
School of Allied Health
Hartford, Connecticut

Marcia A. Armstrong, MS, MLS
Director Emeritus, Medical Laboratory Technician and Phlebotomy Programs
University of Hawaii–Kapiolani Community College
Health Sciences Department
Honolulu, Hawaii

Carol E. Becker, MS, MLS(ASCP)
Program Director
OSF Saint Francis Medical Center
School of Clinical Laboratory Science
School of Histotechnology
Peoria, Illinois

Wilbert S. Ching, BSMT, CPT (NPA)
Phlebotomy Instructor
Quinebaug Valley Community College
Putnam, Connecticut
Program Coordinator and Instructor (Health Services)
American Red Cross of Central Massachusetts
Worcester, Massachusetts

Susan Lynne Day, BSMT(ASCP)
Adjunct Professor/Instructor
Florida State College at Jacksonville
Medical Lab Technology Department
Jacksonville, Florida

Cheri Goretti, MA, BSMT(ASCP), CMA (AAMA)
Professor & Director, Medical Assisting and Allied Health Programs
Quinebaug Valley Community College
Allied Health Department
Danielson, Connecticut

W. Anne Mitchell-Hinton, MT(ASCP), MA, EdD, EMT-B
Professor, Medical Laboratory Technology
Southwest Tennessee Community College
Allied Health Sciences Department
Memphis, Tennessee

Travis Miles Price, MS, MT(ASCP)
Assistant Professor
Clinical Laboratory Sciences Program
Weber State University
College of Health Professions
Ogden, Utah

Sharon Theresa Scott, BS, CLA (ASCP)
Assistant Professor
Ivy Tech Community College
School of Health Sciences
Michigan City, Indiana

Cathy Soto, PhD, MBA, CMA
Director, Medical Assisting Program
El Paso Community College
El Paso, Texas

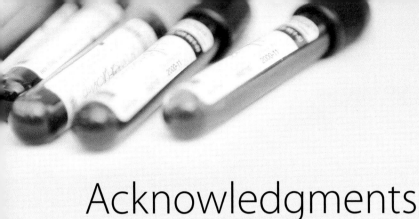

Acknowledgments

We wish to thank the many individuals who have spent much time and effort toward the success of this book and accompanying student and instructor CDs.

We are greatly indebted to the many dedicated professionals at Methodist Hospital for their enthusiasm and willingness in providing us with technical expertise and photographic opportunities. We would particularly like to thank Diane Wolff, MLT(ASCP), Phlebotomy Team Leader, for always being available to share her expertise; to provide charts, forms, and procedures; and to organize the photographic component; and Brenda Franks, MLS(ASCP), POCT Coordinator, for her invaluable resources. Peggy Simpson, MS, MLS(ASCP), Laboratory Director, Danville Memorial Hospital, has been a valuable resource for the updated quality management chapter.

We also appreciate the encouragement and dedication from the supportive team at F. A. Davis. Special thanks go to Christa Fratantoro, Senior Acquisitions Editor, Health Professions; George Lang, Manager of Content Development; Karen Carter, Developmental Editor; Yvonne Gillam, Developmental Editor; Elizabeth Egan, Marketing Manager; Elizabeth Stepchin, Developmental Associate; David Orzechowski, Managing Editor; Cassie Carey, Project Manager at Graphic World Publishing Services; and Tim McCormick at Billings Photography.

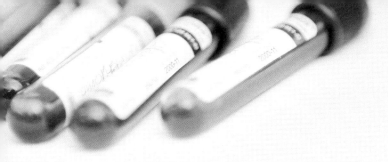

Contents in Brief

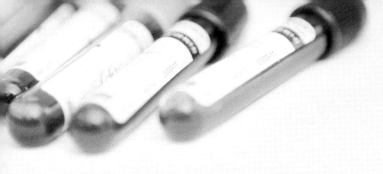

Contents

Phlebotomy and the Health-Care Field

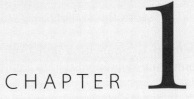

CHAPTER 1

Phlebotomy and the Health-Care Delivery System

Learning Objectives

Upon completion of this chapter, the reader will be able to:

1. State the traditional and expanding duties of the phlebotomist.
2. Describe the professional characteristics that are important for a phlebotomist.
3. Discuss the importance of communication and interpersonal skills for the phlebotomist within the laboratory, with patients, and with personnel in other departments of the hospital.
4. State and describe the three components of communication.
5. List the barriers to communication and methods to overcome them.
6. Describe a phlebotomist using correct listening and body language skills.
7. State six rules of proper telephone etiquette.
8. Define cultural diversity and discuss the actions needed by a phlebotomist when encountering cultural diversity.
9. State the competencies expected of a certified phlebotomist.
10. Describe the functions of the nursing, support, fiscal, and professional hospital service areas and the functions of the departments contained in these services.
11. Describe the different types of health-care settings in which a phlebotomist may be employed.

Key Terms

Accreditation
Alternative medicine
Certification
Confidentiality
Continuing education
Cross-training
Cultural diversity
Decentralization
Diagnostic related groups (DRGs)
Phlebotomy
Professionalism
Samples
Specimens
Zone of comfort

Defined as "an incision into a vein," phlebotomy is one of the oldest medical procedures, dating back to the early Egyptians. The practice of "bloodletting" was used to cure disease and maintain the body in a state of well-being. Hippocrates believed that disease was caused by an excess of body fluids, including blood, bile, and phlegm, and that removal of the excess would cause the body to return to or maintain a healthy state. Techniques for bloodletting included suction cup devices with lancets that pulled blood from the incision; the application of blood-sucking worms, called "leeches," to an incision; and barber surgery, in which blood from an incision produced by the barber's razor was collected in a bleeding bowl. The familiar red and white striped barber pole symbolizes this last technique and represents red blood and white bandages and the pole that the patients held on to during the procedure. Bloodletting is now called "therapeutic phlebotomy" and is used as a treatment for only a small number of blood disorders. It is performed using equipment designed to minimize patient discomfort and with aseptic techniques.

PHLEBOTOMY NOW

At present, the primary role of *phlebotomy* is the collection of blood *samples* for laboratory analysis to diagnose and monitor medical conditions. Because of the increased number and complexity of laboratory tests, phlebotomy has become a specialized area of clinical laboratory practice and has brought about the creation of the job title "phlebotomist." This development supplements, but does not replace, the previous practice, in which laboratory employees both collected and analyzed the *specimens*. Phlebotomy still remains a part of laboratory training programs for medical laboratory technicians and scientists because phlebotomists are not available at all times and in all situations.

The specialization of phlebotomy has expanded rapidly and with it the role of the phlebotomist, who is no longer just someone who "takes blood" but is recognized as a key player on the health-care team. In this expanded role, the phlebotomist must be familiar with the health-care system, the anatomy and physiology related to laboratory testing and phlebotomy, the collection and transport requirements for tests performed in all sections of the laboratory, documentation and patient records, and the interpersonal skills needed to provide quality patient care.

These changes have brought about the need to replace on-the-job training with structured phlebotomy training programs leading to certification in phlebotomy. Because the phlebotomist is often the only personal contact a patient has with the laboratory, he or she can leave a lasting impression of the quality of the laboratory and the entire health-care setting.

DUTIES OF THE PHLEBOTOMIST

A phlebotomist is a person trained to obtain blood samples primarily by venipuncture and microtechniques. In addition to technical, clerical, and interpersonal skills, the phlebotomist must develop strong organizational skills to handle a heavy workload efficiently and maintain accuracy, often under stressful conditions.

Traditional Duties

Major traditional duties and responsibilities of the phlebotomist include:

1. Correct identification and preparation of the patient before sample collection
2. Collection of the appropriate amount of blood by venipuncture or dermal puncture for the specified tests
3. Selection of the appropriate sample containers for the specified tests
4. Correct labeling of all samples with the required information
5. Appropriate transportation of samples back to the laboratory in a timely manner
6. Effective interaction with patients and hospital personnel
7. Processing of samples for delivery to the appropriate laboratory departments
8. Performance of computer operations and record-keeping pertaining to phlebotomy
9. Observation of all safety regulations, quality control checks, and preventive maintenance procedures
10. Attendance at continuing education programs

Phlebotomy and the Changing Health-Care System

In recent years, changes to increase the efficiency and cost effectiveness of the health-care delivery system have affected the duties of phlebotomists in many institutions.

Efficiency can be increased by eliminating the need to move patients to centralized testing areas and the necessity for health-care personnel to travel from a central testing area to the patient's room and then back to the testing area. These changes can range from the *cross-training* of persons already located in nursing units to perform basic interdisciplinary bedside procedures to the actual relocation of specialized radiology and clinical laboratory equipment and personnel to the patient-care units. This also may be referred to as patient-focused care.

Considering the amount of time spent by phlebotomists traveling to and from the laboratory to patient-care units, *decentralization* of phlebotomy was one of the first changes to occur. This decentralization has been accomplished by either cross-training personnel working in the patient units to perform phlebotomy or transferring phlebotomists to the patient units and cross-training them to perform basic patient-care tasks. Based on institutional protocol, phlebotomists also may be trained to perform more advanced blood collection procedures.

Additional Duties of Phlebotomists

1. Training other health-care personnel to perform phlebotomy
2. Monitoring the quality of samples collected on the units
3. Evaluation of protocols associated with sample collection
4. Performing and monitoring point-of-care testing (POCT) (see Chapter 15)
5. Performing electrocardiograms
6. Performing measurement of patient's vital signs
7. Collection of arterial blood samples (see Chapter 14)
8. Collection of samples from central venous access devices (CVADs) (see Chapter 11)

PROFESSIONAL AND PERSONAL CHARACTERISTICS FOR PHLEBOTOMISTS

Phlebotomists are part of a service-oriented industry, and specific personal and professional characteristics are necessary for them to be successful in this area.

There are many characteristics associated with *professionalism* as shown in Box 1-1. All of them are important and can be related to any professon. In this

> **BOX 1-1 Characteristics Associated With Professionalism**
>
> Dependable, cooperative, committed
> Compassionate, courteous, respectful
> Integrity, honesty, competence
> Organized, responsible, flexible
> Appearance
> Communication

chapter they are related to phlebotomy. It is important for phlebotomists to understand that they are the actual face of the laboratory because they are the people who interact with the patients. This is why professionalism and personal characteristics are discussed in the first chapter.

Dependable, Cooperative, Committed

Laboratory testing begins with sample collection and relies on the phlebotomist to report to work whenever scheduled and on time. Phlebotomy schedules are designed to accommodate the expected volume of work. Failure to appear or arriving late puts additional pressure on the staff members present. Only a very serious reason should prevent you from not showing up for scheduled work days.

Working in health care is not always routine. Emergencies and other disruptions occur. Be willing to demonstrate your commitment to your job and your cooperation to assist fellow employees. A committed phlebotomist attends staff meetings, reads pertinent memoranda, and observes notices placed on bulletin boards or in newsletters.

Compassionate, Courteous, Respectful

Phlebotomists deal with sick, anxious, and frightened patients every day. They must be sensitive to their needs, understand a patient's concern about a possible diagnosis or just the fear of a needle, and take the time to reassure each patient. A smile and a cheerful tone of voice are simple techniques that can put a patient more at ease. Courteous phlebotomists introduce themselves to the patients before they approach them. This also aids in identifying the patient as you can then ask them to state their name in the same conversation.

Phlebotomists must also understand and respect the *cultural diversity* of their patients. Cultural diversity includes not only language but also religious beliefs, customs, and values. Do not expect every patient to respond to you in the same way and do not force your mannerisms and approach on them. This is discussed later in this chapter under "Communication Skills."

Honesty, Integrity, Competence

The phlebotomist should never hesitate to admit a mistake, because a misidentified patient or mislabeled sample can be critical to patient safety. Patient *confidentiality* must be protected, and patient information is never discussed with anyone who does not have a professional need to know it. Keep in mind that the cafeteria and elevators are used by visitors and relatives not just hospital employees, and hospital employees can have family members and neighbors as patients.

 Technical Tip 1-1. The legal aspects of maintaining patient confidentiality are covered in Chapter 3.

Phlebotomists must demonstrate competence in the procedures they are trained to perform. However, overconfidence in one's abilities can result in serious errors. Never perform a procedure that you have not been trained to perform. When faced with this situation do not hesitate to ask for assistance from someone more experienced.

 Safety Warning 1-1. Studies in which participants rated themselves on their knowledge of a particular subject and then took a test on that subject show that almost everyone overrated themselves.

Organized, Responsible, Flexible

A patient observing a phlebotomist struggling to locate the necessary collection equipment becomes nervous about the phlebotomist's ability. Always maintain an organized and well-stocked collection tray or station. Not only do phlebotomists need to organize their collection equipment, they must also organize and prioritize their work. Phlebotomists on the morning shift receive many collection requisitions when they arrive at work. These collections must be made before the patients can receive breakfast. For efficiency the requisitions must be organized regarding patient location.

 Technical Tip 1-2. The few minutes it takes to organize can save you and others many minutes of anxiety.

 Technical Tip 1-3. When organizing requistitions, check to be sure that you have all of the patient's requisitions. Missing a requistion can result in patient receiving an additional puncture.

 Technical Tip 1-4. The abbreviation for work that must be done immediately, as in an emergency, is STAT or stat.

Appearance

Each organization specifies the dress code that it considers most appropriate, but common to all institutions is a neat and clean appearance that portrays a professional attitude to the patient.

Appearance of the phlebotomist is the first thing noticed by a patient. Remember first impressions are lasting impressions often made within 30 seconds and the phlebotomist represents the entire laboratory staff. In general a sloppy appearance indicates a tendency toward sloppy performance.

General Appearance Guidelines

1. Clothing and lab coats must be clean and unwrinkled. Clothing worn under the laboratory coat should be conservative and meet institutional requirements. Lab coats must be completely buttoned and completely cover clothing.
2. Shoes must be clean, polished, closed toed, and skid-proof.
3. If jewelry is worn, it must be conservative. Dangling jewelry including earrings can be grabbed by a patient or become tangled in bedside equipment. Many institutions do not permit facial piercings and tattoos; if present, they must be completely covered. Makeup must also be conservatively applied.
4. Perfume and cologne are usually not recommended or must be kept to a minimum. Many persons are allergic to certain fragrances. Remember the phlebotomist works in close contact with the patient and the smell of perfume can be particularly disturbing to a sick person.
5. Hair including facial hair must be clean, neat, and trimmed. Long hair must be neatly

pulled back. Like jewelry, long hair can become tangled in equipment or pulled by the patient. Long hair hanging near an infectious patient can transport the infection to your next patient.

6. Personal hygiene is extremely important because of close patient contact, and careful attention should be paid to bathing and the use of deodorants and mouthwashes.

7. Fingernails must be clean and short. Based on the Centers for Disease Control and Prevention (CDC) Handwashing Guidelines, artifical nail extenders are not allowed.

Communication Skills

Good communication skills are needed for the phlebotomist to function as the liaison between the laboratory and the patients, their family and visitors, and other health-care personnel. The three components of communication—verbal skills, listening skills, and nonverbal skills or body language—are needed for effective communication. Of interest is the fact that verbal and listening skills make up approximately 20 percent of communication and nonverbal skills contribute approximately 80 percent. The message you are verbally giving may be totally misinterpreted because of your body language.

Verbal Skills

Verbal skills enable phlebotomists to introduce themselves, explain the procedure, reassure the patient, and help assure the patient that the procedure is being competently performed. The tone of your voice and emphasis on certain words also is important.

Barriers to verbal communication that must be considered include physical handicaps such as hearing impairment; patient emotions; and the level of patient education, age, and language proficiency. The phlebotomist who recognizes these barriers is better equipped to communicate with the patient. Table 1-1 provides methods to use when verbal communication barriers are encountered.

Listening Skills

Listening skills are a key component of communication. Active listening involves:

- Looking directly and attentively at the patient
- Encouraging the patient to express feelings, anxieties, and concerns

TABLE 1-1 • Verbal Communication Barriers

BARRIER	METHODS TO OVERCOME
Hearing impairment	Speak loudly and clearly
	Look directly at patient to facilitate lip-reading
	Communicate in writing
Patient emotions	Speak calmly and slowly
	Do not appear rushed or disinterested
Age and education levels	Avoid medical jargon, you are collecting a blood sample rather than performing a phlebotomy
	Use age-appropriate phrases
Non–English-speaking	Locate a hospital-based interpreter
	Use hand signals, show equipment, etc.
	Remain calm, smiling, and reassuring

- Allowing the patient time to describe why he or she is concerned
- Providing feedback to the patient through appropriate responses
- Encouraging patient communication by asking questions

Nonverbal Skills

Nonverbal skills (body language) include facial expressions, posture, and eye contact. If you walk briskly into the room, smile, and look directly at the patient while talking, you demonstrate positive body language. This makes patients feel that they are important and that you care about them and your work (Fig. 1-1). Conversely, shuffling into the room, avoiding eye contact, and gazing out the window while the patient is talking are examples of negative body language and indicate boredom and disinterest in patients and their tests.

Allowing patients to maintain their *zone of comfort* (space) is important in phlebotomy even though you must be close to them to collect the sample. Table 1-2 shows the acceptable zones of comfort for Americans.

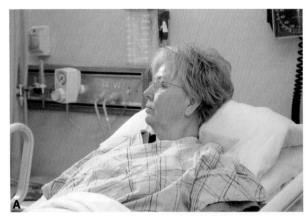
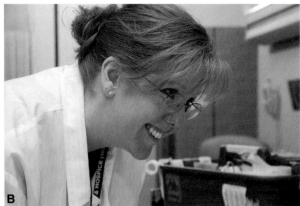
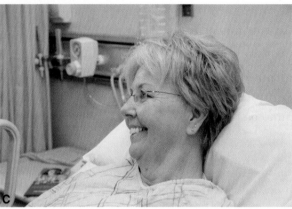

FIGURE 1-1 Patient reactions. A, Notice the unhappy face on the patient as she waits for the phlebotomist to enter. B, Smiling phlebotomist greets the patient. C, Patient reacts to phlebotomist's greeting.

TABLE 1-2 ● American Zones of Comfort	
ZONE	AMOUNT OF DISTANCE
Intimate	2 feet
Personal	2 to 4 feet
Social	4 to 12 feet
Public	Greater than 12 feet

The zones will vary among different cultures. Notice in Figure 1-2 the phlebotomist does not closely appoach the patient during his or her introduction and maintains a reasonable distance even when the patient first extends his or her arm.

Cultural Diversity

Diversity in our population includes more than just the diversity encountered with verbal communication. In addition to language, culture includes the integration of customs, beliefs, religion, and values. All of these differences can affect patient care and communication. Understanding of these cultural differences is important for phlebotomists as they are the laboratory member with the most patient contact.

The Joint Commission (JC) has develped guidelines for health-care organizations to integrate cultural competence into their facilities. Providing employees with seminars, workshops, and materials addressing cultural diversity is included in the guidelines.

General Cultural Diversity Guidelines for Phlebotomists

1. Approach all patients with a smile and use a friendly tone of voice.
2. Be alert to patient reactions to your approach and direct your actions to accommodate them. Do not force your style on them.
3. Do not stereotype a particular culture; not all people of same ethnic culture react in the same manner.

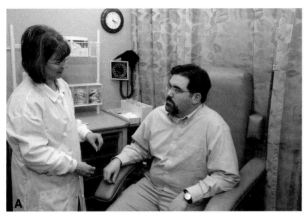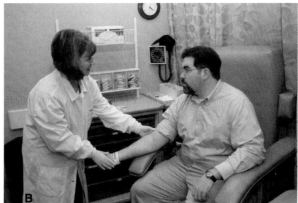

FIGURE 1-2 Phlebotomist greeting a patient. A, Phlebotomist standing away from the patient to introduce herself. B, Phlebotomist explaining the procedure and still maintaining distance.

4. Remember the amount of personal space varies not only among people but also among cultures. Certain cultures are not as welcoming to touching as we might expect them to be. Other cultures may reach for you while you are talking.
5. Plan to spend additional time explaining procedures and patient instructions. Be sure instructions are understood by asking the patient to repeat the instructions to you. In some cultures nodding is considered a sign of politeness and not understanding.
6. Above all, show respect for their diversity.

Telephone Skills

Telephone skills are essential for phlebotomists. The phlebotomy department frequently acts as a type of switchboard for the rest of the laboratory because of its location in the central processing area. This is a prime example of the phlebotomist's role as a liaison for the laboratory, and poor telephone skills affect the image of the laboratory. Phlebotomists should have a thorough understanding of the telephone system regarding transferring calls, placing calls on hold, and paging personnel.

To observe the rules of proper telephone etiquette:

- Answer the phone promptly and politely, stating the name of the department and your name.
- Always check for an emergency before putting someone on hold, and return to calls that are on hold as soon as possible. This may require returning the current call after you have collected the required information.
- Keep writing materials beside the phone to record information such as the location of emergency blood collections, requests for test results, and numbers for returning calls.
- Make every attempt to help callers, and if you cannot help them, transfer them to another person or department that can. Give callers the number to which you are transferring them in case the call is dropped during the transfer.
- Provide accurate and consistent information by keeping current with laboratory policies, looking up information published in department manuals, or asking a supervisor.
- Speak clearly and make sure you understand what the caller is asking and that he or she understands the information you are providing. This is done by repeating what the caller has asked and asking the caller to repeat the information you have given.
- Goal 2 of the National Patient Safety Goals is to improve effectiveness of communication among caregivers. The goal states that for verbal or telephone orders or telephone reporting of critical test results, the individual giving the order or test result verifies the complete order or test result by having the person receiving the information record and read back the complete order or test result.

PHLEBOTOMY EDUCATION AND CERTIFICATION

Structured phlebotomy education programs have been developed by hospitals, accredited colleges, and technical institutions and are also a part of medical laboratory technician and clinical laboratory science/medical technology programs. The length and format of these programs vary considerably. However, the goal of providing the health-care field with phlebotomists who are knowledgeable in all aspects of phlebotomy is universal. The training programs are designed to incorporate a combination of classroom instruction and clinical practice. Most of them follow guidelines developed by national phlebotomy organizations to ensure the quality of the program, to meet national *accreditation* requirements, and to prepare graduates for a national *certification* examination (Box 1-2).

All phlebotomists should obtain certification from a nationally recognized professional organization because it serves to enhance their position within the health-care field and documents the quality of their skills and knowledge. Certification examinations can be taken on completion of a structured educational program that meets the standards of the certifying organization or by documentation of experience that meets specified standards. Certification examinations are offered by the organizations listed in Table 1-3. Phlebotomists who attain a satisfactory score can indicate this achievement by placing the initials of the certifying agency behind their names. Some states require phlebotomists to be licensed. Based on the state, this is accomplished by passing a national certifying exam

or a state licensure exam. Membership in a professional organization enhances the professionalism of a phlebotomist by providing increased opportunities for *continuing education*. Professional organizations present seminars and workshops, publish journals containing information on new developments in the field, and represent the profession at state and national levels to influence regulations affecting the profession.

All health-care professionals are expected to participate in continuing education (CE) activities. Attendance at many workshops and seminars is documented by the issuing of certificates containing continuing education units (CEUs). Certifying organizations and state licensure agencies require documentation of CE to maintain certification.

HEALTH-CARE DELIVERY SYSTEM

As members of the health-care delivery system, phlebotomists should have a basic knowledge of the various health-care settings in which they may be employed. Many phlebotomists are employed by hospitals. Other employment settings include physician office laboratories (POLs), health maintenance organizations (HMOs), reference laboratories, urgent care centers, nursing homes, home health-care agencies, clinics, and blood donor centers. In our rapidly changing health-care system, additional areas of employment are continually developing for phlebotomist employment. Laboratory testing plays a vital role in the diagnosis and management of patients in any health-care setting.

Hospital Organization

Hospitals vary in both size and the extent of the services they provide. They may range in size from fewer than 50 beds to more than 300 beds. Smaller hospitals are usually equipped to provide general surgical and medical procedures and emergency procedures. Patients may need to be referred or transferred to a larger hospital if specialized care is needed. As the size and specialization of a hospital increases, so does the need for more phlebotomists. Many hospitals also support clinics and primary care physician offices to serve patients on an outpatient basis. This service also increases the phlebotomy workload. Phlebotomists may be scheduled to work at one of these areas or patients from these areas may be referred to the laboratory for sample collection.

BOX 1-2 Outline of the National Accrediting Agency for Clinical Laboratory Sciences's Phlebotomy Competencies

1. Knowledge of the health-care system and medical terminology
2. Knowledge of infection control
3. Knowledge of basic anatomy and physiology and anatomic terminology related to the laboratory and the pathology of body systems
4. Understanding of the importance of sample collection and integrity for patient care
5. Knowledge of collection equipment, tube additives, special precautions, and interfering substances associated with laboratory tests
6. Performance of standard operating procedures in collecting samples
7. Understanding of requisitions, sample transport, and sample processing
8. Understanding of quality assurance and quality control in phlebotomy
9. Use of effective and appropriate communication skills

TABLE 1-3 • Phlebotomist Certifications

CERTIFYING ORGANIZATION	PHLEBOTOMIST DESIGNATION
American Medical Technologists (AMT) www.amt1.com 847-823-5169	Registered Phlebotomy Technician, RPT (AMT)
American Society for Clinical Pathology (ASCP) www.ascp.org 312-541-4999	Phlebotomy Technician, PBT (ASCP)
American Society of Phlebotomy Technicians (ASPT) www.aspt.org 828-294-0078	Certified Phlebotomy Technician, CPT (ASPT)
National Phlebotomy Association (NPA) www.nationalphlebotomy.org 301-386-200	Certified Phlebotomy Technician, CPT (NPA)
National Healthcareer Association (NHA) www.nhanow.com 800-499-9092	Certified Phlebotomy Technician, CPT (NHA)

Hospitals vary not only in size but also by the type of services offered and their overall mission. Hospitals are classified in different terms such as community hospitals, teaching hospitals (university-based), and nonprofit and for-profit hospitals. There are hospitals that specialize in a particular type of patient or illness, such as children, mental health, rehabilitation, and cancer treatment.

The traditional hospital contains many different patient areas and departments to which the phlebotomist must travel to collect samples. Patient-care areas are listed and described in Table 1-4. The location of these patient areas is an important part of the orientation of newly hired phlebotomists.

Hospital Services and Departments

A hospital organizational chart is shown in Figure 1-3. Organizational charts are designed to define the position of each employee with regard to authority, responsibility, and accountability. Hospital organizational charts are further broken down into department organizational charts. Job descriptions are based on organizational structure.

As shown in Figure 1-3 the four traditional hospital services are nursing services, support services, fiscal

TABLE 1-4 • Hospital Patient-Care Areas

AREA	DESCRIPTION
Emergency department (ED)	Immediate care
Intensive care unit (ICU)	Critically ill patients
Cardiac care unit (CCU)	Patients with acute cardiac disorders
Pediatrics	Children
Nursery	Infants
Neonatal intensive care nursery	Newborns experiencing difficulty
Labor and delivery (L & D)	Childbirth
Operating room (OR)	Surgical procedures
Recovery room	Postoperative patients
Psychiatric unit	Mentally disturbed patients
Dialysis unit	Patients with severe renal disorders
Medical/surgical units	General patient care
Oncology center	Cancer treatment
Short-stay unit	Outpatient surgery

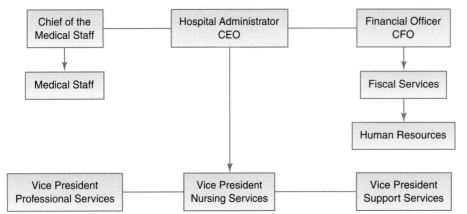

FIGURE 1-3 **Hospital organizational chart.**

services, and professional services. Many departments are located within these four services. Depending on the size and mission of the hospital some departments may be grouped together into a separate category with one director who reports to a large service. An example of this would be a Human Resource Department reporting to the Chief Financial Officer, as shown in Figure 1-3.

Nursing Services

This service deals directly with patient care. It consists of the cardiac care unit (CCU), central supply, emergency department (ED), hospital patient-care units, infection control, intensive care unit (ICU), nursery, social services, and the operating room (OR). Health-care team members associated with this service are registered nurses (RNs), licensed practical nurses (LPNs), certified nursing assistants (CNAs), and the unit secretary. Phlebotomists interact most often with this service and, in decentralized organizations, may be included in it.

Support Services

Support services maintain the hospital and include communications systems, food service/dietary, housekeeping/environmental services, laundry, engineering and maintenance, and security.

Fiscal Services

Fiscal services manage the business aspect of a hospital. Included in this service are accounting, admitting, the business office, credit and collection, data processing, health information management, planning, and public relations departments that include marketing and outreach programs. Table 1-5 describes the departments contained in the support and fiscal services.

Professional Services

This service consists of the departments of the hospital that assist the physician in the diagnosis and treatment of disease. The clinical laboratory, radiology/medical imaging, radiation therapy, nuclear medicine, occupational therapy, pharmacy, physical therapy, respiratory therapy, and cardiovascular testing are the main departments in this service. The phlebotomist is included in this group as part of the clinical laboratory staff.

In addition to patient-care areas, phlebotomists may be asked to collect samples from patients who have been transported to a specialized treatment or testing department. The phlebotomist must be familiar with the location of each department, the nature of the procedures performed there, and the safety precautions pertaining to it.

PROFESSIONAL SERVICES DEPARTMENTS

Radiology and Diagnostic Imaging

The radiology department uses various forms of radiant energy to diagnose and treat disease. Some of the techniques include x-rays of teeth and bones, computerized axial tomography (CAT or CT scan), contrast studies using barium sulfate, cardiac catheterization, fluoroscopy, ultrasound, magnetic resonance imaging (MRI), and positron emission tomography (PET scan). A radiologist, who is a physician, administers diagnostic procedures and interprets radiographs. The allied health-care professional in this department is a radiographer. Phlebotomists must observe radiation exposure precautions when in this department.

TABLE 1-5 • Support and Fiscal Services Departments	
DEPARTMENT	**PRIMARY FUNCTIONS**
Engineering and Maintenance	Maintains hospital's physical plant including communications and clinical equipment
Housekeeping/Environmental Services	Maintains a sanitary and safe hospital including laundry, cleaning of patient rooms, and disposal of biological waste
Dietary/Food Service	Prepares and serves food and provides nutrition care and education
Business Office	Performs daily business functions including patient accounts, paying bills, and payroll
Admitting	Processes patient admissions and discharges
Marketing/Public Relations	Promotes hospital services to the community
Health Information Management	Maintains patient records and hospital legal and regulatory documents
Human Resources	Recruits, interviews, and orients new employees. Provides employee benefit and salary information
Volunteer Services	Coordinates activities of hospital volunteers
Central Supply	Sterilizes, stores, and distributes sterile supplies

Radiation Therapy

The radiation therapy department uses high-energy x-rays or ionizing radiation to stop the growth of cancer cells. Radiation therapy technologists perform these procedures. Because radiation therapy may affect the bone marrow, blood tests are often performed by the laboratory to monitor the patients. Radiation exposure precautions should be observed.

Nuclear Medicine

The nuclear medicine department uses the characteristics of radioactive substances in the diagnosis and treatment of disease. Radioactive materials, called radioisotopes, emit rays as they disintegrate, and the rays are measured on specialized instruments. Two types of tests are used. In vitro tests analyze blood and urine samples using radioactive materials to detect levels of hormones, drugs, and other substances. In vivo tests involve administering radioactive material to the patient by intravenous (IV) injection and measuring the emitted rays to examine organs and evaluate their function. Examples of these procedures are bone, brain, liver, and thyroid scans. Therapeutic doses of radioactive material also can be given to a patient to treat diseases. Nuclear medicine technologists perform these procedures under the supervision of a physician. Radiation exposure precautions should be observed.

Occupational Therapy

The occupational therapy (OT) department teaches techniques that enable patients with physical, mental, or emotional disabilities to function within their limitations in daily living. Occupational therapists and technicians provide this instruction.

Pharmacy

The pharmacy department dispenses the medications prescribed by physicians. The phlebotomist is often responsible for the collection of specifically timed samples used to monitor the blood level of certain medications. Persons trained to dispense medications are called pharmacists who may be assisted by pharmacy technicians.

Physical Therapy

The physical therapy (PT) department provides treatment to patients who have been disabled as a result of illness or injury by using procedures involving water, heat, massage, ultrasound, and exercise. Physical therapists and physical therapy assistants are the professionals trained to provide this therapy.

Respiratory Therapy

Respiratory therapists provide treatment in breathing disorders and perform testing to evaluate lung function.

They may also perform the arterial punctures used to evaluate arterial blood gases, which are discussed in Chapter 14.

Cardiovascular Testing

Cardiac technicians under the supervision of a cardiologist evaluate cardiac function using electrocardiograms, stress tests, and imaging techniques. Patients must be closely monitored for adverse reactions.

Clinical Laboratory

The clinical laboratory provides data to the health-care team to aid in determining the diagnosis, treatment, and prognosis of a patient. The organization and functions of the clinical laboratory are discussed in detail in Chapter 2. The phlebotomist must interact with all hospital professionals in each department and project the professional image of the laboratory to the rest of the hospital staff and the patients.

OTHER HEALTH-CARE SETTINGS

The health-care delivery system has experienced many changes in recent years. As a result of technological advances and the increasing cost of health care, a variety of health-care settings has been created. This development has produced additional places of employment for phlebotomists and, in many settings, also has expanded their duties to include sample processing, performance of waived test procedures (see Chapter 15), and additional record-keeping related to processing of insurance claims (see Chapter 13).

Physicians Office Laboratories (POLs) and Group Practices

POLs have progressed from single practitioners doing simple screening tests to large group medical practices employing both phlebotomists and clinical laboratory personnel authorized to perform tests that are more specialized.

Group practices may consist of several primary care physicians or may specialize in a particular medical specialty such as pediatrics or cardiology. They also may be made up of a combination of family practice physicians and specialists. Group practices may be associated with a particular hospital that services their area. Phlebotomists employed in a group practice may be responsible for processing and packaging samples to be sent to the hospital laboratory. Other group practices contract with a large reference laboratory to perform their laboratory testing and this also requires the phlebotomist to perform sample processing and packaging.

Health Management Organizations (HMOs)

HMOs are managed care group practice centers that provide a large variety of services. Physicians' offices, a clinical laboratory, radiology, physical therapy, and outpatient surgery are often available at one location. Members are charged a prepaid fee for all services performed during a designated time period. They must receive all of their care through services approved by the HMO. Phlebotomists are employed as part of the clinical laboratory staff.

Reference Laboratories

Large, independent reference laboratories contract with health-care providers and institutions to perform both routine and highly specialized tests. Phlebotomists are hired to collect samples from patients referred to the reference laboratory. They may be stationed at the laboratory or at off-site designated collection facilities. Phlebotomists also may be assigned to process samples received in the reference laboratory from its contracted outside health-care facilities.

Government and Hospital Clinics

Veterans Administration clinics are located throughout the country to provide medical care for military veterans. Veterans receive both primary and secondary care at the clinics and this includes the collection of samples for laboratory testing.

Hospital-sponsored specialty clinics, such as cancer, urology, and pediatric clinics, provide more cost-effective delivery of health care to more patients. Increased emphasis on preventive medicine and *alternative medicine* has resulted in the establishment of wellness clinics for health screening. Phlebotomists may be employed in these settings.

Home Health Care

Cost effectiveness has reduced the length of time patients stay in a hospital, and more care is being performed on an outpatient basis. The implementation of *diagnostic related groups (DRGs)* by the federal government to control the rising costs of Medicare and

Medicaid has limited the length of hospital stays and the number of diagnostic procedures that can be performed. The DRG system classified patients into diagnostic categories related to body systems and the illnesses associated with them. Patients are classified based on primary and secondary diagnoses, age, treatment performed, and status on discharge. The system originally determined the amount of money the government will pay for a patient's care and the number of procedures or tests performed. The DRG system was soon adopted by state health insurers and other health-care insurance companies. Therefore, the length of a hospital stay, laboratory tests, and other procedures must be kept within the specified DRG guidelines or the health-care institution or the patient

must absorb the additional cost. Because of the decreased time of hospital stays, home health care has increased to accommodate patients whose conditions are not compatible with frequent outpatient visits to caregivers. Nurses and other health-care providers, including phlebotomists, make scheduled visits to patients requiring home health care. Hospitals may contract with long-term care facilities or nursing homes to provide phlebotomists to perform routine daily blood collections.

In summary, the current health-care delivery system offers a variety of employment opportunities for phlebotomists. Phlebotomists must have the motivation to explore these opportunities and the flexibility to adapt to them.

Key Points

- ✦ The duties of a phlebotomist have expanded to include more than just collection of blood samples.
- ✦ Professional characteristics needed by a phlebotomist include compassion, dependability, honesty, organization, and appropriate appearance.
- ✦ The three components of communication are verbal, listening, and nonverbal (body language).
- ✦ Barriers to verbal communication include hearing impairment, emotions, age, education level, and language other than English.
- ✦ Body language includes facial expressions, posture, providing a zone of comfort, and eye contact.
- ✦ Cultural diversity affects the interactions between a patient and the health-care worker. Phlebotomists

should adapt their actions to the reactions of the patient.
- ✦ Observing correct telephone etiquette by phlebotomists is essential for maintaining the professional image of their workplace.
- ✦ Phlebotomists demonstrate competence in their fields by becoming certified.
- ✦ The basic structure of a hospital includes professional, nursing, support and fiscal services, and the many departments contained within these services that phlebotomists will encounter.
- ✦ Phlebotomists may be employed in POLs, HMOs, reference laboratories, home health care, off-site clinics, and sample collection facilities.

BIBLIOGRAPHY

Joint Commission, National Patient Safety Goals. http://www.jointcommission.org/PatientSafety.
Kruger J, and Dunning, D: Unskilled and Unaware of It: How Difficulties in Recognizing One's Own Incompetence Lead to Inflated Self-Assessments. *Journal of Personality and Social Psychology* 1999;77:1121–1134.
National Accrediting Agency for Clinical Laboratory Sciences. Phlebotomist Competencies. http://www.naacls.org/approval/phleb.

Study Questions

1. Which of the following may be an additional duty of phlebotomists in today's health-care system?
   a. performing patient vital signs
   b. transporting samples to the laboratory
   c. performing dermal punctures
   d. selecting sample collection equipment

2. The primary benefit of hospital decentralization is:
   a. increased efficiency
   b. increased training of personnel
   c. decreased patient complaints
   d. decreased diagnostic testing

3. Which of the following **DOES NOT** represent a professional phlebotomist?
   a. attending a continuing education program
   b. organizing requisitions before leaving the laboratory
   c. exhibiting overconfidence
   d. volunteering to take on an extra duty

4. A phlebotomist who is responding appropriately to cultural diversity will:
   a. speak in the patient's native language
   b. be able to stereotype patients
   c. be sensitive to the patient's reactions
   d. quickly examine the patient's arm

5. Effective communication includes:
   a. verbal
   b. nonverbal
   c. listening
   d. all of the above

6. All of the following actions make patients feel that you care about them **EXCEPT:**
   a. smiling at them
   b. introducing yourself
   c. looking directly at them
   d. avoiding eye contact

Study Questions—cont'd

7. All of the following are barriers to verbal communication **EXCEPT:**
   a. hand signals
   b. hearing impairment
   c. using medical jargon
   d. non–English-speaking patient

8. Good telephone etiquette includes all of the following **EXCEPT:**
   a. checking for an emergency before putting someone on hold
   b. stating your name and department when answering the phone
   c. repeating a request back to the caller before hanging up
   d. immediately transferring a call to the correct department

9. A phlebotomist who takes an examination prepared by a national phlebotomy agency is seeking:
   a. continuing education
   b. certification
   c. accreditation
   d. membership

10. The hospital department that is responsible for sterile supplies is:
   a. housekeeping
   b. central supply
   c. engineering
   d. sterilization

11. A phlebotomist working for an organization that performs highly specialized testing is employed by a:
   a. group practice
   b. health maintenace organization
   c. specialty clinic
   d. reference laboratory

12. The implementation of DRGs has:
   a. increased the length of hospital stays
   b. increased the need for home health care
   c. decreased the opportunities for phlebotomists
   d. decreased the need for rehabilitation facilities

Clinical Situations

1 The phlebotomy supervisor at Healthy Hospital holds a meeting to tell the staff that the phlebotomy department is going to be decentralized.
   a. How could this affect the working location of the phlebotomists?
   b. How might this affect the duties of the phlebotomists?
   c. What is the major benefit for Healthy Hospital of decentralizing phlebotomy?
   d. The phlebotomy supervisor will be teaching classes on phlebotomy. Who might be attending the classes?

2 The phlebotomy supervisor receives the following complaints. State possible causes for the complaints.
   a. A very sick person mistakenly calls the laboratory instead of the emergency department and is put on hold for 10 minutes.
   b. The emergency department calls the laboratory requesting a STAT blood culture. The phlebotomist arrives in the emergency department without the necessary equipment.
   c. A patient's daughter overhears a phlebotomist talking about her mother in the cafeteria.
   d. A patient with limited understanding of English is given instructions to return to the laboratory the next morning for a fasting blood collection. The patient shows up drinking a high-carbohydrate energy drink.

CHAPTER 2

The Clinical Laboratory

Learning Objectives

Upon completion of this chapter, the reader will be able to:

1. Describe the qualifications and functions of the personnel employed in a clinical laboratory.
2. Discuss the basic functions of the hematology, chemistry, blood bank (immunohematology), serology (immunology), microbiology, and urinalysis sections.
3. Describe the appropriate collection and handling of samples analyzed in the individual clinical laboratory sections.
4. Identify the most common tests performed in the individual clinical laboratory sections and state their functions.

The clinical laboratory is divided into two areas, anatomical and clinical. The anatomical area is responsible for the analysis of surgical specimens, frozen sections, biopsies, cytological specimens, and autopsies. Sections of the anatomical area include cytology, histology, and cytogenetics.

CYTOLOGY SECTION

In the cytology section, cytologists (CTs) process and examine tissue and body fluids for the presence of abnormal cells, such as cancer cells. The Papanicolaou (Pap) smear is one of the most common tests performed in cytology.

HISTOLOGY SECTION

In the histology section, histology technicians (HTs) and technologists (HTLs) process and stain tissue obtained from biopsies, surgery, autopsies, and frozen sections. A pathologist then examines the tissue.

CYTOGENETICS

Cytogenetics is the section in which chromosome studies are performed to detect genetic disorders. Blood, amniotic fluid, tissue, and bone marrow specimens are analyzed.

CLINICAL AREA

The clinical area is divided into specialized sections: hematology, coagulation, chemistry, blood bank (immunohematology), serology (immunology), microbiology, urinalysis, phlebotomy, and sample processing. In the clinical sections, blood, bone marrow, microbiology samples, urine, and other body fluids are analyzed.

Many laboratories have a separate section for the laboratory information system (LIS). The LIS department is responsible for laboratory computer operations, maintaining records, and documentation for compliance with accrediting regulations.

Figure 2-1 shows a sample organizational chart of a traditional clinical laboratory. In some institutions,

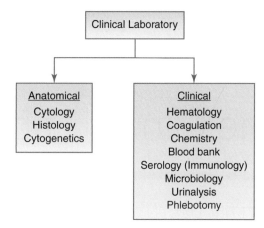

FIGURE 2-1 Clinical laboratory organizational chart.

certain sections, such as hematology, coagulation, chemistry, and urinalysis, may be combined in a core laboratory for more efficient use of personnel.

CLINICAL LABORATORY PERSONNEL

The laboratory employs a large number of personnel, whose qualifications vary with their job descriptions. Most personnel are required to be certified by a national organization. Some states require an additional state licensure, and the number of these states is increasing. See Figure 2-2 for an organizational chart of clinical laboratory personnel.

Laboratory Director (Pathologist)

The director of the laboratory is usually a pathologist, a physician who has completed a 4- to 5-year pathology residency. A pathologist is a specialist in the study of disease and works in both clinical pathology and anatomical pathology.

The pathologist is the liaison between the medical staff and the laboratory staff and acts as a consultant to physicians regarding a patient's diagnosis and treatment. Direct responsibility for the anatomical and clinical areas of the laboratory lies with the pathologist. His or her responsibilities include working with the laboratory administrator to establish laboratory policies, interpret test results, perform bone marrow biopsies and autopsies, and diagnose disease from tissue specimens or cell preparations.

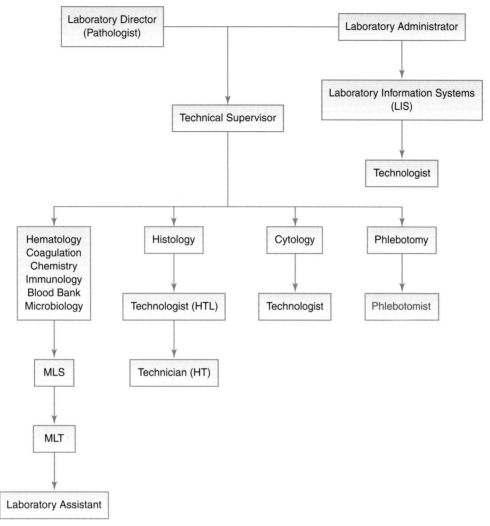

FIGURE 2-2 **Clinical laboratory personnel organizational chart.**

Often the laboratory director has one or more associate pathologists to assist with the laboratory responsibilities. The laboratory director may also be a laboratory specialist who possesses a doctorate degree.

Laboratory Manager (Administrator)

The laboratory manager is responsible for overall technical and administrative management of the laboratory, including personnel and budgets. The laboratory manager is usually a medical laboratory

---

Alert of Changes in Personnel Title Changes

In October 2009, the American Society for Clinical Laboratory Pathology (ASCP) Board of Registry (BOR) and the National Accrediting Agency for Clinical Laboratory Science (NCA) combined to form the ASCP Board of Certification (BOC). Because of this unification the designations of certain laboratory personnel have changed. These changes are:
1. Clinical laboratory technicians, CLT (NCA), and medical laboratory technicians, MLT (ASCP), are now both MLT(ASCP).

Continued

Alert of Changes in Personnel Title Changes—cont'd

2. Clinical laboratory scientists, CLS (NCA), and medical technologists, MT (ASCP), are now both medical laboratory scientists, MLS(ASCP)^{cm}.
3. Certification maintenance (cm) through documentation of a required amount of continuing education has been required of all previously certified clinical laboratory scientists and medical technologists

certified in 2004 and later. Medical technologists certified prior to 2004 must complete the required continuing education or their designation will remain MT (ASCP).
4. For continuity the term medical laboratory scientist (MLS) is used throughout this textbook.

---

scientist (MLS) with a master's degree and 5 or more years of laboratory experience. The additional education is often in either administration or business. The laboratory manager acts as a liaison among the laboratory staff, the administrator of professional services, and the laboratory director.

Technical Supervisor

The technical supervisor is an MLS with experience and expertise related to the particular laboratory section or sections. Many technical supervisors have a specialty certification in hematology, chemistry, blood banking, immunology, or microbiology. The technical supervisor is accountable to the laboratory administrator. Responsibilities of the technical supervisor include reviewing all laboratory test results; consulting with the pathologist on abnormal test results; scheduling personnel; maintaining automated instruments by implementing preventive maintenance procedures and quality control measures; preparing budgets; maintaining reagents and supplies; orienting, evaluating, and teaching personnel; and providing research and development protocols for new test procedures.

Medical Laboratory Scientist

The MLS has a bachelor's degree in medical technology or in a biological science and 1 year of training in an accredited medical technology / clinical laboratory science program. The scientist performs laboratory procedures that require independent judgment and responsibility with minimal technical supervision; maintains equipment and records; performs quality assurance and preventive maintenance activities related to test performance; and may function as a supervisor, educator, manager, or researcher within a medical laboratory setting. Additional duties of the MLS are to evaluate and solve problems related to the collection of samples, perform complex laboratory procedures,

analyze quality control data, report and answer inquiries regarding test results, troubleshoot equipment, participate in the evaluation of new test procedures, and provide education to new employees and students.

Medical Laboratory Technician

A medical laboratory technician (MLT) usually has a 2-year associate degree from an accredited college medical laboratory program. An MLT performs routine laboratory procedures according to established protocol under the supervision of a technologist, supervisor, or laboratory director. The duties of the MLT include collecting and processing biological samples for analysis, performing routine analytic tests, recognizing factors that affect test results, recognizing abnormal results and reporting them to a supervisor, recognizing equipment malfunctions and reporting them to a supervisor, performing quality control and preventive maintenance procedures, maintaining accurate records, and demonstrating laboratory technical skills to new employees and students.

Laboratory Assistant

The laboratory assistant has training in phlebotomy, sample receiving and processing, quality control and preventive maintenance of instruments, and computer data entry and can perform basic "waived" laboratory testing. The laboratory assistant aids the MLS or MLT by preparing samples for testing.

Phlebotomist

The phlebotomist collects blood from patients for laboratory analysis. The phlebotomist must have a high school diploma and usually has completed a structured phlebotomy training program. Certified phlebotomy technicians have passed a national certifying examination. The phlebotomist is trained to identify the patient properly, obtain the correct amount of blood by venipuncture or microtechnique, use the correct equipment and collection tubes, properly label and transport samples to the laboratory, prepare samples to be delivered to the laboratory sections, and observe all safety and quality control policies. Possible additional duties of the phlebotomist are addressed in Chapter 1. Test collection requirements vary with each department; therefore, the phlebotomist must interact with and have knowledge of all the sections in the laboratory.

Additional Laboratory Personnel

Additional laboratory personnel may include an educational coordinator to direct a medical technology or clinical laboratory science program and continuing professional development for staff. With the increased performance of point of care testing (POCT) (see Chapter 15), a point of care coordinator with a clinical laboratory science background evaluates new point of care procedures and protocols, reviews quality assessment, and conducts competency assessments. This person works closely with nurses and other laboratory personnel performing POCT. The LIS manager usually has a clinical laboratory science background and education in computer operations and programming for the laboratory computer system. A quality assessment coordinator collects and evaluates quality control data.

HEMATOLOGY SECTION

Key Terms

Anemia (a NE me a)
Anticoagulant (AN ti ko AG u lant)
Leukemia (loo KE me a)
Plasma
Serum

Hematology is the study of the formed (cellular) elements of the blood. In this section, the cellular elements, red blood cells (RBCs), white blood cells (WBCs), and platelets (Plts) are enumerated and classified in all body fluids and in the bone marrow. These cells, which are formed in the bone marrow, are released into the bloodstream as needed to carry oxygen, provide immunity against infection, and aid in blood clotting.

By examining the cells in a blood specimen, the MLT or MLS can detect disorders such as *leukemia*, *anemia*, other blood diseases, and infection and monitor their treatment (Fig. 2-3).

Sample Collection and Handling

The most common body fluid analyzed in the hematology section is whole blood (a mixture of cells and plasma). A whole blood specimen is obtained by using a collection tube with an *anticoagulant* to prevent clotting of the sample. Most tests performed in the hematology section require blood that has been collected in tubes with a lavender stopper that contain the anticoagulant ethylenediaminetetraacetic acid (EDTA) (see Chapter 8). Immediate inversion of this tube eight times is critical to prevent clotting and ensure accurate blood counts.

Blood is analyzed in the form of whole blood, *plasma,* or *serum.* The liquid portion of blood is called plasma if it is obtained from a sample that has been anticoagulated. If the sample is allowed to clot, the liquid portion is called serum. The major difference between plasma and serum is that plasma contains the protein fibrinogen and serum does not. Refer to Chapter 7 to see the role of fibrinogen in the clotting process. Figure 2-4 illustrates the differences between plasma and serum. It is important to differentiate between plasma and serum because many laboratory tests are designed to be performed specifically on either plasma or serum.

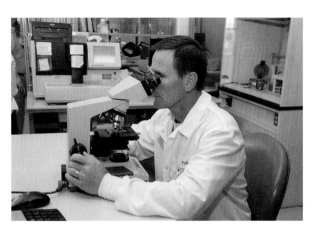

FIGURE 2-3 A technician examining blood cells in the hematology section.

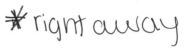

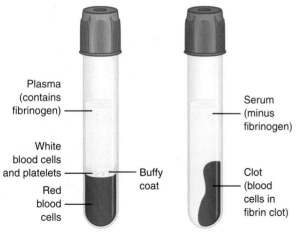

FIGURE 2-4 **Differences between plasma and serum.**

Tests Performed in the Hematology Section

A complete blood count (CBC) is the primary analysis performed in the hematology section. Very often it is ordered on a STAT basis. Table 2-1 lists the tests performed in the hematology section, including components of the CBC, which may also be ordered separately. Many of the tests in hematology are performed on automated instruments.

COAGULATION SECTION

Key Terms

Hemostasis (he MOS ta sis)

TABLE 2-1 • **Tests Performed in the Hematology Section**	
TEST	**FUNCTION**
Complete blood count	
Differential (Diff)	Determines the percentage of the different types of white blood cells and evaluates red blood cell and platelet morphology (may be examined microscopically on a peripheral blood smear stained with Wright's stain)
Hematocrit (Hct)	Determines the volume of red blood cells packed by centrifugation (expressed as a percent)
Hemoglobin (Hgb)	Determines the oxygen-carrying capacity of red blood cells
Indices	Calculations to determine the size of red blood cells and amount of hemoglobin
Mean corpuscular hemoglobin (MCH)	Determines the amount of hemoglobin in a red blood cell
Mean corpuscular hemoglobin concentration (MCHC)	Determines the weight of hemoglobin in a red blood cell and compares it with the size of the cell (expressed as a percent)
Mean corpuscular volume (MCV)	Determines the size of red blood cells
Platelet (PLT) count	Determines the number of platelets in circulating blood
Red blood cell (RBC) count	Determines the number of red blood cells in circulating blood
Red cell distribution width (RDW)	Calculation to determine the differences in the size of red blood cells (expressed as a percent)
White blood cell (WBC) count	Determines the number of white blood cells in circulating blood
Body fluid analysis	Determines the number and type of cells in various body fluids
Bone marrow	Determines the number and type of cells in the bone marrow
Erythrocyte sedimentation rate (ESR)	Determines the rate of red blood cell sedimentation (nonspecific test for inflammatory disorders)
Reticulocyte (Retic) count	Evaluates bone marrow production of red blood cells
Sickle cell	Screening test for Hgb S (sickle cell anemia)
Special stains	Determine the type of leukemia or other cellular disorders

Tests included in the complete blood count (CBC) are shaded in blue.

The coagulation laboratory is sometimes a part of the hematology section, but in larger laboratories it is a separate section. In this area, the overall process of *hemostasis* is evaluated; this includes platelets, blood vessels, coagulation factors, fibrinolysis, inhibitors, and anticoagulant therapy (heparin and Coumadin). Plasma from a sample drawn in a tube with a light blue stopper that contains the anticoagulant sodium citrate is the specimen analyzed. Coagulation tests are performed on automated instruments.

Tests Performed in the Coagulation Section

The tests most frequently performed in the coagulation area of the hematology section and their function are presented in Table 2-2.

CHEMISTRY SECTION

Key Terms

Centrifuge (SEN tri fuj)
Electrolyte (e LEK tro lit)
Electrophoresis (e LEK tro for E sis)
Enzyme (EN zim)

Hemolyzed (HE mo liz)
Icteric (ik TER ik)
Immunochemistry (IM u no KEM is tre)
Lipemic (li PE mik)
Toxicology (TOKS i KOL o je)

The clinical chemistry section is the most automated area of the laboratory. Instruments are computerized and designed to perform single and multiple tests from small amounts of specimen. Figures 2-5 and 2-6 provide examples of the instrumentation and computerization used in the chemistry section.

The chemistry section may be divided into several areas such as general or automated chemistry, *electrophoresis, toxicology,* and *immunochemistry.* The electrophoresis area performs hemoglobin electrophoresis and protein electrophoresis on serum, urine, and cerebrospinal fluid.

In toxicology, therapeutic drug monitoring (TDM) and the identification of drugs of abuse are performed. Immunochemistry uses *enzyme* immunoassay (EIA) techniques to measure substances such as digoxin, thyroid hormones, cortisol, vitamin B_{12}, folate, carcinoembryonic antigen, and creatine kinase (CK) isoenzymes.

TABLE 2-2 ● Tests Performed in the Coagulation Section	
TEST	**FUNCTION**
Activated partial thromboplastin time (APTT [PTT])	Evaluates the intrinsic system of the coagulation cascade and monitors heparin therapy
Antithrombin III	Screening test for increased clotting tendencies
Anti-Xa heparin assay	Monitors unfractionated heparin therapy
Proteins C and S	Evaluate venous thrombosis
Bleeding time (BT)	Evaluates the function of platelets
D-dimer	Measures abnormal blood clotting and fibrinolysis
Factor assays	Detect factor deficiencies that prolong coagulation
Fibrin degradation products (FDP)	Test for increased fibrinolysis (usually a STAT test drawn in a special tube)
Fibrinogen	Determines the amount of fibrinogen in plasma
Platelet aggregation	Evaluates the function of platelets
Prothrombin time (PT) and international normalized ratio (INR)	Evaluates the extrinsic system of the coagulation cascade and monitors Coumadin therapy
Thrombin time (TT)	Determines if adequate fibrinogen is present for normal coagulation

✱ light blue tube - filled to the top - no exceptions!

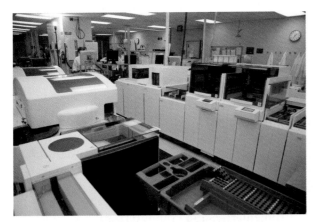

FIGURE 2-5 Automated robotic chemistry instrument.

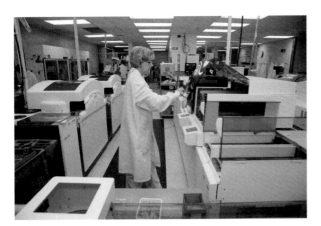

FIGURE 2-6 Medical laboratory scientist programming the automated chemistry analyzer.

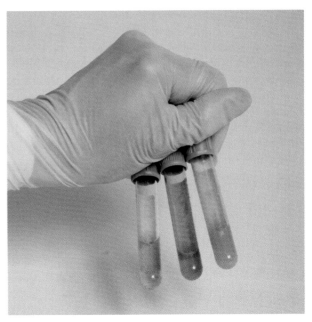

FIGURE 2-7 Normal, icteric, and lipemic serum.

Sample Collection and Handling

Clinical chemistry tests are performed primarily on serum collected in gel barrier tubes, but the serum may also be collected in tubes with red, green, gray, or royal blue stoppers. Tests are also performed on plasma, urine, and other body fluids. Serum and plasma are obtained by *centrifugation,* which should be performed within 1 to 2 hours of collection.

Because many tests are performed on instruments that take photometric readings, differences in the appearance or color of a specimen may adversely affect the test results. Specimens of concern include *hemolyzed* specimens that appear red because of the release of hemoglobin from RBCs, *icteric* specimens that are yellow because of the presence of excess bilirubin, and *lipemic* specimens that are cloudy because of increased lipids (Fig. 2-7). Fasting samples drawn from patients who have not eaten for 8 to 12 hours are preferred. Serum separator tubes contain an inert gel that prevents contamination of the specimen by RBCs or their metabolites. Samples must be allowed to clot fully before centrifugation to ensure complete separation of the cells and serum. Many chemistry tests require special collection and handling procedures, such as chilling and protection from light, and these tests are discussed in Chapter 11.

Tests Performed in the Chemistry Section

The tests most frequently performed in the chemistry section and their functions are presented in Table 2-3.

Chemistry profiles or panels are groups of tests used to evaluate a particular organ, body system, or the general health of a patient. The specific tests included in a profile vary among institutions. Payment for chemistry panels is regulated by the CMS. An example of common chemistry panels is shown in Table 2-4.

BLOOD BANK SECTION

Key Terms

Antibody (AN ti BOD e)
Antigen (AN ti jen)

TABLE 2-3 • Tests Performed in the Chemistry Section

TEST	FUNCTION
Alanine aminotransferase (ALT)	Elevated levels indicate liver disorders
Albumin	Decreased levels indicate liver or kidney disorders or malnutrition
Alcohol	Elevated levels indicate intoxication
Alkaline phosphatase (ALP)	Elevated levels indicate bone or liver disorders
Ammonia	Elevated levels indicate severe liver disorders
Amylase	Elevated levels indicate pancreatitis
Arterial blood gases (ABGs)	Determine the acidity or alkalinity and oxygen and carbon dioxide levels of blood
Aspartate aminotransferase (AST)	Elevated levels indicate myocardial infarction or liver disorders
Bilirubin	Elevated levels indicate liver or hemolytic disorders
Blood urea nitrogen (BUN)	Elevated levels indicate kidney disorders
Brain natriuretic peptide (BNP)	Elevated levels indicate congestive heart failure
Calcium (Ca)	Mineral associated with bone, musculoskeletal, or endocrine disorders
Cholesterol	Elevated levels indicate coronary risk
Creatine kinase (CK)	Elevated levels indicate myocardial infarction or other muscle damage
Creatine kinase (CK) isoenzymes	Determine the extent of muscle or brain damage (elevated in myocardial infarction)
Creatinine	Elevated levels indicate kidney disorders
Creatinine clearance	Urine and serum test to measure glomerular filtration rate
Drug screening	Detects drug abuse and monitors therapeutic drugs
Electrolytes (CO_2, Cl, Na, K)	Evaluate body fluid balance
Gamma-glutamyltransferase (GGT)	Elevated levels indicate early liver disorders
Glucose	Elevated levels indicate diabetes mellitus
Glucose tolerance test (GTT)	Detects diabetes mellitus or hypoglycemia
Haptoglobin	Used to evaluate hemolytic anemia and certain chronic diseases
Hemoglobin A_1C	Monitors diabetes mellitus
Hemoglobin (Hgb) electrophoresis	Detects abnormal hemoglobins
High-density lipoprotein (HDL)	Assesses coronary risk
Iron	Decreased levels indicate iron deficiency anemia
Lactic dehydrogenase (LD [LDH])	Elevated levels indicate myocardial infarction or lung or liver disorders
Lead	Elevated levels indicate poisoning
Lipase	Elevated levels indicate pancreatitis
Lithium (Li)	Monitors antidepressant drug
Low-density lipoprotein (LDL)	Assesses coronary risk
Magnesium	Cation involved in neuromuscular excitability of muscle tissue
Myoglobin	Early indicator of myocardial infarction
Phosphorus (P)	Mineral associated with skeletal or endocrine disorders
Prostate-specific antigen (PSA)	Screening for prostatic cancer
Protein	Decreased levels associated with liver or kidney disorders

Continued

TABLE 2-3 • Tests Performed in the Chemistry Section—cont'd

TEST	FUNCTION
Total protein (TP)	Decreased levels indicate liver or kidney disorders
Triglycerides	Used to assess coronary risk
Troponin I and T	Early indicators of myocardial infarction
Uric acid	Elevated levels indicate kidney disorders or gout

TABLE 2-4 • Common Chemistry Organ/Disease Panels

PANEL	TESTS
Comprehensive	Glucose, BUN, creatinine, sodium (Na), potassium (K), carbon dioxide (CO_2), chloride (Cl), AST, ALT, total protein, albumin, bilirubin, Ca, and ALP
Hepatic	ALP, ALT, AST, bilirubin total and direct, total protein, albumin
Lipid	Cholesterol, triglycerides, HDL, LDL, and cholesterol/HDL ratio
Basic metabolic	Glucose, BUN, creatinine, Na, Cl, K, CO_2, and ionized calcium
Renal	Glucose, BUN, creatinine, CO_2, Cl, NA, K, total protein, albumin, calcium, phosphorous

ALP = alkaline phosphatase; ALT = alanine aminotransferase; AST = aspartate aminotransferase; BUN = blood urea nitrogen; HDL = high-density lipoproteins; LD = lactic dehydrogenase; LDL = low-density lipoproteins.

Blood group
Compatibility (crossmatch)
Cryoprecipitate (KRI o pre SIP i tat)
Fresh frozen plasma
Immunohematology (i mu no HEM a TOL o je)
Packed cells
Rh type
Unit of blood

The blood bank (BB) is the section of the laboratory where blood may be collected, stored, and prepared for transfusion. It is also called the *immunohematology* section because the testing procedures involve RBC *antigens* (Ag) and *antibodies* (Ab). In the blood bank, blood from patients and donors is tested for its *blood group* (ABO) and *Rh type* (see Figure 7-16 in Chapter 7), the presence and identity of abnormal antibodies, and its *compatibility* (*crossmatch*) for use in a transfusion (Fig. 2-8). *Units of blood* are collected from donors, tested for the presence of bloodborne pathogens such as hepatitis viruses and human immunodeficiency virus (HIV), and stored for transfusions (Fig. 2-9). Donor blood may also be separated into components including *packed cells,* platelets, *fresh frozen plasma,* and *cryoprecipitate.*

These components are stored separately and used for patients with specific needs. Patients may come to the blood bank to donate their own blood so that they can receive an **autologous transfusion** if blood is needed during surgery.

Sample Collection and Handling

Blood bank samples are collected in plain red (serum), lavender, or pink (plasma) stopper tubes. Serum separator tubes containing gel are not acceptable because the gel will coat the RBCs and interfere with testing. Hemolysis also interferes with the interpretation of test results.

Patient identification is critical in the blood bank, and phlebotomists must carefully follow all patient identification and sample labeling procedures to ensure that a patient does not receive a transfusion with an incompatible blood type.

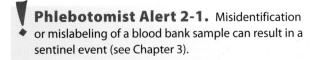

Phlebotomist Alert 2-1. Misidentification or mislabeling of a blood bank sample can result in a sentinel event (see Chapter 3).

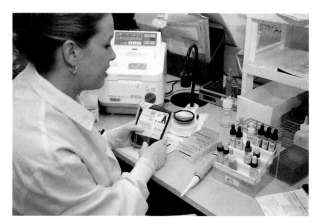

FIGURE 2-8 A medical laboratory scientist tests a unit of blood before it is transfused.

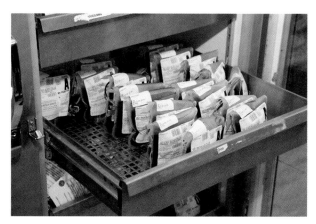

FIGURE 2-9 A blood bank refrigerator.

SEROLOGY (IMMUNOLOGY) SECTION

Key Terms

Autoimmunity (AW to im MU ni te)
Immunoglobulin (IM u no GLOB u lin)
Immunology (IM u NOL o je)
Serology (se ROL o je)

The *serology* (*immunology*) section performs tests to evaluate the body's immune response; that is, the production of antibodies (*immunoglobulins*) and cellular activation. Because most tests performed in this section analyze for the presence of antibodies in serum, the section is frequently called serology rather than by the broader term immunology.

Tests in the serology section detect the presence of antibodies to bacteria, fungi, parasites, viruses, and antibodies produced against body substances (*autoimmunity*).

Sample Collection and Handling

Blood for serological testing is collected in tubes with red stoppers. Serum separator tubes are not used when the gel will interfere with the antigen-antibody reactions.

Tests Performed in the Blood Bank Section

The tests most frequently performed in the blood bank section and their function are presented in Table 2-5.

Tests Performed in the Serology (Immunology) Section

The tests most frequently performed in the serology (immunology) section and their functions are presented in Table 2-6.

TABLE 2-5 • Tests Performed in the Blood Bank Section	
TEST	**FUNCTION**
Antibody (Ab) screen (indirect antiglobulin test)	Detects abnormal antibodies in serum
Direct antihuman globulin test (DAT) or direct Coombs	Detects abnormal antibodies on red blood cells
Group and type	ABO and Rh typing
Panel	Identifies abnormal antibodies in serum
Type and crossmatch (T & C)	ABO, Rh typing, and compatibility test
Type and screen	ABO, Rh typing, and antibody screen

TABLE 2-6 • **Tests Performed in the Serology (Immunology) Section**	
TEST	**FUNCTION**
Anti-HIV	Screening test for human immunodeficiency virus
Antinuclear antibody (ANA)	Detects nuclear autoantibodies
Antistreptolysin O (ASO) screen	Detects a previous *Streptococcus* infection
C-reactive protein (CRP)	Elevated levels indicate inflammatory disorders
Cold agglutinins	Elevated levels indicate atypical (*Mycoplasma*) pneumonia
Complement levels	Evaluate the function of the immune system
Cytomegalovirus antibody (CMV)	Detects cytomegalovirus infection
Febrile agglutinins	Detect antibodies to microorganisms causing fever
Fluorescent antinuclear antibody (FANA)	Detects and identifies nuclear autoantibodies
Fluorescent treponemal antibody-absorbed (FTA-ABS)	Confirmatory test for syphilis
Hepatitis A antibody	Detects hepatitis A current or past infection
Hepatitis B surface antigen (HBsAg)	Detects hepatitis B infection
Hepatitis C antibody	Detects hepatitis C infection
Human chorionic gonadotropin (HCG)	Hormone found in the urine and serum during pregnancy
Immunoglobulin (IgG, IgA, IgM) levels	Evaluate the function of the immune system
Monospot	Screening test for infectious mononucleosis
Rapid plasma reagin (RPR)	Screening test for syphilis
Rheumatoid arthritis (RA)	Detects autoantibodies present in rheumatoid arthritis
Rubella titer	Evaluates immunity to German measles
Venereal Disease Research Laboratory (VDRL)	Screening test for syphilis
Western blot	Confirmatory test for human immunodeficiency virus

MICROBIOLOGY SECTION

Key Terms

Bacteria (bak TE re a)
Bacteriology (bak TE re OL o je)
Culture and sensitivity
Gram stain
Microbiology (MI kro bi OL o je)
Microorganism (mi kro OR gan izm)
Mycology (mi KOL o je)
Parasitology (PAR a sī TOL o je)
Virology (vi ROL o je)

The *microbiology* section is responsible for the identification of pathogenic microorganisms and for hospital infection control. In large laboratories, the section may be divided into *bacteriology, mycology, parasitology,* and *virology.*

A *culture and sensitivity* (C & S) test is the primary procedure performed in microbiology. It is used to detect and identify *microorganisms* and to determine the most effective antibiotic therapy. Results are available within 2 days for most bacteria; however, cultures for tuberculosis and fungi may require several weeks for completion.

Identification of *bacteria* is based on morphology, *Gram stain* reactions, oxygen and nutritional requirements, and biochemical reactions. Fungi are identified primarily by culture growth and microscopic morphology. Stool samples are concentrated and examined microscopically for the presence of parasites, ova, or larvae. Viruses must be cultured in living cells, and most laboratories send viral specimens for culturing to specialized reference laboratories. The clinical laboratory performs serological testing for detection of antibodies against the virus in the patient's serum.

Sample Collection and Handling

Most microbiology samples are obtained from the blood, urine, throat, sputum, genitourinary tract, wounds, cerebrospinal fluid, and feces. Correct identification of pathogens depends on proper collection and prompt transport to the laboratory for processing. Figures 2-10 and 2-11 provide examples of specimen processing in the microbiology section.

Phlebotomists are responsible for collecting blood cultures and may be required to obtain throat cultures (TCs) and instruct patients in the procedure for collecting urine samples for culture. Specific sterile techniques must be observed in the collection of culture samples to prevent bacterial contamination. These procedures are covered in Chapters 10 and 16.

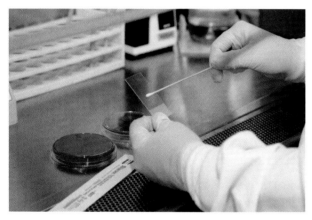

FIGURE 2-10 Medical laboratory scientist plating a culture and preparing a Gram stain.

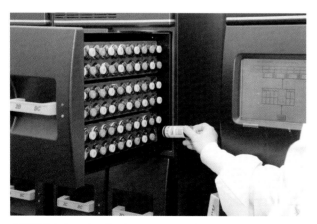

FIGURE 2-11 Blood culture specimen being placed in the automated blood culture incubator.

Tests Performed in the Microbiology Section

The tests most frequently performed in the microbiology section and their functions are presented in Table 2-7.

URINALYSIS SECTION

Key Terms

Cast
First morning sample
Glycosuria (GLI ko SU re a)
Hematuria (HEM a-TU re a)
Hemoglobinuria (HE mo glo bin U re a)
Ketonuria (ke to NU re a)
Proteinuria (PRO te in U re a)
Reagent strip (dipstick)
Urinalysis (U ri NAL i sis)

Urinalysis (UA) may be a separate laboratory section or a part of the hematology or chemistry sections. UA is a routine screening procedure to detect disorders and infections of the kidney and to detect metabolic disorders such as diabetes mellitus and liver disease.

TABLE 2-7 • Tests Performed in the Microbiology Section	
TEST	**FUNCTION**
Acid-fast bacillus (AFB) culture	Detects acid-fast bacteria, including *Mycobacterium tuberculosis*
Blood culture	Detects bacteria and fungi in the blood
Culture and sensitivity (C & S)	Detects microbial infection and determines antibiotic treatment
Fungal culture	Detects the presence of and determines the type of fungi
Gram stain	Detects the presence of and aids in the identification of bacteria
Occult blood	Detects nonvisible blood (performed on stool samples)
Ova and parasites (O & P)	Detects parasitic infection (performed on stool samples)

A routine UA consists of physical, chemical, and microscopic examination of the urine. The physical examination evaluates the color, clarity, and specific gravity of the urine. The chemical examination is performed using chemical *reagent strips* (*dipsticks*) to determine pH, glucose, ketones, protein, blood, bilirubin, urobilinogen, nitrite, and leukocytes. The microscopic examination identifies the presence of cells, *casts,* bacteria, crystals, yeast, and parasites. Automated systems can perform a complete UA (Fig. 2-12).

Sample Collection and Handling

Phlebotomists may be requested to deliver urine samples to the laboratory. This should be done promptly because many changes can take place in a urine sample that sits at room temperature for longer than 2 hours. Different types of samples are required for testing. Random samples are most frequently collected for routine screening; however, a *first morning sample* is more concentrated and may be required for certain tests. Other types of urine samples include timed or 24-hour collections for quantitative chemistry tests, and midstream clean-catch and catheterized samples for cultures (see Chapter 16).

Tests Performed in the Urinalysis Section

The primary test performed in the urinalysis section is the routine urinalysis. As shown in Table 2-8, the test has multiple parts.

TABLE 2-8 ● **Routine Urinalysis**	
TEST	**FUNCTION**
Color	Detects blood, bilirubin, and other pigments
Appearance	Detects cellular and crystalline elements
Specific gravity (SG)	Measures the concentration of urine
pH	Determines the acidity of urine
Protein	Elevated levels indicate kidney disorders (**proteinuria**)
Glucose	Elevated levels indicate diabetes mellitus (**glycosuria**)
Ketones	Elevated levels indicate diabetes mellitus or starvation (**ketonuria**)
Blood	Detects red blood cells or hemoglobin (**hematuria/ hemoglobinuria**)
Bilirubin	Elevated levels indicate liver disorders
Urobilinogen	Elevated levels indicate liver or hemolytic disorders
Nitrite	Detects bacterial infection
Leukocyte esterase	Detects white blood cells
Microscopic	Determines the number and type of cellular elements

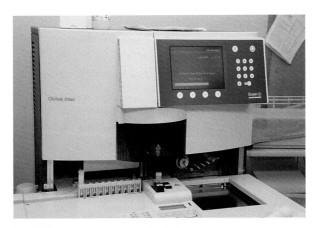

FIGURE 2-12 **Automated urinalysis system.**

Key Points

- The two main areas of the clinical laboratory are anatomical and clinical. The anatomical area consists of the histology, cytology, and cytogenetics sections.
- The laboratory director is a pathologist (MD). The laboratory administrator often has a master's degree and courses in business. Technical supervisors have bachelor's degrees or higher and manage laboratory sections and report to the laboratory administrator. Medical laboratory scientists have bachelor's degrees and technicians have associate degrees.
- The laboratory director acts as a liaison for the medical staff and the laboratory and performs autopsies, interprets test results, and analyzes anatomical specimens. The laboratory administrator is responsible for laboratory personnel, budgeting, and technical administrative duties. Testing is performed by medical laboratory scientists and technicians. Blood samples are collected by phlebotomists and processed by laboratory assistants.
- The major sections of the clinical laboratory are hematology, coagulation, chemistry, blood bank/immunohematology, serology/immunology, microbiology, and urinalysis.
- The hematology sections analyzes anticoagulated whole blood specimens for the counting and examination of red blood cells (RBCs), white blood cells (WBCs), and platelets.
- Plasma is the liquid portion of anticoagulated blood. Serum is the liquid portion of clotted blood. Plasma contains fibrinogen and serum does not contain fibrinogen. Plasma and serum specimens are obtained by sample centrifugation.
- The coagulation section analyzes plasma coagulation factors and the function of platelets in maintaining hemostasis. Anticoagulation therapy is monitored by tests performed in coagulation.
- The clinical chemistry section analyzes serum and plasma for chemical constituents to evaluate general health and disorders of body systems and organs.
- The blood bank/immunohematology prepares blood and blood products for transfusions. Patient identification and sample labeling are extremely critical in preparing blood for transfusions.
- The serology/immunology section evaluates the body's immune system. Serum is tested for the presence of antibodies to infectious agents and autoimmune antibodies.
- The microbiology section detects and identifies bacteria, fungi, parasites, and viruses. Microorganisms are Gram stained, cultured, and tested for antibiotic susceptibility. When collecting samples for microbiology such as blood cultures, sterile technique very important.
- The urinalysis section tests urine samples for physical, chemical, and microscopic characteristics. Urinalysis screens for kidney disorders and infections and other metabolic disorders.

Study Questions

1. Which of the following laboratory sections is included in the anatomical area of the laboratory?
   a. microbiology
   b. histology
   c. immunology
   d. urinalysis

2. Which of the following laboratory personnel is an MD?
   a. pathologist
   b. laboratory administrator
   c. technical supervisor
   d. medical technician

3. A phlebotomist reports first to the:
   a. laboratory administrator
   b. technical supervisor
   c. medical technician
   d. laboratory director

4. Which of the following tests would be delivered to the chemistry section?
   a. CBC
   b. Gram stain
   c. bilirubin
   d. type and screen

5. A prothrombin time (PT) test is performed in:
   a. coagulation
   b. immunology
   c. microbiology
   d. chemistry

6. Which of the following tests is **NOT** part of a CBC?
   a. red blood cell count
   b. platelet count
   c. sedimentation rate
   d. differential

7. Plasma differs from serum in that:
   a. serum contains fibrinogen
   b. serum is obtained by centrifugation
   c. plasma contains fibrinogen
   d. plasma is obtained by centrifugation

8. The clinical laboratory section that performs serum testing to detect antibodies to hepatitis viruses is:
   a. hematology
   b. chemistry
   c. blood bank
   d. immunology

9. The routine urinalysis includes all of the following **EXCEPT:**
   a. physical examination
   b. culture and sensitivity
   c. chemical testing
   d. microscopic examination

10. All of the following are found in whole blood **EXCEPT:**
    a. casts
    b. white blood cells
    c. red blood cells
    d. platelets

11. Testing of stools for parasites is performed in:
    a. hematology
    b. microbiology
    c. immunology
    d. urinalysis

12. A sentinel event would be most likely caused by delivery of a mislabeled tube to:
    a. coagulation
    b. hematology
    c. immunology
    d. blood bank

Clinical Situations

1 A phlebotomist with a high school diploma has completed a structured phlebotomy program and obtained national certification. After working in a hospital for a year, the phlebotomist asks the phlebotomy supervisor how he or she can continue with a clinical laboratory career.

   a. What would be the quickest education and training route the supervisor could recommend?
   b. What would be the next step in education and training for this person's advancement?
   c. How might specialist certification help this person's career?
   d. Name two categories of educational courses that could help this person's advancement to a laboratory manager.

2 State whether the following situations are acceptable or not acceptable procedure and explain your answer.

   a. A phlebotomist delivering a sample to the urinalysis section is instructed to place the sample in the refrigerator.
   b. A histology technician is examining Pap smears to detect cancerous cells.
   c. A phlebotomist delivers a gel serum separator tube to the blood bank for a type and crossmatch.
   d. A phlebotomist is asked to deliver a urine sample to microbiology for a C & S.
   e. A phlebotomist working in a POL is performing dipstick urinalysis.
   f. A phlebotomist delivers a CBC to the chemistry section.

CHAPTER 3

Regulatory, Ethical, and Legal Issues

Learning Objectives

Upon completion of this chapter, the reader will be able to:

1. Discuss the roles of the Clinical Laboratory Improvement Amendments (CLIA), Clinical and Laboratory Standards Institute (CLSI), the Joint Commission (JC), and the College of American Pathology (CAP) in the regulation of health care.
2. Discuss the JC Patient Safety Goals that relate to the laboratory and the phlebotomist.
3. Explain the role of the phlebotomist in complying with the Patient's Bill of Rights.
4. Differentiate between ethics and medical law.
5. State the primary role of the phlebotomist in complying with Health Insurance Portability and Accountability Act (HIPAA).
6. Define assault, battery, and defamation.
7. Describe how a phlebotomist could be involved in a malpractice suit.
8. State examples of how informed consent is obtained.
9. Describe how a phlebotomist should respond to a patient who refuses a venipuncture.
10. Describe the methods required for obtaining consent for collection of a sample for HIV testing.
11. Discuss the goals of a risk management department.
12. Define sentinel event and give examples of how a phlebotomist could be involved in an event.

Key Terms

Assault
Battery
Civil lawsuit
Code of ethics
Confidentiality
Criminal lawsuit
Defamation
Defendant
Health Insurance Portability and Accountability Act
Incident report
Informed consent
Invasion of privacy
Libel
Malpractice
Negligence
Opt-out screening
Patient Care Partnership
Patient Safety Goals
Patient's Bill of Rights
Plaintiff
Risk management
Root cause analysis
Sentinel event
Slander
Standard of care
Tort

This chapter is designed to stress to phlebotomists the important role they play in the health-care system. Along with importance comes responsibility. Therefore, phlebotomists must understand the regulatory, ethical, and legal aspects associated with the performance of phlebotomy.

REGULATORY ISSUES

The health-care regulation systems include both governmental and public agencies. All agencies have the same goal, which is to provide safe and effective health care.

Clinical Laboratory Improvement Amendments of 1988 (CLIA'88) ✷

CLIA is a governmental regulatory agency administered by the Centers for Medicare and Medicaid Services (CMS) and the Food and Drug Administration (FDA). CLIA stipulates that all laboratories that perform testing on human specimens for the purposes of diagnosis, treatment, monitoring, or screening must be licensed and obtain a certificate from the CMS. This includes all independent and hospital laboratories, physician-office laboratories, rural health clinics, mobile health screening entities such as health fairs, and public health clinics.

CLIA classifies laboratory tests into four categories: waived, provider performed microscopy, and non-waived testing. Nonwaived testing is separated in to the categories of moderate and high complexity with regard to requirements for personnel performing the tests (Box 3-1). Phlebotomists are subject to CLIA regulations when they are performing point-of-care testing (POCT) covered in Chapter 15. Laboratories with CLIA certification are inspected to document compliance with the regulations. The inspections may be performed by CMS personnel or an accrediting agency recognized by CMS including the College of American Pathologists (CAP), the Joint Commission (JC), and the Commission on Laboratory Assessment (COLA).

Clinical and Laboratory Standards Institute (CLSI)

The CLSI is a nonprofit organization that publishes recommendations by nationally recognized experts for the performance of laboratory testing. CLSI

BOX 3-1 CLIA Test Classifications

Waived Testing

Tests considered easy to perform by following the manufacturer's instructions and have little risk of error. No special training or education is required.
Example: Urine pregnancy test

Provider Performed Microscopy

Microscopy tests performed by a physician, midlevel practitioner, or a dentist.
Example: Microscopic urinalysis

Moderate Complexity Tests

Tests that require documentation of training in test principles, instrument calibration, periodic proficiency testing, and on-site inspections.
Example: Automated complete blood count (CBC)

High Complexity Tests

Tests that require sophisticated instrumentation and a high degree of interpretation. Proficiency testing and on-site inspections are required.
Example: Urine culture and susceptibility

---

standards are considered the ***standard of care*** for laboratory procedures. These standards are referred to throughout the text. In a legal situation, they would be considered the standard of care that should have been met.

Joint Commission (JC)

The JC is an independent, not-for-profit organization that accredits and certifies more than 15,000 health-care organizations and programs in the United States. The mission of the JC is to continuously improve the safety and quality of care provided to the public through the provision of health-care accreditation and related services that support performance improvement in health-care organizations.

The JC has recently published the Joint Commission ***Patient Safety Goals.*** It is essential that health-care organizations adhere to these goals to maintain their accreditation. Goals pertaining to the laboratory are:

Goal 1 Improving the Accuracy of Patient Identification
Goal 2 Improving the Effectiveness of Communication among Healthcare Givers

Goal 7 Reduce the Risk of Healthcare-Associated Infections

Goal 13 Encourage Patients' Active Involvement in Their Own Case as a Patient Safety Strategy

All of these goals are important to phlebotomy and are included throughout the text.

College of American Pathologists (CAP)

The CAP is an organization of board-certified pathologists that advocates high-quality and cost-effective medical care. The CAP provides laboratory accreditation and proficiency testing for laboratories.

For accreditation purposes, CAP-trained pathologists and laboratory managers and technologists perform on-site laboratory inspections on a biennial basis. Inspectors examine the laboratory's records and quality control of procedures for the preceding 2 years. Also examined are the qualifications of the laboratory staff including continuing education attendance, the laboratory's equipment, facilities, safety program, and laboratory management. CAP accreditation is accepted by both the CMS and the JC and fulfills Medicare/Medicaid requirements.

Laboratories that subscribe to the proficiency program receive periodic samples to analyze and return their results to the CAP. The laboratory receives a report on how its results compared with other laboratories performing the procedures in a similar manner.

Failure to perform satisfactorily on a proficiency test can result in a laboratory losing its CLIA certificate to perform the failed test.

Phlebotomists are included in a CAP inspection and also in proficiency testing when performing POCT.

ETHICAL AND LEGAL ISSUES

Principles of right and wrong, called the *code of ethics,* provide the personal and professional rules of performance and moral behavior as set by members of a profession. Medical ethics or bioethics focus on the patient to ensure that all members of a health-care team possess and exhibit the skill, knowledge, training, professionalism, and moral standards necessary to serve the patient. Professional agencies such as the American Society for Clinical Pathology (ASCP), American Society for Clinical Laboratory Science (ASCLS), and the National Phlebotomy Association (NPA) have developed codes of ethics for laboratory personnel. Phlebotomists are

expected to follow this code by performing the duties specified in their job description, adhering to established standards of performance, and continuing to improve their knowledge and skills (Box 3-2).

The Patient's Bill of Rights

A document first published by the American Hospital Association (AHA) in 1973 and amended in 1992 called the *Patient's Bill of Rights* specified what the patient has a right to expect during medical treatment. A patient's rights and dignity must be protected in the process of providing quality care. It was provided to patients upon hospital admission. The document addresses the following 12 areas:

1. Patients have the right to considerate and respectful care.
2. Patients have the right to obtain from their health-care provider complete current information about their diagnosis, treatment, and prognosis in terms that patients can be reasonably expected to understand.
3. Patients have the right to receive from a health-care provider the information necessary to give *informed consent* before a procedure. The information should include knowledge of the proposed procedure, with risks and probable duration of incapacitation. In addition, the patient has a right to information about medically significant alternatives.
4. Patients have the right to refuse treatment to the extent permitted by law and to be informed of the medical consequences of their action.
5. Patients have the right to privacy in their medical care. Case discussion, consultation, examination, and treatment should be conducted discreetly. Those not directly involved with a patient's care must have the patient's permission to be present.

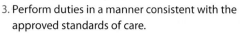

BOX 3-2 Conduct Included in Medical Codes of Ethics

1. First do no harm.
2. Respect patients' rights.
3. Perform duties in a manner consistent with the approved standards of care.
4. Continue to enhance knowledge and apply new techniques.
5. Demonstrate commitment to the profession and coworkers.

6. Patients have the right to expect that all communication and records pertaining to their care be treated as confidential.

7. Patients have the right to expect the hospital to make a reasonable response to their request for services and to provide evaluation, service, and referral as indicated.

8. Patients have the right to obtain information as to any relationship of their hospital with other health-care and educational institutions, insofar as their care is concerned, and to the professional relationship among individuals who are treating them.

9. Patients have the right to be advised if the hospital proposes to engage in or perform human experimentation affecting their care or treatment. Patients have the right to refuse to participate in research projects.

10. Patients have the right to expect continuity of care, including future appointments and instructions on continuing health-care requirements after discharge.

11. Patients have the right to examine and receive an explanation of their bill, regardless of the source of payment.

12. Patients have the right to know what hospital rules and regulations apply to their conduct as a patient (Box 3-3).

The Patient Care Partnership

In 2003 the AHA published a revision to the Patient's Bill of Rights titled *The Patient Care Partnership*: Understanding Expectations, Rights and Responsibilities. This revision is published as a brochure to be given to patients. A major goal of the revision was to provide information in plain, straightforward language to better communicate with patients. Notice the emphasis on improving communication that is in the JC Patient Safety Goal 2. All of the patients' rights from the original documents are covered in the brochure under new headings shown in Box 3-4.

 Technical Tip 3-1. The Patient Care Partnership brochure can be accessed at http://www.aha.org. On the home page click on "About" and then on "Patient Care Partnership."

Legal Issues Relating to Medicine

Failure to respect patients' rights and performing beneath the standard of care can result in legal action initiated by the patient or the patient's family. Medical law regulates the conduct of members of the health-care professions. It differs from ethics, which are recommended standards, by being legally required conduct. Litigation initiated because of illegal actions can be at the local, state, or national level and can result in criminal or civil prosecution. Penalties may include revocation of professional licenses, monetary fines, or imprisonment.

A *criminal lawsuit* is an action initiated by the state for committing an illegal act against the public welfare and can be punishable by imprisonment. A *civil lawsuit* is a court action between parties seeking monetary compensation for an offense.

BOX 3-3 The Phlebotomist is Directly Involved with the Following Sections of the Patient's Bill of Rights.

1. Patients may be difficult to deal with because they are afraid to be in the hospital or are angry because they have just received an unfavorable diagnosis. However, the phlebotomist must still treat them with respect and consideration.

2. Notice that it is the health-care provider, not the phlebotomist, who must provide information concerning the purpose of test procedures. When questioned, phlebotomists should refer the patient to the health-care provider.

3. The patient has the right to refuse to have blood drawn. If the patient still refuses after you have explained the procedure and explained that it was requested by the health-care provider to provide treatment, do not forcibly obtain the sample. Notify the nursing staff or the health-care provider of the patient's refusal and note this information on the requisition form.

4. The patient's condition and laboratory test results are confidential and must not be discussed with anyone who is not directly involved with the patient's care or testing. Do not discuss patient information in elevators or in the cafeteria where bystanders may overhear it.

5. Reports of laboratory test results are given only to the patient's health-care providers or their designated representatives. Family or friends requesting information should be referred to the patient's health-care provider.

BOX 3-4 The Patient Care Partnership

What to expect during your hospital stay
High-quality hospital care
A clean and safe environment
Involvement in your care
Protection of your privacy
Help when leaving the hospital
Help with your billing claims

In a lawsuit, the person who brings the lawsuit or action is the *plaintiff,* and the health-care worker or institution against whom the action or lawsuit is filed is the *defendant.*

Tort Law

A wrongful act committed by one person against another that causes harm to the person or his or her property is called a **tort.** Torts are classified as intentional and unintentional. **Assault, battery,** and **defamation** are considered intentional torts, whereas negligence and malpractice are considered unintentional torts.

- Assault is the threat to touch another person without his or her consent and with the intention of causing fear of harm.
- Battery is the actual harmful touching of a person without his or her consent.
- Defamation is spoken or written words that can injure a person's reputation.
- **Libel** is false defamatory writing that is published.
- **Slander** is false and malicious spoken word.
- **Invasion of privacy** is the violation of the patient's right to be left alone and the right to be free from unwanted exposure to public view.
- Release of confidential information is considered an invasion of privacy. Entering a patient's room without asking permission may be considered a physical intrusion and an invasion of privacy.

Other examples of invasion of privacy would be using a patient's laboratory requisition for classroom

> ❗ **Phlebotomist Alert 3-1.** Charges of
> ◆ assault and battery could be initiated against a phlebotomist who ignores the refusal or forcibly tries to collect a sample from a patient who refuses to have blood drawn.

> ❗ **Phlebotomist Alert 3-2.** Defamation
> ◆ relates to confidentiality. A patient can claim defamation if you release or are overheard saying any confidential information.

instruction purposes without removing the identification criteria or releasing patient information to a local newspaper or television reporter.

The Health Insurance Portability and Accountability Act of 1996

The Health Insurance Portability and Accountability Act of 1996 (HIPAA) legislation encompasses a variety of health-care issues, not all of which directly affect the laboratory. Primary goals of the legislation are to:

- Protect workers with pre-existing conditions from losing health insurance when changing jobs
- Provide easier detection of fraud and abuse
- Reduce paperwork by requiring electronic data transactions
- Guarantee the privacy of individual health information

In addition to developing approved methods of data transmission, health-care workers are most affected by the requirement to guarantee privacy of individual health information. The release of patient test results now falls under the HIPAA. In general, release of patient information, even between health-care providers, must be kept to the minimum required for care, and written patient consent to release the information must be obtained. Standards for complying with HIPAA continue to be developed. Phlebotomists can expect to encounter continually evolving methods and regulation of data transfer.

Confidentiality

Long before HIPAA was enacted health-care workers were legally responsible to respect the *confidentiality* of patient information. This information includes patient or health-care provider communications, the patient's verbal statements, or the patient's chart or laboratory results. All information acquired through the care of a patient must be kept confidential and given only to health professionals who have a medical need to know. Laboratory results may be given only to the health-care provider, and the patient must give permission to release the test results.

Phlebotomists collect samples for employee or athlete drug or alcohol screening, as well as screening for human immunodeficiency virus (HIV) or other sexually transmitted diseases. Care must be taken that this information not be discussed where it can be overheard by unauthorized people.

> **Phlebotomist Alert 3-3.** Unauthorized includes your coworkers not involved with the patient.

With the use of computers in health care, confidentiality and accessibility must be addressed. HIPAA has mandated that health-care professionals become familiar with information security standards and ensure that policies exist to control access to and release of patient-identifiable health information.

Malpractice

Medical ***malpractice*** is misconduct or lack of skill by a health-care professional that results in injury to the patient. ***Negligence,*** which is defined as failure to give reasonable care by the health-care provider, must be proven in a malpractice suit. Reasonable care requires that the health-care professional understand and practice a specific standard of care, which essentially means that he or she performs the duties with the same skill and knowledge as other workers with the same training and experience would.

State statutes, licensing requirements, and regulatory and professional agencies establish standards of care.

Four factors must be proven to claim negligence:

1. Duty: Indicates that there was an established standard of care and proof that it was not followed. The standard of care can be for the procedure and for the training and evaluating protocols of the phlebotomist performing the procedure.
2. Breach of Duty: The plaintiff (patient) must show what actually happened and that the defendant (phlebotomist) failed to perform. It has to be proven that the defendant knew or should have known that this failure could cause harm.
3. Causation: Indicates that the breach of duty directly caused the injury and that no other factors could have contributed.
4. Damages: Actual physical, emotional, or financial injury had to occur to the plaintiff (patient) because of the negligent act.

The most common phlebotomy events that may initiate litigation are nerve injury, hemorrhage from an accidental arterial puncture or inadequate pressure to the vein, drawing from inappropriate locations such as the same side as a mastectomy, injuries occurring when a patient faints, or death of a patient caused by misidentification of a patient or sample and wrong diagnosis or mistreatment of a patient due to sample collection errors. Examples of actual phlebotomist involvement in malpractice suits that resulted in awards to the plaintiff are shown in Box 3-5.

BOX 3-5 Examples of Medical Malpractice Involving Phlebotomists

Duty: Phlebotomists must have training, demonstrate competency when hired, have institutional policies available to them, and have periodic competency assessments.

1. Breach of Duty: Misidentification of a patient when collecting a sample for the blood bank
   Causation: Hemolytic transfusion reaction
   Damages:
   Patient 1. Death
   Patient 2. Lengthy treatment for acute renal failure
2. Breach of Duty:
   Patient 1. Phlebotomist performs a venipuncture at an excessive angle
   Patient 2. Vigorous probing during a second venipuncture
   Patient 3. Phlebotomist performs an unauthorized arterial puncture
   Causation:
   Patient 1. Nerve damaged during the puncture
   Patients 2 and 3. Formation of a large hematoma compressing the nerves in the arm
   Damages: Loss of function in the punctured arms
3. Breach of Duty: Phlebotomist assists patient out of bed to go the bathroom
   Phlebotomist is not trained to assist bedridden patients
   Causation: Patient falls
   Damages: Patient breaks hip
4. Breach of Duty: Phlebotomist does not place patient who states previous fainting episodes in a reclining chair or bed and observe patient following the venipuncture
   Causation: Patient stands up and falls
   Damages: Patient breaks arm

Technical Tip 3-2. To avoid becoming involved in a malpractice litigation, the phlebotomist must practice blood collection techniques following procedures that are written according to the CLSI standards at all times.

Patient Consent

Patients must give consent prior to any procedure and the type of consent depends on the type of procedure to be performed. Different types of patient consent in health care include informed consent, expressed consent, minor consent, implied consent, and HIV consent.

Informed Consent

Informed consent requires that the health-care professional explain what the medical procedure is; how it is to be performed, including possible risks; and the expected results. The procedure must be explained in a manner that the patient will understand. Vital to consent is the patient's belief that the health-care professional is competent to perform the procedure. Health-care professionals may be legally liable for failing to offer information to patients and for not obtaining informed consent. Consent may be expressed or implied.

Expressed Consent

Expressed consent is primarily required for invasive procedures but can include phlebotomy. The health-care worker explains the procedure as discussed under informed consent. The patient then gives consent in writing or verbally. The most commonly used and safest method for obtaining expressed consent is in writing. Verbal consent must be documented in the patient's chart.

Implied Consent

Implied consent is very common in blood collection. The phlebotomist must explain the procedure that will be used to collect the blood sample, stressing that the patient's health-care provider ordered the test. The patient expects that the phlebotomist is competent in blood collection procedures and gives consent to collect the blood samples by extending the arm or rolling up the sleeve.

Implied consent also exists when emergency procedures must be performed to save a person's life or prevent permanent impairment to the patient. The law implies consent for treatment for these patients without consent from the responsible party. Implied consent is a state statute, and the limitations vary from state to state.

Phlebotomist Alert 3-4. A patient has the right to refuse medical treatment, and this decision should be documented in the medical record.

Consent for Minors and Incapacitated Patients

Blood collection in minors requires consent of their parents or legal guardians. A legally responsible person must give consent for patients who cannot communicate, persons who are mentally incompetent, patients in shock or trauma, demented patients, or those under the influence of drugs or alcohol. A legal guardian who can give consent may have to be appointed by the courts.

Consent for Testing for Human Immunodeficiency Virus

State legislation may require informed consent be obtained before HIV testing is performed. The laws dictate what type of information must be provided to the patient. The patient may have to receive an explanation of the test and its purpose, possible uses of the test, the limitations of the test, and the meaning of the test results.

In 2006 the Centers for Disease Control and Prevention (CDC) issued a new screening recommendation for HIV testing on all persons between the ages of 13 and 64 receiving treatment at health-care facilities. The procedure is called ***opt-out screening*** or opt-out testing. This means that the patient is told that the HIV screening test is part of their routine care and covered by their general consent for treatment. Patients have the right to ask questions about the procedure and the right to decline (opt-out of) the procedure. This differs from opt-in testing where the health-care provider recommends that the patient have the test and the patient must give written consent. Based on state laws the procedure of opt-out screening may vary or not be an option for the facility to use.

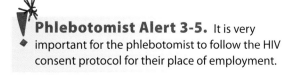
Phlebotomist Alert 3-5. It is very important for the phlebotomist to follow the HIV consent protocol for their place of employment.

In some states an accidental needlestick is considered a significant exposure to the health-care worker, and HIV testing can be ordered by a health-care provider without patient consent. In this situation, the HIV results are not entered into the patient's chart.

Respondeat Superior

The Latin phrase *respondeat superior*, "let the master answer," establishes that employers are responsible for their own acts of negligence as well as their employees' acts. Institutions are responsible for ensuring that their employees perform only those tasks that are within the scope of their knowledge and training. However, this does not diminish the responsibility of the employee. Both the institution and the employee can be found liable if injury occurs to the patient because of the employee's actions. Professional liability should be a concern for all health-care workers.

Malpractice Insurance

Most institutions have policies covering all workers, and the phlebotomist should confirm this coverage at the time of employment. Phlebotomists who work independently for insurance companies or home health-care agencies may need to be covered by personal malpractice insurance. Liability insurance can be purchased at a reduced rate through professional organizations.

By consistently practicing good patient care standards, the phlebotomist can avoid the trauma of a lawsuit (Box 3-6).

Risk Management

The potential for injury exists in the health-care profession, and the phlebotomist should be aware of these risks and the precautions necessary to minimize them. Risk is inherent with every venipuncture. **Risk management** departments develop policies to protect patients and employees from preventable injuries and the employer from financial loss. Risk management programs must identify the risk; determine policies and procedures to prevent the risk; educate employees, patients, and visitors; and evaluate changes that may be necessary for improvement.

Various tools are available to identify risks and determine methods for reducing risk and the financial loss incurred by paying for the occurrences after they have happened. One commonly used tool

---

BOX 3-6 Guidelines to Preventing a Lawsuit

- Obtain informed consent before collecting samples.
- Perform within the scope of training and education.
- Comply with state statutes and federal regulations (OSHA and JC regulations).
- Adhere to standard blood collection techniques as determined by CLSI guidelines, procedure manuals, and package inserts.
- Practice aseptic phlebotomy techniques.
- Correctly use personal protection equipment including safety devices and containers.
- Practice standard precautions.
- Keep patient information confidential.
- Practice good communication skills and genuine caring for the patient.
- Accurately record information concerning patients.
- Relay patient reports to the proper supervisor.
- Document incidents immediately and report them to a supervisor.
- Document any deviations from the standard care of practice.
- Avoid unethical criticism of other health-care professionals.
- Regularly participate in continuing education to maintain proficiency.
- Ensure that continuing education records are maintained.

---

in the phlebotomy department is the ***incident report*** (Fig. 3-1). The employee who detects the incident describes both the incident and the corrective action taken. Each step of the follow-up should be clearly documented. This form is used to investigate the occurrence and is signed by the employee's supervisor and reviewed by the quality assessment (QA) coordinator.

New policies and procedures are continually being developed and instituted as incidents are investigated. Effective communication and education in the new policies must be available for employees for successful implementation.

Preventing Medical Errors

In November 1999, the National Academy of Sciences' Institute of Medicine (IOM) issued a report entitled "To Err is Human: Building a Safer Health System." The report stimulated considerable public and governmental concern by stating that most

The Pathology Center at Methodist Hospital
PATHOLOGY INCIDENT REPORT

PART 1. TO BE COMPLETED BY EMPLOYEE DETECTING OCCURRENCE

Date of incident _____ Time of incident _____

Employee initiating report _____ Date of report _____

Patient Name _____ Patient ID_____ Room Number _____

Description of occurrence. Include any attachments, pertinent details, any supporting evidence or documentation, and immediate corrective action taken. Attach additional pages if necessary.

_____

_____

_____

_____

_____

_____

_____

_____

_____

_____

Immediate Corrective Action _____

_____

_____

_____

_____

_____

_____

_____

Employee signature (or initials)

Forward to Team Leader or Employee for additional comments
Page 1 of 2

The Pathology Center at Methodist Hospital

PART 2. TO BE COMPLETED BY EMPLOYEE (If different than employee initiating report)
(Forward to Team Leader)
Additional Comments

_____

_____

_____

_____

_____

_____

Signature/Date_____

Part 3. To be completed by Team Leader (Forward to Service Leader)
Patient Condition : Changed_____   Unchanged_____
Physician Notifed? Y   N   Name _____ Time_____ Date_____

Corrective Action Taken (if additional to immediate corrective action)

_____

_____

_____

_____

_____

Team Leader signature/date

PART 4: Classification of Incident (To be completed by Service Leader or Quality Assurance Coordinator)

Pathology Incident	Methodist Hospital Incident	Client Incident
A. __Specimen Problem	A. __Specimen Problem	A. __Specimen Problem
B. __Specimen ID	B. __Specimen ID	B. __Specimen ID
C. __Patient ID	C. __Patient ID	C. __Patient ID
D. __Order Error	D. __Order Error	D. __Order Error
E. __Safety Violation	E. __Safety Violation	E. __Safety Violation
F. __Complaint	F. __Complaint	F. __Complaint
G. __Communication	G. __Communication	G. __Communication
H. __Failure to respond to a STAT	H. __Lack of required information	H. __Lack of required information
I. __Test performed improperly	I. __Technical/procedural error	I. __Technical/Procedural error
J. __Result entry error	J. __Miscellaneous	J. __Miscellaneous
K. __Miscellaneous		

_____ Courier   _____ Tube system   Service Leader review _____

_____ Other   QA Coordinator review _____

Copy of report sent to:

Name _____ Title _____ Dept _____

Name _____ Title _____ Dept _____

Name _____ Title _____ Dept _____

Page 2 of 2

FIGURE 3-1 Pathology incident report. *(Courtesy of Diane Wolff, MLT (ASCP), Phlebotomy Team Leader, Nebraska Methodist Hospital, Omaha, NE.)*

adverse medical events were caused by preventable medical errors. Health-care institutions, accrediting agencies, and government agencies are placing increased emphasis on the designing of safe medical practices. The IOM report stresses that most of the medical errors are system related and are not caused by individual negligence or misconduct.

 Technical Tip 3-3. Systems should be designed to make it easy to do the right thing and hard to do the wrong thing.

Sentinel Events

As part of the JC's mission to improve safety and quality of health care, the commission has adopted a standard referred to as Sentinel Event Policies and Procedures.

A *sentinel event* is defined as an unexpected occurrence involving death or serious physical or psychological injury, or the risk thereof. Serious injury specifically includes loss of limb or function. A list of sentinel events designated by the JC is shown in Box 3-7. The list is updated periodically as the JC becomes aware of additional events.

BOX 3-7 Types of Reportable Sentinel Events

Patient suicide

Medication error

Procedural complication (patient identification)

Hemolytic transfusion reaction (patient identification)

Unauthorized absence

Wrong site/side surgery

Treatment delay

Abduction

Assault, rape, homicide

Fall related

Unanticipated full-term infant death

Unintended retention of a postsurgery foreign body

Sentinel events must be documented for the JC. The report must include a ***root cause analysis*** and an action plan. Acceptable root cause analyses identify basic or causal factors that underlie variation in performance, including the occurrence or possible occurrence of a sentinel event and focus primarily on systems and processes rather than individual performance.

A report concerning the event must be prepared for the JC. It can be sent at the time of the event and must be available for the JC for an accreditation renewal. Format for the report includes:

1. The event
2. A root cause analysis of the processes leading to the event
3. An action plan to be taken as a result of the event

As the JC analyzes sentinel event reports, it periodically publishes lists of specific sentinel event causes to alert the health-care community of areas to evaluate in their institutions.

A significant number of sentinel events involve incorrect patient identification. This problem directly affects the phlebotomist and serves to stress again the importance of this first step in any phlebotomy procedure. Remember that the first Patient Safety Goal addresses patient identification. Of equal concern to the phlebotomist should be the improper labeling of samples delivered to the laboratory and in particular the blood bank, because this can be the root cause of a hemolytic transfusion reaction.

Key Points

✦ Agencies regulating the laboratory and phlebotomy include:
  ✦ CLIA—Requirements for persons performing waived, provider-performed microscopy, moderate-complexity, and high-complexity testing
  ✦ JC—Accreditation and certification of health-care organizations
  ✦ CAP—Laboratory accreditation and provision of proficiency testing
  ✦ CLSI—Agency that develops written standards and guidelines for sample collection, handling and processing, and laboratory testing and reporting
✦ The JC Patient Safety Goals affecting the phlebotomist include patient identification, communication, health-care–associated infection and patient involvement in their care.
✦ The Patient's Bill of Rights and the Patient Care Partnership require phlebotomists to be respectful of their patients, refer patients to their health-care provider for information on their tests and condition, recognize that a patient can refuse treatment, and maintain the confidentiality of patient information.
✦ Ethics are recommended standards of right and wrong. Medical law specifies legally required conduct of health-care providers.
✦ HIPAA requires that patient information only be provided to designated persons.
✦ A phlebotomist who ignores a patient who refuses a procedure and continues to prepare for the procedure can be accused of assault. A phlebotomist who performs a procedure on a patient who refuses the procedure can be accused of battery. A phlebotomist discussing a patient's condition in a public place can be accused of defamation or breach of confidentiality.
✦ All of the following can put phlebotomists in danger of a malpractice suit:
  ✦ Patient or sample misidentification resulting in harm to the patient
  ✦ Performing a venipuncture incorrectly and causing nerve damage to the patient's arm
  ✦ Failure to follow Occupational Safety and Health Administration (OSHA) standard precautions resulting in an infected patient
  ✦ Performing an unauthorized arterial puncture resulting in loss of function to the patient's arm
  ✦ Failure to return a bed rail to its original position or assisting a patient to perform an activity for which the phlebotomist is not trained to perform resulting in patient injury
✦ A patient has the right to refuse treatment, including phlebotomy. When a patient refuses to allow a blood sample to be collected, the phlebotomist should contact the patient's health-care provider and document the incident.
✦ Informed consent requires the health-care worker to thoroughly explain the procedure. Expressed consent may be given verbally or in writing. Written consent is needed for invasive procedures. Implied consent is commonly seen in phlebotomy. After the phlebotomist explains the procedure, the patient extends his or her arm. A parent or legal guardian's consent is required for minors or patients incapable of speaking for themselves.
✦ Based on state laws, patient consent for HIV testing may require certain information regarding the purpose, possible uses, limitations, and meaning of the test be provided to the patient. CDC recommends opt-out testing be performed on all patients between the ages of 13 and 64 as a routine procedure. Consent for HIV testing will vary among states and place of employment.
✦ The goal of a risk management department is to identify risks and develop policies to protect patients and employees from preventable injuries.
✦ A sentinel event is an unexpected occurrence resulting in death or serious physical (such as loss of a limb) or psychological injury. A report including the event, a root cause analysis, and an action plan must be developed for the JC. Phlebotomists can cause a sentinel event by patient misidentification and sample mislabeling.

BIBLIOGRAPHY

Clinical Laboratory Improvement Amendments. http://www.cdc.gov/clia/.

College of American Pathologists. http://www.cap.org.

Health Information Portability and Accountability Act. http://www.cms.hhs.gov/HIPAAGenInfo.

National Academy of Sciences' Institute of Medicine: To Err Is Human: Building a Safer Health System. National Academy Press, 1999, Washington, DC.

National Patient Safety Goals. http://www.jointcommission.org/PatientSafety/.

Sentinel Events. http://www.jointcommission.org/SentinelEvents/.

Study Questions

1. Which of the following laboratory regulatory agencies classifies laboratory tests by their complexity?
   a. CAP
   b. JC
   c. HIPAA
   d. CMS

2. A phlebotomist who fails to change gloves and wash hands between patients is not observing the:
   a. Clinical Laboratory Improvement Amendments
   b. Joint Commission Patient Safety Goals
   c. College of American Pathology Safety Rules
   d. Patient's Bill of Rights

3. Phlebotomists' involvement with the Patient's Bill of Rights includes all of the following **EXCEPT** the patient's right to:
   a. refuse treatment
   b. respectful care
   c. receive diagnostic information from their health-care provider
   d. examine their hospital bill

4. Ethics are defined as:
   a. standards of right and wrong
   b. legally required conduct
   c. the patient's right to know
   d. the standard of care

5. The law that specifically addresses privacy of health information is the:
   a. Patient's Bill of Rights
   b. Clinical Laboratory Improvement Amendments
   c. Health Insurance Portability and Accountability Act
   d. JC Patient Safety Goals

6. A phlebotomist who tells a patient who is refusing to have blood drawn to calm down or they will get someone to hold them down is committing:
   a. assault
   b. negligence
   c. defamation
   d. battery

7. Performing an unauthorized arterial puncture that results in damage to the patient's use of the arm is termed:
   a. malpractice
   b. negligence
   c. unethical
   d. battery

8. Implied consent for a venipuncture on an adult requires the:
   a. patient's signature
   b. patient extending an arm
   c. presence of a witness
   d. signature of a witness

9. When a patient refuses to have blood drawn, the phlebotomist should:
   a. notify the patient's health-care provider
   b. ask another phlebotomist to collect the sample
   c. document the refusal
   d. both A and C

10. Consent for HIV testing:
    a. must adhere to state laws
    b. must be done on an opt-out basis
    c. must be done on an opt-in basis
    d. requires written consent

Study Questions—cont'd

11. Risk management departments develop policies to protect the:
  a. employees
  b. patients
  c. employer
  d. all of the above

12. An unexpected patient death that is not related to the patient's illness is termed a:
  a. root cause error
  b. human error
  c. sentinel event
  d. professional liability

Clinical Situations

1 A hometown professional football player was admitted to the hospital for blood work. Tests to rule out Hodgkin's disease were ordered. The phlebotomist obtained the blood samples and delivered them to the laboratory. After work, the phlebotomist told friends about drawing blood from the famous person and the sad reason why he was in the hospital.

  a. Could the phlebotomist face legal charges? Why or why not?
  b. If the football coach calls the laboratory for the test results, can a phlebotomist release the results? Why or why not?
  c. Under what conditions would HIPAA permit release of these results to the coach?

2 Indicate whether a phlebotomist would be accused of libel, slander, assault, battery, invasion of privacy, negligence, or malpractice in the following situations.

  a. A phlebotomist tells a patient who refuses to have blood drawn that help will be summoned to forcibly obtain the blood.
  b. A nurse reports that a patient was found sleeping with a bed rail lowered after the phlebotomist had drawn blood.
  c. A phlebotomist, angry over recently receiving a speeding ticket, tells a local reporter that the police officer has been to the hospital for an HIV test and it was positive. The hospital has no record of this.
  d. A phlebotomist pretends to be checking on a celebrity patient who is recovering from surgery.

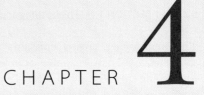

Safety and Infection Control

Learning Objectives

Upon completion of this chapter, the reader will be able to:

1. List and describe the six components of the chain of infection and the safety precautions that will break the chain.
2. Define nosocomial and health-care–associated infections.
3. Describe the correct procedure for performing routine hand hygiene.
4. List and state the purpose of the personal protective equipment used by phlebotomists.
5. Describe the symptoms of latex allergy.
6. Describe the procedures for donning and removing personal protective equipment (PPE).
7. List and describe Standard Precautions.
8. List and describe the transmission-based precautions.
9. Describe the procedures followed by phlebotomists in isolation areas.
10. Name a common blood and body fluid disinfectant.
11. Describe the requirements mandated by the Occupational Exposure to Bloodborne Pathogens Compliance Directive.
12. List in order the actions to be taken if an exposure to bloodborne pathogens occurs.
13. Describe safety precautions used when handling chemicals and the purpose of an MSDS.
14. State when a phlebotomist should avoid areas marked with a radiation symbol.
15. Discuss electrical safety and the procedure to follow in cases of electrical shock.
16. Define the acronyms RACE and PASS.
17. Identify the types of fire extinguishers and the NFPA hazardous materials symbols.
18. List six precautions observed by phlebotomists to avoid physical hazards.

Key Terms

Airborne precautions
Biohazard
Chain of infection
Contact precautions
Droplet precautions
Health-care–acquired infection
Infection control
Nosocomial infection
Personal protective equipment
Postexposure prophylaxis
Radioactivity
Standard Precautions
Transmission-based precautions

The health-care setting contains a wide variety of safety hazards, many capable of producing serious injury or life-threatening disease. To work safely in this environment, the phlebotomist must learn what hazards exist and the basic safety precautions associated with them and finally apply the basic rules of commonsense required for everyday safety. Some hazards are unique to the health-care environment and others are encountered routinely throughout life. One must also keep in mind that these hazards affect not only the phlebotomist but also the patient. Therefore, phlebotomists must be prepared to protect both themselves and the patients (Table 4-1).

BIOLOGICAL HAZARDS

The health-care setting provides an abundant source of potentially harmful microorganisms. All health-care facilities have developed procedures to control and monitor infections occurring within their facilities. This is referred to as *infection control.*

The Chain of Infection

The *chain of infection* requires a continuous link between six components (Fig. 4-1). To prevent infection it is necessary to understand the components that make up the chain and the methods by which the chain can be broken. The components in the chain are:

1. Infectious Agent
   Infectious agents consist of bacteria, fungi, parasites, and viruses.

Breaking the Chain: Early detection and treatment of infectious agents.

2. Reservoir
   The reservoir must be a place where the infectious agent can live and possibly multi-ply. Humans and animals make ideal reservoirs. Equipment and other soiled objects often called fomites will serve as reservoirs particularly if they contain blood or other body fluids. Some microorganisms form spores or become inactive when conditions are not ideal such as in dried blood. They wait patiently until a suitable reservoir is available.
   Breaking the Chain: Disinfecting the work area kills the infectious agent and eliminates the reservoir.

3. Portal of Exit
   The infectious agent must have a way to exit the reservoir to continue the chain of infection. When the reservoir is a human or an animal this can be through the nose, mouth, and mucous membranes and in blood or other body fluids. Phlebotomists provide a portal of exit when they collect blood.
   Breaking the Chain: Disposing of needles and lancets in sealed sharps containers and other contaminated materials in biohazard containers and keeping tubes and sample containers sealed. When contaminated materials are in the appropriate containers, the infectious agent still has a reservoir but no means to exit as long as the container remains sealed.

TABLE 4-1 • Types of Safety Hazards		
TYPE	**SOURCE**	**POSSIBLE INJURY**
Biological	Infectious agents	Bacterial, fungal, viral, or parasitic infections
Sharp	Needles, lancets, and broken glass	Cuts, punctures, or bloodborne pathogen exposure
Chemical	Preservatives and reagents	Exposure to poisonous, caustic, or carcinogenic agents
Radioactive	Equipment and radioisotopes	Damage to a fetus or generalized overexposure to radiation
Electrical	Ungrounded or wet equipment and frayed cords	Burns or shock
Fire/explosive	Open flames and organic chemicals	Burns or dismemberment
Physical	Wet floors, heavy boxes, and patients	Falls, sprains, or strains

4. Means of Transmission
Once the infectious agent has left the reservoir it must have a way to reach a susceptible host. Means of transmission include:

- Direct contact: unprotected host touches or is touched by the reservoir
- Droplet: the host inhales material from the reservoir such as aerosol droplets from an infected person

- Airborne: inhalation of dried aerosol nuclei circulating on air currents or attached to dust particles
- Vehicle: ingestion of contaminated food or water
- Vector: parasites such as malaria transmitted by a mosquito bite

Technical Tip 4-1. For phlebotomists the means of transmission can be an accidental needlestick.

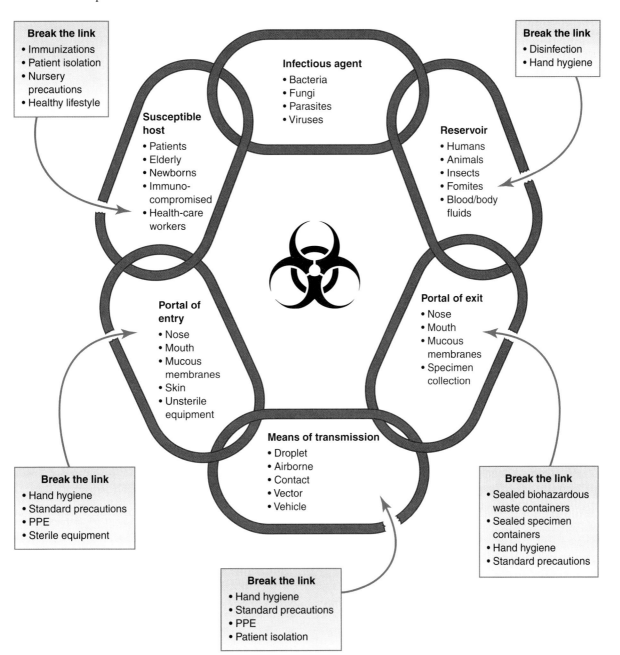

FIGURE 4-1 Chain of infection and safety practices related to the biohazard symbol.

Breaking the Chain: Hand washing, *Standard Precautions* and *transmission-based precautions* are covered later in this chapter.

5. Portal of Entry

After the infectious agent has been transmitted to a new reservoir it must have a means to enter the reservoir. The portal of entry can be the same as the portal of exit. This includes the nose, mouth, mucous membranes, and open wounds. Medical and surgical procedures provide a very convenient portal of entry for infectious agents. This is why all needles used in phlebotomy are packaged individually in sterile containers and a needle is never used more than once or from a container that has been opened.
Breaking the Chain: Disinfection and sterilization and strict adherence to Standard Precautions and transmission-based precautions are used to block the portal of entry.

6. Susceptible Host

This can be another patient or the health-care provider. Patients are ideal susceptible hosts because their immune systems that normally provide defense against infection are already involved with the patient's illness. Patients receiving chemotherapy and immunocompromised patients are very susceptible hosts. The immune system is still developing in newborns and infants and begins to weaken as people age, making these groups of patients more susceptible to infection. The immune system also is depressed by stress, fatigue, and lack of proper nutrition. These factors contribute to the susceptibility of the health-care provider.
Breaking the Chain: Observation of special precautions when working in the nursery and in isolation rooms designated for protection of susceptible patients. Workers must stay current with the required health-care workers' immunizations and tests (Box 4-1). Maintenance of a healthy lifestyle is very important for the health-care worker.

Nosocomial/Health-Care–Acquired Infections

The term *nosocomial infection* has been used to designate an infection acquired by a patient during a hospital stay. A newer term *health-care–acquired infection* **(HAI)** refers to an infection acquired by a patient as

---

BOX 4-1 Health-Care Worker Immunizations/ Tests
Hepatitis B vaccination
Completion of three-shot immunization protocol
Positive antibody titer
Measles, mumps, and rubella (MMR)
Immunization
Current positive antibody titer
Varicella (chickenpox)
Immunization
Current positive antibody titer
Tetanus
Immunization within the past 10 years
Annual tuberculosis skin test (purified protein derivative [PPD])
Positive tests followed by chest radiograph

---

the result of a health-care procedure that may or may not require a hospital stay. For example, an HAI could occur following an outpatient phlebotomy procedure if proper precautions were not followed.

 Technical Tip 4-2. It is not uncommon for people to use either of these terms for all health-care–acquired infections. The abbreviation HAI may also be translated into a hospital acquired or associated infection.

The number of HAIs has been increasing in recent years. Estimates have raised the number from 5 percent to 8 percent of hospital admissions. The number of HAIs is estimated at 1.7 million per year with 99,000 deaths occuring as a result of the infection. The Hospital Infection Control Practices Advisory Committee (HICPAC) of the Centers for Disease Control and Prevention (CDC) monitors and analyzes infection control.

Although some HAIs are caused by visitors, the majority are the result of personnel not following infection control practices.

In addition to observing infection control procedures, phlebotomists must report all cases of personal illness to a supervisor and keep immunizations current. A phlebotomist with a contagious disease can easily transmit it to a patient, and institutions have regulations limiting patient contact in certain conditions.

Conditions limiting phlebotomist-patient contact are shown in Box 4-2.

Transmission Prevention Procedures

Preventing the transmission of microorganisms from infected reservoirs to susceptible hosts is critical in controlling the spread of infection. Procedures used to prevent microorganism transmission include hand hygiene, the wearing of **personal protective equipment** (**PPE**), isolation of highly infective or highly susceptible patients, and proper disposal of contaminated materials. Strict adherence to guidelines published by the CDC and the Occupational Safety and Health Administration (OSHA) is essential. These procedures are designed to protect the phlebotomist when encountering infectious patients, prevent the phlebotomist from transferring microorganisms among patients, and protect highly susceptible patients.

Hand Hygiene

Hand contact represents the number one method of infection transmission. Phlebotomists circulate from one patient to another throughout their working hours, and without the observance of proper precautions, such contact can provide an unlimited vehicle for the transmission of infection.

Hand hygiene includes both hand washing and the use of alcohol-based antiseptic cleansers (Fig. 4-2). Alcohol-based cleansers can be used when hands are not visibly contaminated. They are not recommended after contact with spore-forming bacteria including *Clostridium difficile* and *Bacillus sp.*

 Technical Tip 4-3. *C. difficile* has become a major source of HAIs.

When using alcohol-based cleansers, the cleanser is applied to the palm of one hand. The hands are rubbed together and over the entire cleansing area, including between the fingers and thumbs. The rubbing is continued until the alcohol dries.

The importance of hand hygiene extends away from the patient setting to include the protection of

---

BOX 4-2 Conditions That Can Limit Phlebotomist-Patient Contact

Chickenpox
Conjunctivitis
Diarrheal disorders
Hepatitis A
Herpes zoster/shingles
Impetigo
Influenza
Mumps
Pediculosis/lice
Pertussis/whooping cough
Respiratory synctial virus (RSV)
Rubella
Scabies
Streptococcus group A/strep throat
Tuberculosis/active
Work status varies with institutional regulations determined by the employee health department and may require physician clearance.

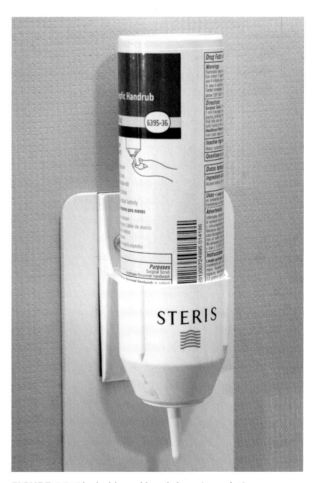

FIGURE 4-2 **Alcohol-based hand cleansing solution.**

coworkers, family and friends, and the phlebotomist. Hands should always be washed:

- Before patient contact
- When gloves are removed
- Before leaving the work area
- At any time when they have been knowingly contaminated
- Before going to designated break areas
- Before and after using bathroom facilities

The CDC has developed hand washing guidelines to be followed for correct routine hand washing. Procedure 4-1 demonstrates the CDC routine hand washing guidelines. More stringent procedures are used in surgery and in areas with highly susceptible patients such as immunocompromised and burn patients and newborns.

PROCEDURE 4-1 ✦ **Hand Washing Technique**

EQUIPMENT:

Antimicrobial soap
Paper towels
Running water
Waste container

PROCEDURE:

Step 1. Wet hands with warm water. Do not allow parts of body to touch the sink.

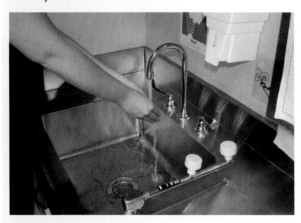

Step 2. Apply soap, preferably antimicrobial.

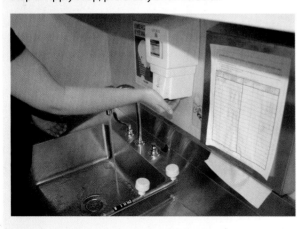

Step 3. Rub to form a lather, create friction, and loosen debris. Thoroughly clean between the fingers and under the fingernails for at least 20 seconds; include thumbs and wrists in the cleaning.

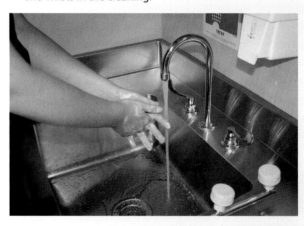

Step 4. Rinse hands in a downward position to prevent recontamination of hands and wrists.

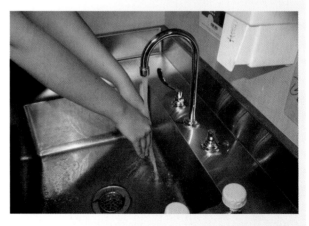

PROCEDURE 4-1 ✦ **Hand Washing Technique** (Continued)

Step 5. Obtain paper towel from dispensor.

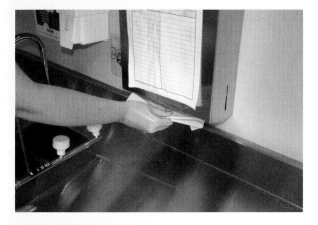

Step 7. Turn off faucets with a clean paper towel to prevent recontamination.

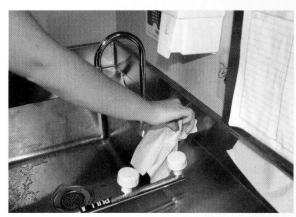

Step 6. Dry hands with paper towel.

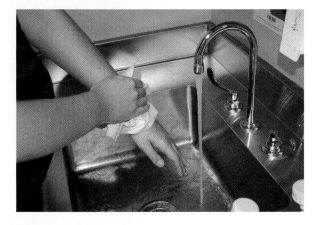

 Technical Tip 4-4. Scrubbing the hands for 20 seconds is approximately the time it will take you to sing the ABCs or 2 rounds of "Happy Birthday."

Personal Protective Equipment (PPE)

PPE encountered by the phlebotomist includes gloves, gowns, masks, goggles, face shields, and respirators.

Gloves

Gloves are worn to protect the health-care worker's hands from contamination by patient body substances and to protect the patient from possible microorganisms on the health-care worker's hands. They are mandated by the National Institute of Occupational Safety and Health (NIOSH) for phlebotomy procedures. Wearing gloves is not a substitute for hand washing. Hands must always be washed before putting on gloves and after removing gloves. A variety of gloves is available including sterile and nonsterile, powdered and unpowdered, and latex and nonlatex.

Latex Allergy

Allergy to latex is increasing among health-care workers, and phlebotomists should be alert for symptoms of reactions associated with latex contact. Reactions to latex include irritant contact dermatitis that produces patches of dry, itchy irritation on the hands, delayed hypersensitivity reactions resembling poison ivy that appear 24 to 48 hours following exposure, and true immediate hypersensitivity reactions often characterized by respiratory difficulty. Hand washing immediately after removal of gloves and avoiding powdered gloves may aid in preventing the development of latex allergy. Replacing latex gloves with nitrile or vinyl gloves provides an acceptable alternative. Phlebotomists should report any signs of a latex reaction to a supervisor because true latex allergy can be life-threatening.

 Safety Tip 4-1. Be alert for warnings of latex allergy in patients and take appropriate precautions.

Gowns

Gowns are worn to protect the clothing and skin of health-care workers from contamination by patient body substances and to prevent the transfer of microorganisms out of patient rooms. Fluid-resistant gowns should be worn when the possibility of encountering splashes or large amounts of body fluids is anticipated. Gowns tie in the back at the neck and the waist and have tight-fitting cuffs. They should be large enough to provide full body coverage, including closing completely at the back.

 Technical Tip 4-5. It may be necessary to use two gowns if one gown will not cover the back. Put the first gown on and tie it in the back. Put the second gown on and tie it in the front.

Masks, Goggles, and Face Shields

Masks are worn to protect against inhalation of droplets containing microorganisms from infective patients. Masks and goggles are worn to protect the mucous membranes of the mouth, nose, and eyes from splashing of body substances (Fig. 4-3). Face shields also protect the mucous membranes from splashes.

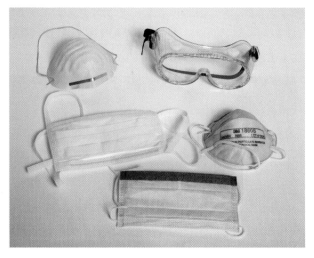

FIGURE 4-3 Face protective equipment.

Respirators

Respirators may be required when collecting blood from patients who have airborne diseases, such as tuberculosis. The NIOSH approved respirator is the N95. With the increased incidents of antibiotic-resistant tuberculosis and the appearance of new strains of influenza viruses, respirators have become more routinely used. The N95 respirators are individually fitted for each person who will be wearing one.

Donning and Removing PPE

Specific procedures must be followed when putting on and removing protective apparel (see Procedures 4-2 and 4-3). To prevent contact with or the spread of infectious microorganisms, apparel is put on before entering a room and removed and disposed of before leaving the room. An exception to these procedures is observed for patients requiring sterile conditions and is discussed later in this chapter. Care must be taken to avoid touching the outside of contaminated areas of apparel when it is being removed.

EQUIPMENT:

Gown
Mask
Face shield
Gloves
Biohazard waste container

PROCEDURE:

Step 1. The gown is put on first and tied at the neck and waist.

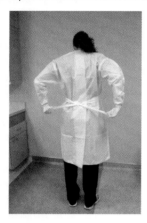

Step 2. Place face protection over the nose and mouth.

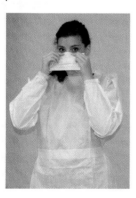

Step 3. Masks with ties are fastened first at the top, adjusted to the nose and mouth, tied at the neck and refitted. Masks with straps are fitted to the nose and mouth. The mask is held in place with one hand while the other hand places the straps over the head and a final adjustment is made.

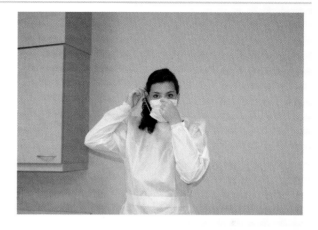

Step 4. When needed, goggles and face shields are put on after the mask and adjusted for fit.

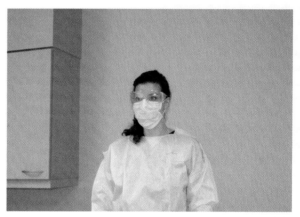

Respirators are individually fitted for the wearer and are donned just prior to entering the room.

Step 5. Gloves are donned last and securely pulled over the cuffs of the gown.

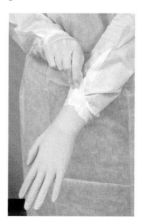

PROCEDURE 4-3 ✦ **Removing Personal Protective Equipment**

EQUIPMENT:

Gloves
Gown
Face shield
Biohazard container

PROCEDURE:

Step 1. Gloves are the most contaminated. They are removed first.

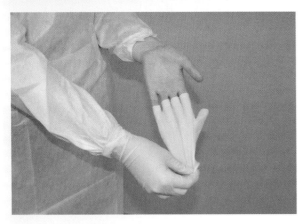

Step 2. The first glove is pulled off using the gloved hand so that it will end up inside out in the still gloved hand.

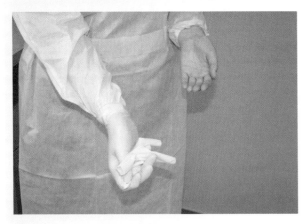

Step 3. Remove the second glove by sliding the ungloved finger inside the glove of the other hand and remove the glove without touching the outside of the glove.

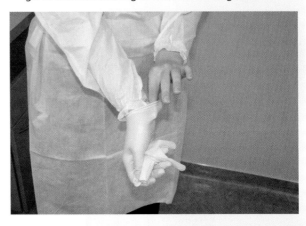

Step 4. Dispose of gloves in a biohazard container.

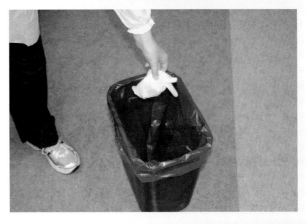

Step 5. Untie the gown and remove it by touching only the inside of the gown.

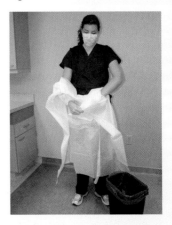

PROCEDURE 4-3 ✦ **Removing Personal Protective Equipment** (Continued)

Step 6. Dispose of the gown in a biohazard container.

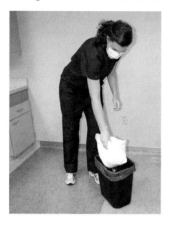

Step 7. Remove the mask touching only the ties or bands.

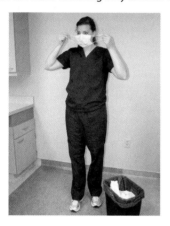

Step 8. Unfasten the lower tie first so that the mask will not fall forward while removing the lower tie. Dispose of the mask in a biohazard container.

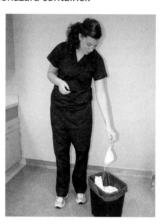

Standard Precautions

Standard Precautions (SP) were developed by the CDC by combining the recommendations of Universal Precautions and Body Substance Isolation procedures. CDC consistently modifies SP as changes occur in the health-care environment. SP assumes that every person in the health-care setting is potentially infected or colonized by an organism that could be transmitted. SP applies to all blood and body fluids, mucous membranes, and nonintact skin and stresses hand washing (Fig. 4-4).

 Technical Tip 4-6. The continual emergence of antibiotic-resistant bacteria will result in modifications to Standard Precautions.

Transmission-Based Precautions

In addition to the protective barriers provided by PPE, the spread of infection can be controlled by placing highly infectious or highly susceptible patients in private isolation rooms. Guidelines for isolation practices are published by the CDC and have been periodically revised to meet the ever-changing health-care environment. Phlebotomists will find these guidelines regarding PPE posted on the outside of doors to isolation rooms.

Safety Tip 4-2. Pay strict attention to all warning signs posted outside or inside patient rooms.

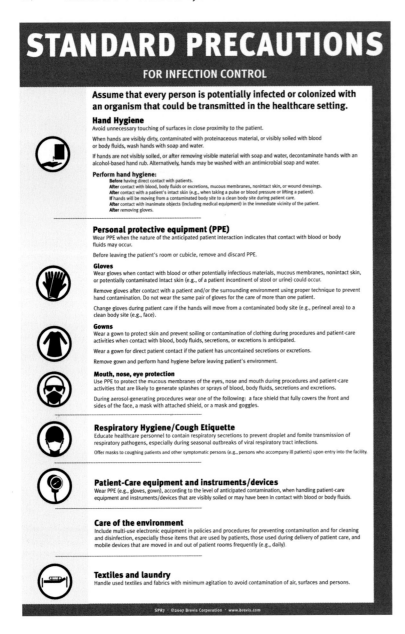

FIGURE 4-4 **Standard precautions.** *(Courtesy of Brevis Corporation. http://www.brevis.com.)*

Classification of isolation has evolved from category-specific isolation to disease-specific isolation to the current practice of transmission-based precautions instituted in 1995. The type of PPE worn by phlebotomists when entering an isolation room is determined by the isolation classification. Warning signs containing specific instructions for the type of PPE required are posted on the doors of isolation rooms. The three isolation categories used in transmission-based precautions are airborne, droplet, and contact. They are implemented in addition to SP for patients known or suspected to be infected by certain microorganisms that are transmitted by these routes (see Table 4-2).

Airborne precautions are necessary when microorganisms can remain infective while being carried through the air on the dried residue of a droplet or on a dust particle. PPE may include a respirator. Filtration systems may be required in the patient's room (Fig. 4-5).

Droplet precautions are required for persons infected with microorganisms that can be transmitted on moist particles such as those produced during coughing and sneezing. Droplets are capable of traveling only short

TABLE 4-2 • **Transmission-Based Precautions Classifications**		
TYPE	**POSSIBLE CONDITIONS**	**PPE**
Airborne	Tuberculosis, measles, chickenpox, herpes zoster/shingles, mumps, adenovirus	Standard Precautions Mask or respirator
Droplet	Infection with *Neisseria meningitides, Haemophilus sp.,* pertussis/whooping cough, Group A streptococcus, influenza, rhinovirus, scarlet fever, parvovirus B19, respiratory syncytial virus, and diphtheria	Standard Precautions Mask
Contact	*Clostridium difficile,* rotavirus, draining wounds, antibiotic-resistant infections, scabies, impetigo, herpes simplex, respiratory syncytial virus, and herpes zoster	Standard Precautions Gown and gloves

PPE = personal protective equipment.

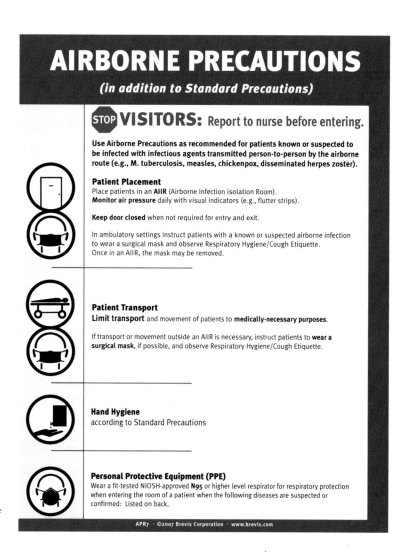

FIGURE 4-5 **Airborne precautions.** *(Courtesy of Brevis Corporation. http://www.brevis.com.)*

distances through the air, less than 3 feet; therefore, masks are worn when procedures requiring close patient contact are performed (Fig. 4-6).

 Technical Tip 4-7. Respiratory hygiene is a recent addition to Standard Precautions (see Fig. 4.4).

Contact precautions are used when patients have an infection that can be transmitted by direct skin-to-skin contact or by indirect contact by touching objects in the patient's room. Gloves should be worn even if no contact with moist body substances is anticipated. Gowns are worn when entering the room and removed before leaving the room. After removing the gown and washing the hands, care must be taken to avoid touching objects in the room (Fig. 4-7).

Phlebotomy Procedures in Isolation

Special precautions must be taken with phlebotomy equipment and samples collected in isolation areas. Bring only necessary equipment (not the phlebotomy tray) into isolation rooms. Be sure, however, to include duplicate collection tubes and enough supplies to perform a second venipuncture if necessary. All equipment, including PPE, taken into the room must be left in the room and, when appropriate, deposited in labeled waste containers. Tourniquets, gauze, alcohol pads, and pens may already be present in the room.

Samples taken from the room should be cleaned of any blood contamination and placed in plastic bags located near or just outside the door. Bags should be folded open to allow tubes to be added to the bag without touching the outside of the bag with contaminated

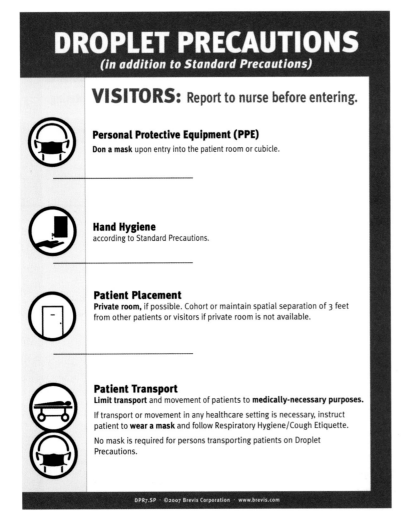

FIGURE 4-6 Droplet precautions. *(Courtesy of Brevis Corporation. http://www.brevis.com.)*

CONTACT PRECAUTIONS
(in addition to Standard Precautions)

STOP VISITORS: Report to nurse before entering.

Gloves
Don gloves upon entry into the room or cubicle.
Wear gloves whenever touching the patient's intact skin or surfaces and articles in close proximity to the patient.
Remove gloves before leaving patient room.

Hand Hygiene
according to Standard Precautions

Gowns
Don gown upon entry into the room or cubicle.
Remove gown and observe hand hygiene before leaving the patient-care environment.

Patient Transport
Limit transport of patients to medically necessary purposes.
Ensure that infected or colonized areas of the patient's body are contained and covered.
Remove and dispose of contaminated PPE and perform hand hygiene prior to transporting patients on Contact Precautions.
Don clean PPE to handle the patient at the transport destination.

Patient-Care Equipment
Use disposable noncritical patient-care equipment or implement patient-dedicated use of such equipment.

CPR7 · ©2007 Brevis Corporation · www.brevis.com

FIGURE 4-7 Contact precautions. *(Courtesy of Brevis Corporation. http://www.brevis.com.)*

gloves or tubes (Fig. 4-8). If double bagging is required, a clean open bag must be available immediately outside the room.

 Technical Tip 4-8. Double-bagging may require a second person to stand outside the room to hold the second bag open.

Protective/Reverse Isolation

In addition to preventing transmission of microorganisms from infected patients to other persons, patients with compromised immunity must be protected from microorganisms routinely encountered by persons with intact immune systems. Protective isolation procedures may be required for severely burned patients, patients receiving chemotherapy, and organ and bone marrow transplant patients and in the nursery.

PPE worn by phlebotomists entering protective isolation includes gowns, gloves, and masks. All PPE must be sterile instead of the routinely used chemically clean PPE that is acceptable in other situations.

When performing phlebotomy under conditions of protective isolation, only necessary equipment is brought in to the room and all equipment brought into the room is taken out of the room. PPE is removed after leaving the room.

 Technical Tip 4-9. Gowns used when entering patient isolation rooms are put on over the laboratory coat.

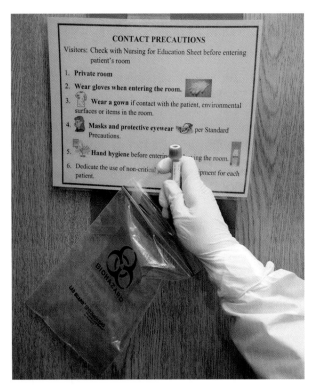

FIGURE 4-8 Example of sample bagging outside of a room.

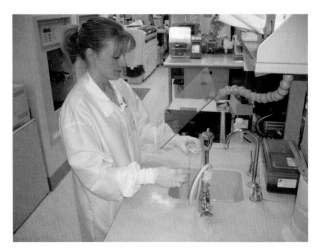

FIGURE 4-9 Technologist using plastic shield to dispose of urine samples. *(From Strasinger, SK, and Di Lorenzo, MS: Urinalysis and Body Fluids, ed. 5. FA Davis, 2008, Philadelphia, with permission.)*

PPE in the Laboratory

PPE used in the laboratory includes gloves, fluid-resistant gowns, eye and face shields, and Plexiglas countertop shields. Gloves should be worn when in contact with patients, samples, and laboratory equipment or fixtures. When samples are collected, gloves must be changed between every patient. In the laboratory, they are changed whenever they become noticeably contaminated or damaged and are always removed when leaving the work area. Wearing gloves is not a substitute for hand washing, and hands must be washed after gloves are removed.

Laboratory coats are worn when processing laboratory samples. Fluid-resistant laboratory coats with wrist cuffs are worn to protect clothing and skin from exposure to patients' body substances. They should always be completely buttoned, and gloves should be pulled over the cuffs. Coats are worn at all times when working with patients or patient samples.

A variety of protective equipment to protect against mucous membrane exposure is available, including goggles, full-face plastic shields, and Plexiglas countertop shields. Particular care should be taken to avoid splashes and aerosols when removing container tops, pouring specimens, and centrifuging samples (Fig. 4-9). Samples must never be centrifuged in uncapped tubes or in uncovered centrifuges. When samples are received in containers with contaminated exteriors, the exterior of the container must be disinfected or, if necessary, a new sample may be requested.

Biological Waste Disposal

Phlebotomy equipment and supplies contaminated with blood and body fluids must be disposed of in containers clearly marked with the *biohazard* symbol or red or yellow color coding (Fig. 4-10). These items include alcohol pads, gauze, bandages, disposable tourniquets, gloves, masks, gowns, and specimens except urine. Urine can be poured out in the laboratory sink. Disposal of needles and other sharp objects is discussed in the next section.

Contaminated nondisposable equipment, blood spills, and blood and body fluid processing areas must be disinfected. The most commonly used disinfectant is a 1:10 dilution of sodium hypochlorite (household bleach) prepared weekly and stored in a plastic, not a glass, bottle. The bleach should be allowed to air dry on the contaminated area before removal (Box 4-3).

SHARP HAZARDS

A primary concern for phlebotomists is possible exposure to bloodborne pathogens caused by accidental puncture with a contaminated needle or lancet. Although

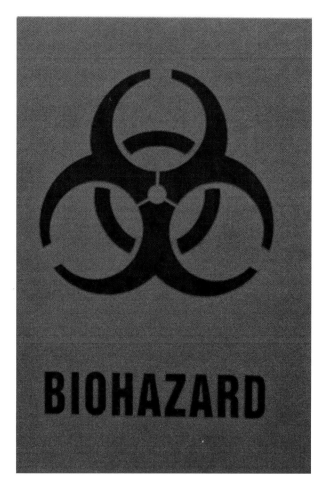

FIGURE 4-10 **Biohazard symbol.**

BOX 4-3 Transmission Prevention Guidelines for Phlebotomists

Wear appropriate PPE.

Change gloves between patients.

Wash hands after removing gloves.

Dispose of biohazardous material in designated containers.

Properly dispose of sharps in puncture-resistant containers.

Do not recap needles.

Do not activate needle safety device using both hands.

Follow institutional protocol governing working during personal illness.

Maintain personal immunizations.

Decontaminate work areas and equipment.

Do not centrifuge uncapped tubes.

Do not eat, drink, smoke, or apply cosmetics in the work area.

be carried on phlebotomy trays or placed at specified blood collection areas. Containers may be attached to the walls in patient rooms (Fig. 4-11).

 Safety Tip 4-3. Do not reach into sharps disposal containers when discarding material. Containers must always be replaced when the safe capacity mark is reached.

Bloodborne Pathogens

Bloodborne pathogens are of particular concern to health-care workers because of their exposure to blood and sharp objects such as needles. Of primary concern are human immunodeficiency virus (HIV), hepatitis B virus (HBV), and hepatitis C virus (HCV). This does not mean that safety precautions are only in place for these diseases as other bloodborne pathogens including those causing syphillis, malaria, and other viral diseases can also be contacted from blood exposure.

HIV attacks the human immune system by infecting and destroying the T-lymphocyte subset referred to as CD4 cells that are needed for protection against foreign substances (pathogens) entering the body. As the destruction of T cells increases, a person progresses from having HIV to being diagnosed with acquired immunodeficiency syndrome (AIDS). In recent years, progress has been made to control the progression of HIV to AIDS. Phlebotomists may receive requisitions to

bloodborne pathogens also are transmitted through contact with mucous membranes and nonintact skin, a needle or lancet used to collect blood has the capability to produce a very significant exposure to bloodborne pathogens. It is essential that safety precautions be followed at all times when sharp hazards are present.

The number one personal safety rule when using needles is to *never* recap a needle. Many safety devices are available for needle disposal, and they provide a variety of safeguards, including needle holders that become a sheath, needles that automatically resheath or become blunt, and needles with attached sheaths (see Chapter 8). Needle safety devices must be activated before disposing of the entire blood collection assembly. All sharps must be disposed of in puncture-resistant, leak-proof containers labeled with the biohazard symbol. Containers should be located in close proximity to the phlebotomist's work area. Portable containers can

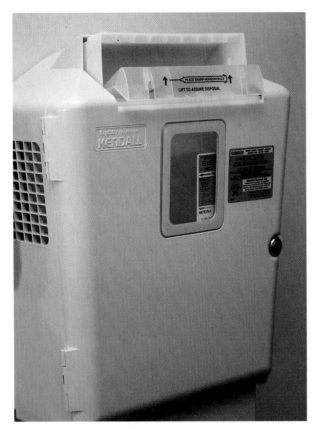

FIGURE 4-11   **Wall unit for sharps disposal.**

collect samples to measure a patient's CD4 count or HIV viral load or for antibiotic resistance tests.

HBV attacks the liver causing mild to severe to chronic (carrier) disorders. Patients may develop jaundice along with flu-like symptoms in the early stages of the disease. Persons with chronic infections frequently develop fatal liver cancer or cirrhosis of the liver. The development of the HBV vaccine has provided a much needed protection for health-care workers against acquiring HBV. OSHA requires that employers of health-care workers exposed to blood provide the vaccine free of charge to their employees. The vaccine consists of three to four spaced shots over a period of several months.

Safety Tip 4-4. A person can refuse the vaccine with a signed statement that remains in his or her file. This is not recommended as the vaccine has a good safety record. The vaccine is so effective that CDC now recommends that the vaccination series be started on all newborns.

HCV also attacks the liver and is now the leading bloodborne pathogen cause of chronic liver disease progressing to cirrhosis and liver cancer. Infected persons are closely monitored and frequently require liver transplantation. Phlebotomists may receive requisitions to collect samples to monitor the HVC viral load.

Occupational Exposure to Bloodborne Pathogens Standard

The Occupational Exposure to Bloodborne Pathogens Standard was first published by OSHA in 1991 to protect health-care workers from exposure to the bloodborne pathogens. In 1999, OSHA issued a new compliance directive, called the Enforcement Procedures for the Occupational Exposure to Bloodborne Pathogens Standard. The new directive placed more emphasis on the use of engineering controls to prevent accidental exposure to bloodborne pathogens. Additional changes to the directive were mandated by passage of the Needlestick Safety and Prevention Act, signed into law in 2001.

In June 2002, OSHA issued a revision to the Bloodborne Pathogens Standard compliance directive. In the revised directive, the agency requires that all blood holders with needles attached be immediately discarded into a sharps container after the device's safety feature is activated. The rationale for the new directive is based on the exposure of workers to the unprotected stopper-puncturing end of evacuated tube needles, the increased needle manipulation required to remove it from the holder, and the possible worker or patient exposure from the use of contaminated holders.

OSHA requires all employers to have a written Bloodborne Pathogen Exposure Control Plan and to provide necessary protection, free of charge for employees. The components of the current Bloodborne Pathogens Exposure Control Plan that is required of all institutions are shown in Box 4-4.

 Technical Tip 4-10. Always become thoroughly proficient with the operation of new devices before using them to draw blood from patients.

Use of Glass Capillary Tubes

Accidental breakage of glass capillary tubes used by phlebotomists when collecting samples from a dermal puncture can present a major risk of bloodborne

---

BOX 4-4 Components of the OSHA Bloodborne Pathogen Standard

Engineering Controls
1. Providing sharps disposal containers and needles with safety devices.
2. Requiring discarding of needles with the safety device activated and the holder attached.
3. Labeling all biohazardous materials and containers.

Work Practice Controls
4. Requiring all employees to practice Standard Precautions.
5. Prohibiting eating, drinking, smoking, and applying cosmetics in the work area.
6. Establishing a daily work surface disinfection protocol.

Personal Protective Equipment
7. Providing laboratory coats, gowns, face shields, and gloves to employees and laundry facilities for nondisposable protective clothing.

Medical
8. Providing immunization for the hepatitis B virus free of charge.

9. Providing medical follow-up to employees who have been accidentally exposed to bloodborne pathogens.

Documentation
10. Documenting annual training of employees in safety standards.
11. Documenting evaluations and implementation of safer needle devices.
12. Involving employees in the selection and evaluation of new devices and maintaining a list of those employees and the evaluations.
13. Maintaining a sharps injury log including the type and brand of safety device, location and description of the incident, and confidential employee follow-up.

Phlebotomists should be prepared to assist in the evaluation of new safety devices.

---

pathogen exposure. A 1999 government safety advisory recommended using the following items:

1. Capillary tubes wrapped in puncture-resistant film
2. Plastic capillary tubes
3. Sealing methods that do not require pushing the tubes into a sealant to form a plug
4. Methods that do not require centrifuging of capillary hematocrit tubes

Currently there are many varieties of capillary tubes that are made of plastic or glass wrapped in puncture-resistant film. These products can still be used with plug-forming sealant (see Chapter 12).

 Safety Tip 4-5. Be sure to follow institutional protocol when sealing capillary tubes.

Postexposure Prophylaxis

Any accidental exposure to blood through needlestick, mucous membranes, or nonintact skin must be reported to a supervisor and a confidential medical examination must be started immediately. Evaluation of the incident must begin immediately to ensure appropriate *postexposure prophylaxis (PEP)* is initiated within 24 hours. Needlesticks are the most frequently encountered exposure in phlebotomy and place the

phlebotomist in danger of contracting HIV, HBV, and HCV. The CDC has recommended procedures to follow for the initial examination and for any necessary PEP. Procedures are shown in Box 4-5.

 Safety Tip 4-6. Never, never hesitate to report a possible bloodborne pathogen exposure.

CHEMICAL HAZARDS

 Phlebotomists may come in contact with chemicals while accessioning or processing samples in the laboratory and preparing containers for urine samples that require preservatives. Many of these preservatives can be hazardous when they are not properly handled.

General rules for safe handling of chemicals include:

1. Taking precautions to avoid getting chemicals on the body, clothes, and work area.
2. Wearing PPE, such as safety goggles when pouring chemicals.
3. Observing strict labeling practices.
4. Carefully following instructions.

Chemicals should never be mixed together unless specific instructions are followed, and they must be

---

BOX 4-5 Postexposure Prophylaxis

1. Draw a baseline blood sample from the employee and test it for HBV, HCV, and HIV.
2. If possible, identify the source patient, collect a blood sample, and test it for HBV, HCV, and HIV. Patients must usually give informed consent for these tests, and they do not become part of the patient's record. In some states, a physician's order or court order can replace patient consent because a needlestick is considered a significant exposure.
3. Testing must be completed within 24 hours for maximum benefit from PEP.

Source patient tests positive for HIV:

1. Employee is counseled about receiving PEP using zidovudine (ZDV) and one or two additional anti-HIV medications.
2. Medications are started within 24 hours.

3. Employee is retested at intervals of 6 weeks, 12 weeks, and 6 months.
4. Additional evaluation and counseling is needed if the source patient is unidentified or untested.

Source patient tests positive for HBV:

1. Unvaccinated employees can be given hepatitis B immune globulin (HBIG) and HBV vaccine.
2. Vaccinated employees are tested for immunity and receive PEP, if necessary.

Source patient tests positive for HCV:

1. No PEP is available.
2. Employee is monitored for early detection of HCV infection and treated appropriately.

Any exposed employee should be counseled to report any symptoms related to viral infection that occur within 12 weeks of the exposure.

---

added in the order specified. This is particularly important when combining acid and water, because acid should always be added to water to avoid the possibility of sudden splashing caused by heat generated when water and acid combine.

When skin or eye contact occurs, the best first aid is to flush the area immediately with water for at least 15 minutes and then seek medical attention. Do not try to neutralize chemicals spilled on the skin. Phlebotomists must know the location of and how to use the emergency shower and eyewash station in the laboratory (Fig. 4-12 and Fig. 4-13).

> ❗ **Safety Tip 4-7.** Learn how to use the shower and eyewash.

All chemicals and reagents containing hazardous ingredients in a concentration greater than 1% are required to have a Material Safety Data Sheet (MSDS) on file in the work area. By law, vendors must provide these sheets to purchasers; however, it is the responsibility of the facility to obtain and keep them available to employees. An MSDS contains information on physical and chemical characteristics, fire, explosion reactivity, health hazards, primary routes of entry, exposure limits and carcinogenic potential, precautions for safe handling, spill clean-up, and emergency first-aid information (Fig. 4-14). Containers of chemicals that pose a high risk must be labeled with a chemical

hazard symbol representing the possible hazard, such as flammable, poison, or corrosive (Fig. 4-15).

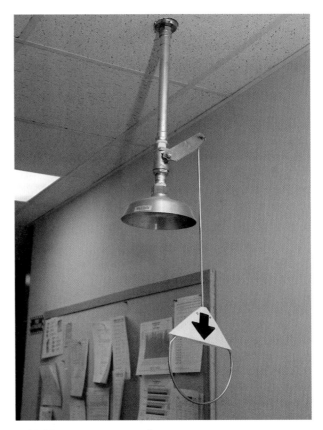

FIGURE 4-12 Emergency shower.

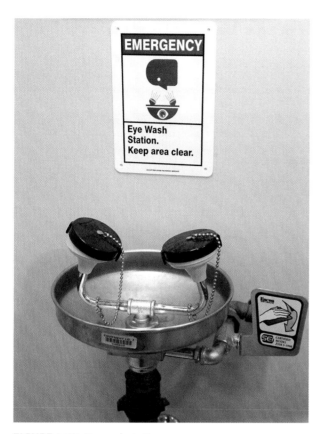

FIGURE 4-13 **Eyewash station.**

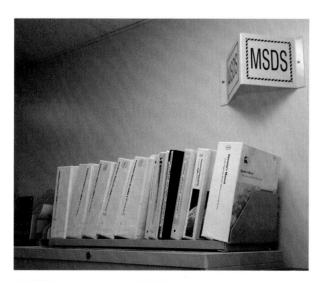

FIGURE 4-14 **Laboratory MSDS manuals.**

RADIOACTIVE HAZARDS

 Phlebotomists may come in contact with *radioactivity* while drawing blood from patients in the radiology department or from patients receiving radioactive treatments and in the laboratory when procedures using radioisotopes are performed. The amount of radioactivity present in most medical situations is very small and represents little danger; however, the effects of radiation are related to the length of exposure and are cumulative. Exposure to radiation is dependent on the combination of time, distance, and shielding. Persons working in a radioactive environment are required to wear measuring devices to determine the amount of radiation they are accumulating.

Phlebotomists should be familiar with the radioactive symbol (Fig. 4-16). This symbol must be displayed on the doors of all areas where radioactive material is present. Exposure to radiation during pregnancy presents a danger to the fetus, and phlebotomists who are pregnant or think they may be should avoid areas with this symbol.

ELECTRICAL HAZARDS

 The health-care setting contains a large amount of electrical equipment with which phlebotomists are in contact, both in patients' rooms and in the laboratory. The same general rules of electrical safety observed outside the workplace apply. Keep in mind that the danger of water or fluid coming in contact with equipment is greater in the hospital setting.

 Safety Tip 4-8. Do not operate electrical equipment with wet hands or while in contact with water.

Electrical equipment is closely monitored by designated hospital personnel. However, phlebotomists should be observant for any dangerous conditions such as frayed cords and overloaded circuits, and they should report these items to the appropriate persons. Equipment that has become wet should be unplugged and allowed to dry completely before reusing. Equipment should also be unplugged before cleaning. It is

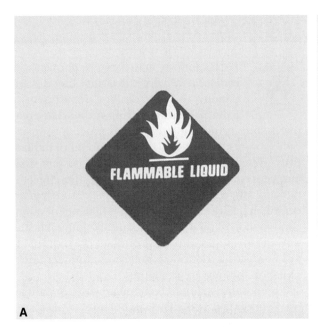

A   **B**

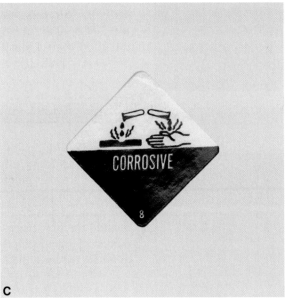

C

FIGURE 4-15   A-C. Chemical hazard symbols.

required that all electrical equipment is grounded with a three-pronged plug.

As an additional precaution when drawing blood or performing other procedures, phlebotomists should avoid contact with electrical equipment in the patient's room because current from improperly grounded equipment can pass through the phlebotomist and metal needle to the patient.

When a situation involving electrical shock occurs, it is important to remove the electrical source immediately. This must be done without touching the person

or the equipment because the current will pass on to you. Turning off the circuit breaker and moving the equipment using a nonconductive glass or wood object are safe procedures to follow. The victim should receive immediate medical assistance following discontinuation of the electricity. Cardiopulmonary resuscitation (CPR) may be necessary.

 Technical Tip 4-11. Phlebotomists should maintain current CPR certification.

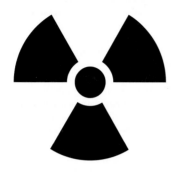

RADIATION

FIGURE 4-16 Radiation symbol.

FIRE/EXPLOSIVE HAZARDS

The Joint Commission (JC) requires that all health-care institutions have posted evacuation routes and detailed plans to follow when a fire occurs. Phlebotomists should be familiar with these procedures and with the basic steps to follow when a fire is discovered. Initial steps to follow when a fire is discovered are identified by the code word RACE.

1. Rescue—anyone in immediate danger
2. Alarm—activate the institutional fire alarm system
3. Contain—close all doors to potentially affected areas
4. Extinguish/Evacuate—extinguish the fire, if possible, or evacuate, closing the door

The laboratory uses many chemicals that may be volatile or explosive, and special procedures for handling and storage are required. Designated chemicals are stored in safety cabinets or explosion-proof refrigerators and are used under vented hoods. Fire blankets may be present in the laboratory. Persons with burning clothes should be wrapped in the blanket to smother the flames.

 Technical Tip 4-12. Always return chemicals to their designated storage area.

The National Fire Protection Association (NFPA) classifies fires with regard to the type of burning material and also classifies the type of fire extinguisher that is used to control them. This information is summarized in Table 4-3. The multipurpose ABC fire extinguishers are the most common, but the label should always be checked before using. Phlebotomists should be thoroughly familiar with the operation of the fire extinguishers. The code word PASS can be used to remember the steps in the operation.

1. Pull pin
2. Aim at base of fire
3. Squeeze handles
4. Sweep nozzle, side to side

The Standard System for the Identification of the Fire Hazards of Materials, NFPA 704, is a symbol system used to inform firefighters of the hazards they may encounter when fighting a fire in a particular area. The color-coded areas contain information relating to health, flammability, reactivity, use of water, and personal protection. These symbols are placed on doors, cabinets, and reagent bottles. An example of the hazardous material symbol and information is shown in Figure 4-17.

TABLE 4-3 • **Types of Fires and Fire Extinguishers**			
FIRE TYPE	**COMPOSITION OF FIRE**	**TYPE OF FIRE EXTINGUISHER**	**EXTINGUISHING MATERIAL**
Class A	Wood, paper, or clothing	Class A	Water
Class B	Flammable organic chemicals	Class B	Dry chemicals, carbon dioxide, foam, or Halon
Class C	Electrical	Class C	Dry chemicals, carbon dioxide, or Halon
Class D	Combustible metals	None	Sand or dry powder
		Class ABC	Dry chemicals
Class K	Grease, oils, fats	Class K	Liquid designed to prevent splashing and cool the fire.

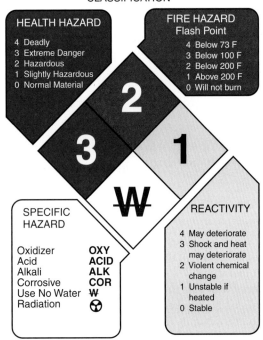

FIGURE 4-17 **NFPA hazardous material symbol.** *(From Strasinger, SK, and Di Lorenzo, MS: Urinalysis and Body Fluids, ed. 5. FA Davis, 2008, Philadelphia, with permission).*

PHYSICAL HAZARDS

Physical hazards are not unique to the health-care setting, and routine safety precautions observed outside the workplace can usually be applied. General precautions that phlebotomists should observe include:

1. Avoid running in rooms and hallways.
2. Be alert for wet floors.
3. Bend the knees when lifting heavy objects or patients.
4. Keep long hair tied back and remove dangling jewelry to avoid contact with equipment and patients.
5. Wear comfortable, closed-toe shoes with non-skid soles that provide maximum support.
6. Maintain a clean, organized work area.

▶ *Technical Tip 4-13.* Additional and up-to-date information on safety and regulations can be found by using CDC, FDA, and OSHA.gov websites and using the search function on the home page. Example: http://www.osha.gov. Search bloodborne pathogens.

Key Points

- The six components of the chain of infection are an infectious agent, reservoir, portal of exit, mode of transmission, portal of entry, and a susceptible host. Methods to break the chain of infection include hand hygiene, disinfection, wearing PPE, using needle safety precautions, patient isolation, following Standard Precautions, using biohazarous waste containers, and maintaining a healthy lifestyle.

- The terms nosocomial and health-care–acquired infections (HAI) indicate infections contracted by patients during a hospital stay or an outpatient procedure.

- Correct hand hygiene requires following the CDC guidelines for hand washing and the use of alcohol-based hand cleansers.

- PPE includes gowns to protect the skin and clothing; masks, goggles, face shields, and respirators to protect the eyes, mouth, nose, and mucous membranes from inhalation or splashing of infectious organisms; and gloves pulled over the sleeves of the gown.

- Allergy to latex produces contact dermatitis type rashes, delayed poison ivy–type rashes, and respiratory symptoms. These symptoms should be reported to a supervisor and nonlatex gloves worn.

- The order of donning PPE is gown, mask, goggles, respirator, face shield, and gloves. PPE is removed in the order of most contaminated first (gloves, gown, face shield, goggles, mask, respirator).

- Standard Precautions assume that everyone is potentially infected or colonized with an organism that can be transmitted in the health-care setting.

- Transmission-based precautions include airborne, droplet, and contact. Phlebotomists should follow the posted instructions for PPE when entering these rooms.

- When entering transmission-based precautions rooms, phlebotomists should bring in only the required equipment (including extra tubes). Everything brought in to the room is disposed of or left in the room. PPE is removed before leaving the room. When entering protective isolation rooms, only the necessary equipment is also brought in to the room, but all equipment is brought out of the room and PPE is removed after leaving the room.

- The most common disinfectant for cleaning blood and body fluid spills in the laboratory is 1:10 sodium hypochlorite.

- The Occupational Exposure to Bloodborne Pathogens Compliance Directive requires a laboratory plan for worker protection that includes engineering and work practice controls, provision of PPE, free immunizations and exposure PEP, documentation of employee input when selecting safety equipment, and a sharps incident log.

- Following an accidental exposure to a bloodborne pathogen, the site must be immediately flushed with water and the incident reported. PEP includes testing the employee for HIV, HBV, and HCV and if possible testing the source patient for HIV, HBV, and HCV. If the source patient is positive, the employee is counseled and provided with appropriate treatment that should be started within 24 hours. Follow-up testing is provided for all exposures.

- Avoid getting chemicals used in the laboratory on skin, clothes, and work surfaces. Wear goggles when pouring chemicals; observe labeling and mixing instructions. Never add water to acid; always add acid to water. When skin or eye contact occurs immediately flush the area with water. Do not try to neutralize chemicals. The MSDS must be available for all employees to warn them of potential chemical hazards and handling procedures.

- A phlebotomist who is pregnant or thinks she might be should avoid areas including patient rooms when a radiation symbol is present.

- Avoid working with electrical equipment that is wet or when you are wet. Be observant for frayed cords, overloaded circuits, and improperly grounded equipment. Avoid coming in contact with electrical equipment in patient rooms. Never touch a person receiving an electrical shock. Turn off the circuit breaker or remove the electical source using nonconductive glass or wood objects. Get medical assistance for the person.

Continued

Key Points—cont'd

✦ The acronym RACE outlines the steps to follow when a fire is discovered. They are (R) rescue any one in danger, (A) activate the fire alarm, (C) contain the fire, (E) extinguish the fire if possible or evacuate closing the door. The acronym PASS outlines the steps for operating a fire extinguisher. They are (P) pull the pin, (A) aim the extinguisher at the base of the fire, (S) squeeze the handles, (S) sweep nozzle from side to side.

✦ Fires and fire extinguishers are classified as Class A (wood, paper, clothing), Class B (organic chemicals), and Class C (electrical). Class D fires are metal and can only be extinguished with substances such as sand. Class K fires are grease, oil,

and fats that use a Class K fire extinguisher designed to cool and smother the flame without causing splashing. The most common type of fire extinguisher is the multipurpose Class ABC. The NFPA hazardous materials symbols classify materials in laboratories that could affect firefighters by their health, fire, reactivity, and specific hazards.

✦ Phlebotomists can prevent physical hazards by not running in rooms and hallways; being alert for wet floors; bending the knees when picking up heavy objects or patients; keeping long hair tied back; and avoiding dangling jewelry, wearing closed toed nonskid shoes, and maintaining an organized work area.

BIBLIOGRAPHY

Centers for Disease Control and Prevention. Guidelines for Infection Control in Healthcare Personnel. http://www.cdc.gov. Search infection control in healthcare personnel.

Centers for Disease Control and Prevention. Updated U.S. Public Health Service Guidelines for the Management of Occupational Exposures to HBV, HCV, and HIV and Recommendations for Post-exposure Prophylaxis. *MMWR* 2001;50(RR11):1–42. http://www.cdc.gov.

Centers for Disease Control and Prevention. Guidelines for Isolation Precautions: Preventing Transmission of Infectious Agents in Healthcare Settings, 2007. http://www.cdc.gov/hicpac/2007IP/2007isolationPrecautions.html.

Food and Drug Administration. Glass Capillary Tubes: Joint Safety Advisory About Potential Risks. FDA, 1999, Rockville, MD. http://www.fda.gov/MedicalDevices/Safety/AlertsandNotices/PublicHealthNotifications/UCM062285.

National Fire Protection Association. Hazardous Chemical Data, No. 49. NFPA, 1991, Boston.

NIOSH Alert. Preventing Allergic Reactions to Natural Rubber Latex in the Workplace. DHHS (NIOSH) Publication 97-135. National Institute for Occupational Safety and Health, 1997, Cincinnati, OH.

Occupational Exposure to Bloodborne Pathogens, Final Rule. *Federal Register* 1991; 29(Dec 6).

Occupational Safety and Health Administration. Revision to OSHA's Bloodborne Pathogens Standard. 2001. http://www.osha.gov/SLTC/bloodbornepathogens.

Study Questions

1. In the chain of infection, the susceptible host can also become the:
   a. reservoir
   b. portal of entry
   c. means of transmission
   d. portal of exit

2. The terms nosocomial and HAI refer to infections:
   a. caused by antibiotic resistant bacteria
   b. contacted by health-care workers
   c. contacted by patients
   d. contacted by visitors

3. Hand hygiene is performed:
   a. before putting on gloves
   b. after removing gloves
   c. when gloves are visibly soiled
   d. all of the above

4. PPE includes all of the following **EXCEPT:**
   a. gloves
   b. gowns
   c. uniforms
   d. masks

Study Questions—cont'd

5. A phlebotomy student who notices a rash on his or her hands after the first week of training should:
   a. tell the instructor
   b. stop wearing gloves
   c. change antiseptic soap
   d. apply antihistamine lotion

6. The order used to put on PPE is:
   a. gloves, gown, mask
   b. mask, gown, gloves
   c. gown, mask, gloves
   d. gloves, mask, gown

7. The current routine infection control policy developed by CDC and followed in all health-care settings is:
   a. Universal Precautions
   b. Isolation Precautions
   c. Blood and Body Fluid Precautions
   d. Standard Precautions

8. Before entering an isolation room, the first thing a phlebotomist should do is:
   a. read the posted instructions
   b. perform hand hygiene
   c. put on a gown and a mask
   d. put on sterile gloves

9. OSHA requires employers of health-care workers to provide the employees with all of the following **EXCEPT:**
   a. PPE
   b. HCV immunization
   c. HBV immunization
   d. needles with safety devices

10. The recommended disinfectant for blood and body fluid contamination is:
    a. sodium hydroxide
    b. antimicrobial soap
    c. hydrogen peroxide
    d. sodium hypochlorite

11. When a chemical is accidentally spilled on the body, the first thing to do is:
    a. notify a supervisor
    b. flush the area with water
    c. refer to the MSDS
    d. neutralize the chemical

12. When a person is receiving an electrical shock, all of the following should be done **EXCEPT:**
    a. pull the person away from the electrical source
    b. turn off the circuit breaker
    c. move the electrical source using a glass object
    d. move the electrical source using a wood object

13. The acronym RACE should be followed:
    a. to determine the type of fire extinguisher to use
    b. when operating a fire extinguisher
    c. to classify fires and fire extinguishers
    d. when a fire is first discovered

14. The acronym PASS should be followed:
    a. to determine the type of fire extinguisher to use
    b. when operating a fire extinguisher
    c. to classify fires and fire extinguishers
    d. when a fire is first discovered

15. The most common type of fire extinguisher is a:
    a. Class A
    b. Class C
    c. Class ABC
    d. Class D

Clinical Situations

1 A phlebotomist with an exceptionally heavy workload decides to save time by not changing gloves and washing his or her hands between patients.
  a. What type of infection could be spread to previously uninfected patients?
  b. Who would be considered the reservoir of these infections?
  c. Who would be considered the host of these infections?
  d. How were these infections transmitted?

2 For each of the following actions taken by a phlebotomist, place a "T" for transmission-based precautions, a "P" for protective isolation, or a "PT" for both situations in the blank.
  a. _____Only necessary equipment is brought into the room.
  b. _____Sterile gloves are worn.
  c. _____PPE is removed and disposed of inside the room.
  d. _____Duplicate tubes are taken into the room.
  e. _____Samples may require double bagging.
  f. _____Equipment taken into the room is taken out of the room.

3 A phlebotomist using a new safety device for the first time receives an accidental needlestick while activating the safety feature on the used needle.
  a. How could this accident possibly have been avoided?
  b. What should the phlebotomist do first?
  c. What tests are performed on the phlebotomist?
  d. If necessary, when should the phlebotomist receive PEP?

Laboratory Safety Exercise

Instructions

Explore the student laboratory or the area designated by the instructor and provide the following information:

1. Location of the fire extinguishers
2. Instructions for operation of the fire extinguisher
3. Location of the fire blanket if present
4. Location of the eyewash station
5. Location of the emergency shower
6. Location of the first aid kit
7. Location of the master electrical panel
8. Location of the fire alarm
9. The emergency exit route
10. Location of the MSDS pertaining to phlebotomy
11. Location of the emergency spill kit
12. Location of the Bloodborne Pathogen Exposure Control Plan
13. Locate an NFPA sign and list the following:
    Location
    Health rating
    Fire rating
    Reactivity rating
14. What disinfectants are available for cleaning work areas?

Evaluation of Hand Washing Competency

RATING SYSTEM:
2 = Satisfactorily Performed,   **1** = Needs Improvement,   **0** = Incorrect/Did Not Perform

_____ 1. Turns on warm water

_____ 2. Dispenses an adequate amount of soap onto palm

_____ 3. Creates a lather

_____ 4. Creates friction, rubbing both sides of hands

_____ 5. Rubs between fingers and thumbs and under nails

_____ 6. Rinses hands in a downward position

_____ 7. Obtains paper towel, touching only the towel

_____ 8. Dries hands with paper towel

_____ 9. Turns off water using a clean paper towel

_____ 10. Does not recontaminate hands

TOTAL POINTS _____

MAXIMUM POINTS = 20

Comments:

Evaluation of Personal Protective Equipment (Gowning, Masking, and Gloving) Competency

RATING SYSTEM:
2 = Satisfactorily Performed,   **1** = Needs Improvement,   **0** = Incorrect/Did Not Perform

_____ **1.** Correctly washes hands

_____ **2.** Puts on gown with opening at the back

_____ **3.** Ensures that gown is large enough to close in the back

_____ **4.** Ties neck strings

_____ **5.** Ties waistband

_____ **6.** Positions mask with proper side facing outward and fastens top tie above the ears

_____ **7.** Securely positions mask over nose

_____ **8.** Fastens bottom tie at back of neck

_____ **9.** Puts on gloves

_____ **10.** Pulls gloves over cuffs of gown

_____ **11.** Removes gloves touching only the inside

_____ **12.** Deposits gloves in biohazard container

_____ **13.** Unties gown at waist and neck

_____ **14.** Removes gown touching only the inside

_____ **15.** Deposits gown in biohazard container

_____ **16.** Unfastens mask at neck and then head

_____ **17.** Touches only the strings of the mask

_____ **18.** Deposits mask in biohazard container

_____ **19.** Correctly performs hand hygiene

TOTAL POINTS _____

MAXIMUM POINTS = 38

Comments:

Body Systems

CHAPTER 5

Basic Medical Terminology

Learning Objectives

Upon completion of this chapter, the reader will be able to:

1. Define and state the purpose of prefixes, word roots, suffixes, and combining forms.
2. Correctly form medical terms using prefixes, word roots, suffixes, and combining forms.
3. State the meaning of the commonly used prefixes, suffixes, and word roots.
4. Associate common word roots with the corresponding body system.
5. State the different plural forms for medical terms.
6. Define the meanings for common medical abbreviations.
7. Name the abbreviations on The Joint Commission "Do Not Use" list.

Key Terms

Combining form
Combining vowel
Prefix
Suffix
Word root

Medical terminology is derived primarily from the classic Greek and Latin languages. However, it is not necessary to master either of these languages to obtain a solid background in basic medical terminology. Medical terms consist of combinations of three major word parts: prefixes, word roots, and suffixes. The same prefixes and suffixes are frequently used with different word roots. Therefore, knowledge of a small number of commonly used prefixes, word roots, and suffixes can provide the phlebotomist with an extensive medical vocabulary and the medical communication skills necessary for successful job performance.

PREFIXES AND SUFFIXES

Prefixes are letters or syllables added to the beginning of a word root to alter its meaning. The prefix usually indicates direction, number, position, size, presence or absence, or time.

Suffixes are letters or syllables added to the end of a word root to alter its meaning. In medical terminology, suffixes often indicate a condition or a type of procedure.

The most commonly used prefixes and suffixes are presented in Tables 5-1 and 5-2. It is necessary to memorize these common prefixes and suffixes. This process is easier if you relate them to terms that are already familiar to you.

EXAMPLE 5-1
In medical terminology, the prefix "post" means "after," just as it does in the term "postgraduate." The suffix "-ectomy" means "surgical removal," and the term "tonsillectomy" is a familiar word to most people.

WORD ROOTS AND COMBINING FORMS

Word roots are the main part of a word and may be combined with prefixes, suffixes, or other roots. The *combining form* of a word root contains a vowel, usually an "o," which is used to facilitate pronunciation

TABLE 5-1 • Common Prefixes			
PREFIX	**MEANING**	**PREFIX**	**MEANING**
a-, an-, ar-	no, not, without	blasto-	growth
ab-	away from	brachy-	short
ac-	pertaining to	brady-	slow
acous-	hearing	cata-	down
ad-	toward	centi-	hundred
af-	to, toward	chromo-	color
alb-	white	circum-, peri-	around
allo-	different or an addition	co-, com-, con-	together, with
ambi-	both	contra-	opposite
ana-	up	cor-	with, together
aniso-	unequal	cyan-	blue
ante-	before	de-	down, from
anti-, contra-	against	di-	two, apart, separation
apo-	separated or derived from	dia-	through, complete
atel-	imperfect, incomplete	dif-	apart, separation
auto-	self	diplo-	double
bi-	two	dis-	apart, away from
bio-	life	dys-	difficult, painful

TABLE 5-1 • Common Prefixes—cont'd

PREFIX	MEANING	PREFIX	MEANING
ec-	out, away	milli-	one thousandth
ecto-, exo-	outside	mono-, uni-	one
edem-	swelling	multi-, poly-	many
endo-, intra-	inside, within	narco-	sleep
epi-	on, over	neo-	new
erythr-	red	non-	not
eu-	normal, good	pachy-	thick
ex-	out, away from	pan-	all
exo-	without, outside of	para-	beside, abnormal
extra-	outside of, in addition to, beyond	per-	through
fasci-	band	peri-	around
fore-	before, in front	poly-	many
haplo-	single, simple	post-, retro-	after
hemi-	half	pre-, ante-	before, in front
hetero-	different	primi-	first
homo-	same	pro-	before, in front of
homeo-	unchanged	pseudo-	false
hydro-	water	quadri-, quadro-	four
hyper-	increased	re-	again, backward
hypo-	decreased	retro-	behind, backward
idio-	distinct, peculiar to an individual	semi-	half
infra-, sub-	below	steno-	narrow
inter-	between	sub-	below
intra-	within	supra-, super-	above
iso-	equal	sym-	together
macro-	large	syn-	together
mal-	bad, ill	tachy-	fast
medi-	middle	tox-	poison
mega-	great	trans-	across
meta-	beyond	tri-	three
micro-	small	ultra-	excessive, extreme

when the word root is combined with another word root or a suffix that does not begin with a vowel.

EXAMPLE 5-2
The word root for "heart" is "cardi."
The combining form is "cardi/o."
The suffix "logy" is "study of."
The study of the heart is "cardiology."

A *combining vowel* is not used when the suffix already begins with a vowel.

EXAMPLE 5-3
The word root for "liver" is "hepat."
The suffix for "inflammation" is "itis."
Inflammation of the liver is "hepatitis."

TABLE 5-2 • Common Suffixes

SUFFIX	MEANING	SUFFIX	MEANING
-ac, -al, -ar, -ary, -ic	pertaining to	-ia	condition
-ad	toward	-iasis	diseased condition
-agon	assemble, gather together	-ile	having qualities of
-algesia	excessive sensitivity to pain	-ion	process
-algia, -dynia	pain	-ism	condition of
-an	characteristic of	-ist	specialist
-ar	relating to	-itis	inflammation
-arche	beginning	-kinesia	movement
-ase	enzyme	-lepsy	seizure
-asthenia	lack of strength	-lith	stone
-ation	process	-logist	one who studies
-atresia	abnormal closure	-logy	study of
-blast	immature cell	-lysis, -rrhexis	rupture
-capnia	carbon dioxide	-malacia	softening
-cele	swelling	-megaly	enlargement
-centesis	surgical puncture	-meter	instrument to measure
-cidal	pertaining to death	-metry	measurement
-cide	kill	-ness	state of, quality
-clast	break	-oid	like, similar to
-coccus	spherical	-ole	small, little
-crine	secrete	-oma	tumor
-cyte	cell	-opia	eye, vision
-cytosis	abnormal condition of cells	-ory	pertaining to
-desis	binding, stabilizing, fusion	-ose	sugar, having qualities of
-dipsia	thirst	-osis, -iasis	abnormal condition
-ectasia, -ectasis	distention, expansion	-ostomy	surgical opening
-ectomy	surgical removal	-otomy	cut into, incision into
-emesis	vomit	-ous	pertaining to
-emia	pertaining to blood	-oxia	oxygen level
-esthesia	nervous sensation	-paresis	weakness
-form	structure	-pathy	disease
-gen	producing	-penia	lack of, deficiency
-genesis	origin of	-pepsia	digestion
-globin, -globulin	protein	-pexy	fixation
-gram	written record	-phagia	eating, swallowing
-graph	an instrument for making records	-philia	increase in cell numbers
-graphy	method of recording	-phobia	fear
-gravida	pregnancy	-phonia	voice

TABLE 5-2 • Common Suffixes—cont'd			
SUFFIX	**MEANING**	**SUFFIX**	**MEANING**
-phylaxis	protection	-sthenia	strength
-physis	growth	-stenosis	narrowing, tightening
-plasia	growth	-stomy	new opening
-plasty	surgical repair	-taxia	muscle coordination
-plegia	paralysis	-tension	pressure
-pnea	breathing	-therapy	treatment
-poiesis	production	-tome	instrument for cutting
-prandial	meal	-tomy	incision
-ptosis	dropping	-tony	tension
-ptysis	spitting	-tripsy	crushing
-rrhage	bursting forth	-trophy	development
-rrhea	discharge	-tropin	stimulation
-scope	instrument for viewing	-tropic	turning toward
-scopy	visual examination	-ula, -ule	small, little
-sis	condition of	-uria	pertaining to urine
-spasm, -stalsis	involuntary contraction	-y	condition, process
-stasis	controlling, to be still, stop		

The combining vowel, however, remains between two word roots even if the second root begins with a vowel.

EXAMPLE 5-4
The word root for "electricity" is "electr."
The combining form is "electr/o."
The word root for "brain" is "encephal."
The suffix for "written record" is "gram."
A written record of the electricity of the brain is an "electroencephalogram."

When defining a medical term, begin at the last part of the word (suffix), then define the first part of the word (prefix), and, last, define the middle of the word (word root).

Word roots frequently refer to body components. Therefore, common word roots are listed with their corresponding body system in Table 5-3.

PLURAL FORMS

In writing and using medical terms, it is important to know that various medical terms have different plural forms. The phlebotomist should become familiar

TABLE 5-3 • Combining Forms and Associated Body Systems		
BODY SYSTEM	**COMBINING FORM**	**MEANING**
Anatomy		
	anter/o	front, before
	dist/o	distant
	dors/o	back
	kary/o	nucleus

Continued

BODY SYSTEM	COMBINING FORM	MEANING
	later/o	side
	medi/o	middle
	poster/o	back, behind
	proxim/o	near
	viscer/o	internal organs
Integumentary		
	albin/o	white
	carcin/o	cancer
	cutane/o, dermat/o, derm/o	skin
	erythemat/o	redness
	hidr/o	sweat
	hist/o	tissue
	hydr/o	water
	kerat/o	hard tissue
	melan/o	black
	onych/o	nail
	seb/o	sebum or oily secretion
	squam/o	scalelike
	trich/o	hair
	xanth/o	yellow
Skeletal		
	arthr/o	joint
	axill/o	armpit
	cephal/o	head
	caud/o	tail
	chrondr/o	cartilage
	cost/o	ribs
	dactyl/o	finger or toe
	fibul/o	fibula
	humer/o	humerus
	mandibul/o	lower jawbone
	maxill/o	upper jawbone
	myel/o	bone marrow
	orth/o	straight
	oste/o	bone
	patell/o	kneecap
	rheumat/o	watery flow

TABLE 5-3 ● **Combining Forms and Associated Body Systems—cont'd**

TABLE 5-3 • Combining Forms and Associated Body Systems—cont'd		
BODY SYSTEM	**COMBINING FORM**	**MEANING**
	sacr/o	sacrum
	scapul/o	shoulder blade
	spondyl/o	vertebrae
	synov/i	synovial membrane
Muscular		
	fibr/o	fibrous connective tissue
	my/o, muscul/o	muscle
	kinesi/o	movement
Nervous		
	cerebell/o	cerebellum
	cerebr/o	cerebrum
	crani/o	skull
	encephal/o	brain
	gli/o	glue
	mening/o	meninges
	neur/o	nerve
Respiratory		
	alveol/o	alveolus, air sac
	bronch/o	bronchus
	cyan/o	blue
	nas/o, rhin/o	nose
	olfact/o	sense of smell
	pector/o, thorac/o	chest
	pleur/o	pleura
	pneum/o	air, lung
	pulmon/o	lung
	spir/o	breathe
	steth/o	chest
	trache/o	trachea, wind pipe
Digestive		
	abdomin/o	abdomen
	adip/o, lip/o, steat/o	fat
	amyl/o	starch
	bil/i, chol/o	bile, gall
	bucc/o	cheek
	celi/o, lapar/o	abdomen
	cholecyst/o	gallbladder
	choledoch/o	common bile duct

Continued

TABLE 5-3 • **Combining Forms and Associated Body Systems—cont'd**		
BODY SYSTEM	**COMBINING FORM**	**MEANING**
	cirrh/o	yellow
	col/o	colon
	dent/i, odont/o	tooth
	enter/o	intestine
	esophag/o	esophagus
	gastr/o	stomach
	gingiv/o	gums
	gloss/o, lingu/o	tongue
	gluc/o, glyc/o	glucose
	hepat/o	liver
	icter/o	jaundice
	lith/o	stone
	or/o, stomat/o	mouth
	proct/o	rectum
	sigmoid/o	sigmoid colon
Urinary		
	cyst/o	urinary bladder
	glomerul/o	glomerulus
	micturit/o	urination
	nephr/o, ren/o	kidney
	noct/i	night
	olig/o	scanty
	pyel/o	renal
	ur/o, urin/o	urine
Endocrine		
	aden/o	gland
	andr/o	male
	cortic/o	cortex
	crin/o	secrete
	kal/o	potassium
	natr/o	sodium
	somat/o	body
	ster/o	solid structure
	thyr/o	thyroid gland
Reproductive		
	amni/o	amnion
	balan/o	glans penis
	colp/o	vagina

TABLE 5-3 • Combining Forms and Associated Body Systems—cont'd

BODY SYSTEM	COMBINING FORM	MEANING
	episi/o	vulva
	gonad/o	sex glands
	gynec/o	female
	hyster/o	uterus, womb
	lact/o	milk
	mamm/o, mast/o	breast
	men/o	menses, menstruation
	nat/o	birth
	oopho/o, ovul/o	ovary
	orch/o	testes
	ovari/o	ovary
	salping/o	fallopian tubes
	spermat/o	spermatozoa
	test/o	testicle
Circulatory		
	angi/o	vessel
	arteri/o	artery
	ather/o	fatty substance
	brachi/o	arm
	cardi/o, coron/o	heart
	cyt/o	cell
	erythr/o	red
	leuk/o	white
	scler/o	hardening
	ser/o	serum
	sphygm/o	pulse
	thromb/o	clot
	vas/o	vessel
	ven/o	vein
Lymphatic		
	immun/o	protection
	lymphaden/o	lymph node
	splen/o	spleen
	tox/o	poison
General		
	aer/o	air
	agglutin/o	clumping

Continued

TABLE 5-3 • Combining Forms and Associated Body Systems—cont'd		
BODY SYSTEM	**COMBINING FORM**	**MEANING**
	ambul/o	to walk
	anis/o	unequal
	audi/o	to hear
	aur/o, ot/o	ear
	bacill/o	rod
	bi/o	life
	coagul/o	clotting
	cry/o	cold
	esthesi/o	feeling
	febr/o	fever
	gen/o	formation
	ger/o	old age
	hem/o, hemat/o	blood
	isch/o	to hold back
	kil/o	thousand
	morph/o	form
	myc/o	fungus
	myring/o	eardrum
	necr/o	death
	nos/o	pertaining to disease
	ocul/o, ophthalm/o	eye
	onc/o	tumor
	opt/o	vision
	path/o	disease
	ped/i	children
	phag/o	eat
	pharmac/o	drug
	phleb/o	vein
	prandi/o	meal
	psych/o	mind
	pur/o, py/o	pus
	radi/o	x-ray, radiant energy

with the common word endings that have an unusual plural ending (Table 5-4).

EXAMPLE 5-5
appendix, singular
appendices, plural

PRONUNCIATION GUIDELINES

Medical terms usually follow the rules of the pronunciation of words in the English language but may seem difficult to pronounce initially. Helpful

TABLE 5-4 ● **Plural Endings**	
SINGULAR WORD ENDING	**PLURAL ENDING**
-a	-ae
-ax	-aces
-en	-ina
-ex, ix	-ices
-is	-es
-ma	-mata
-nx	-nges
-on	-a
-um	-a
-us	-i
-y	-ies

TABLE 5-5 ● **Pronunciation Guidelines**
ae and oe, only the second vowel is pronounced—bursae
c and g are given the soft sound of s and j, before e, i, and y—cell, gel
c and g have a hard sound before other letters—cardiology, gastritis
e and es, when forming the final letter or letters of a word are pronounced as separate syllables—syncope, nares
ch is sometimes pronounced like k—cholesterol
i at the end of a word to form a plural is pronounced "eye"—bronchi
pn in the beginning of a word is pronounced with only the n sound—pneumothorax
pn in the middle of a word is pronounced with a hard p and a hard n—orthopnea
ps is pronounced like s—psychosis

Adapted from Gylys, BA, and Wedding, ME: Medical Terminology: A Body Systems Approach, ed. 6. FA Davis, 2009, Philadelphia.

diacritical marks, the macron and breve, may be used for long and short vowel pronunciations. The macron (¯) indicates the long sound of vowels as in fā - tal The breve (˘) indicates the short sound of vowels as in fā - tăl. Phonetic spelling of syllables also can be used as a pronunciation guideline as in AN-ti-BAH-dee. Capitalization is often used to indicate the emphasis on certain syllables as in MEM - ber.

Spelling a medical term correctly is important because some medical terms are spelled differently but are pronounced the same and have a completely different meaning. For example, ileum is part of the intestine and ilium is part of the hip bone.

Correct pronunciation and spelling of a medical term is essential to communicate the correct meaning. General pronunciation rules are listed in Table 5-5.

ABBREVIATIONS

Abbreviations are used to shorten words, names, or phrases. Numerous abbreviations are used in the medical field to represent terms, names of organizations, or common medical phrases. Laboratory tests are frequently abbreviated, and phlebotomists must become familiar with these abbreviations.

General medical abbreviations are listed in Table 5-6, and a more extensive list of abbreviations can be found in Appendix B.

TABLE 5-6 ● **Common Abbreviations**			
ABBREVIATION	**DEFINITION**	**ABBREVIATION**	**DEFINITION**
a. c.	before meals	cm	centimeter
ad lib	as desired	CPR	cardiopulmonary resuscitation
ASAP	as soon as possible	DOA	dead on arrival
bid	twice a day	DOB	date of birth
BP	blood pressure	Dx	diagnosis
Bx	biopsy	ECG/EKG	electrocardiogram
cc*, cm³	cubic centimeter	ED	emergency department

Continued

TABLE 5-6 • Common Abbreviations—cont'd

ABBREVIATION	DEFINITION	ABBREVIATION	DEFINITION
g, gm	gram	pre-op	before surgery
h	hour	PRN	as needed
h.s.	at bedtime	Pt	patient
Hx	history	q	every
IM	intramuscular	QNS	quantity nonsufficient
IV	intravenous	R/O	rule out
kg	kilogram	R/R	recovery room
mcg	microgram	Rx	prescription/treatment
mg	milligram	stat	immediately
mL	milliliter	Sx	symptoms
mm	millimeter	TPN	total parenteral nutrition (IV feeding)
m	meter	TPR	temperature, pulse, respiration
NB	newborn	Tx	treatment
NPO	nothing by mouth	Wd	wound
OP	outpatient	Wt	weight
oz	ounce	y/o	years old
post-op (p/o)	after surgery		
pp	postprandial		

*On the list of possible future additions to the "Do Not Use" list.

The Joint Commission established a "Do Not Use" list of abbreviations, acronyms, and symbols to avoid confusion and possible medical errors if interpreted incorrectly (Table 5-7). All accredited organizations are required to incorporate this policy. Table 5-8 lists possible future additions to the "Do Not Use" abbreviations list. The lists were developed in response to a Sentinel Event Alert involving medical abbreviations with the intention to reduce medical errors caused by an inaccurate interpretation of medical abbreviations and symbols. The list applies to orders and medication-related documentation that is handwritten including free-text computer entry or on preprinted forms.

TABLE 5-7 • The Joint Commission: Official "Do Not Use" List[1]

DO NOT USE	POTENTIAL PROBLEM	USE INSTEAD
U (Unit)	Mistaken for "0" (zero), the number "4" (four), or "cc"	Write "unit"
IU (International Unit)	Mistaken for IV (intravenous) or the number 10 (ten)	Write "International Unit"
Q.D., QD, q.d., qd (daily)	Mistaken for each other	Write "daily"
Q.O.D., QOD, q.o.d, qod (every other day)	Period after the Q mistaken for "I" and the "O" mistaken for "I"	Write "every other day"

TABLE 5-7 • The Joint Commission: Official "Do Not Use" List[1]—cont'd		
DO NOT USE	**POTENTIAL PROBLEM**	**USE INSTEAD**
Trailing zero (X.0 mg)*	Decimal point is missed	Write X mg
Lack of leading zero (.X mg)		Write 0.X mg
MS	Can mean morphine sulfate or magnesium sulfate	Write "morphine sulfate"
MSO_4 and $MgSO_4$	Confused for one another	Write "magnesium sulfate"

[1]Applies to all orders and all medication-related documentation that are handwritten (including free-text computer entry) or on preprinted forms.
*Exception: A "trailing zero" may be used only where required to demonstrate the level of precision of the value being reported, such as for laboratory results, imaging studies that report size of lesions, or catheter/tube sizes. It may not be used in medication orders or other medication-related documentation.
© The Joint Commission, 2009. Reprinted with permission.

TABLE 5-8 • Possible Future Inclusions to the Official "Do Not Use" List		
DO NOT USE	**POTENTIAL PROBLEM**	**USE INSTEAD**
> (greater than) < (less than)	Misinterpreted as the number "7" (seven) or the letter "L"	Write "greater than" Write "less than"
	Confused for one another	
Abbreviations for drug names	Misinterpreted due to similar abbreviations for multiple drugs	Write drug names in full
Apothecary units	Unfamiliar to many practitioners	Use metric units
	Confused with metric units	
@	Mistaken for the number "2" (two)	Write "at"
cc	Mistaken for U (units) when poorly written	Write "mL" or "ml" or "milliliters" ("mL" is preferred)
µg	Mistaken for mg "milligrams" resulting in one thousand-fold overdose	Write "mcg" or "micrograms"

© The Joint Commission, 2009. Reprinted with permission.

Key Points

✦ Medical terms consist of four word parts:
  ✦ Prefix—a word part that is added at the beginning of a word root that changes the meaning to indicate direction, number, position, size, presence or absence, or time.
  ✦ Suffix—a word part that is added at the end of a word root that changes the meaning to indicate a condition or type of procedure.
  ✦ Word root—the main part of a word that is derived from the Greek or Latin language and usually refers to body components.
  ✦ Combining form—the word root plus a vowel, usually "o" that is used to facilitate pronunciation when the word root is combined with another word root or a suffix that does not begin with a vowel.

✦ When defining a medical term, begin at the last part of the word (suffix), then define the first part of the word (prefix), and last, define the middle of the word (word root).
✦ Various medical terms have different plural forms.
✦ Correct pronunciation and spelling of medical terms is critical to the correct interpretation.
✦ Abbreviations are used to shorten words, names, or phrases and are used to identify laboratory tests, names of organizations, and medical terms. The Joint Commission has adopted an official "Do Not Use" list and a list for possible future inclusions.

BIBLIOGRAPHY

Gylys, BA, and Wedding, ME: Medical Terminology: A Body Systems Approach, ed. 6. FA Davis, 2009, Philadelphia.
Masters, RM, and Gylys, ME: Introducing Medical Terminology Specialties. FA Davis, 2003, Philadelphia.

Scanlon, V, and Sanders, T: Essentials of Anatomy and Physiology, ed. 5. FA Davis, 2007, Philadelphia.
The Joint Commission: The Official "Do Not Use" List. http://www.jointcommission.org/NR/rdonlyres/2329F8F5-6EC5-4E21-B932-54B2B7D53F00/0/dnu_list.pdf.

Study Questions

1. The main foundation of a word that denotes a body component is the:
   a. prefix
   b. word root
   c. suffix
   d. combining vowel

2. In the words cardiology, bradycardia, cardiomegaly, and cardiologist, the word root is:
   a. cardi
   b. brady
   c. logy
   d. logist

3. To define a medical word, first define the:
   a. prefix
   b. word root
   c. combining form
   d. suffix

4. Which word means pertaining to the period around birth?
   a. prenatal
   b. perinatal
   c. postnatal
   d. pronatal

5. In the word, encephalomeningitis, which part of the word is the suffix?
   a. encephal
   b. itis
   c. mening
   d. o

6. The combining form cyt/o means:
   a. cold
   b. secrete
   c. ribs
   d. cell

Study Questions—cont'd

7. The medical word for inflammation of the liver is:
- **a.** nephritis
- **b.** hematoma
- **c.** hepatitis
- **d.** hepatomegaly

8. The plural form for bronchus is:
- **a.** bronchi
- **b.** bronches
- **c.** bronchia
- **d.** bronchis

9. The abbreviation for microgram is:
- **a.** mg
- **b.** mcg
- **c.** mL
- **d.** mm

10. Which abbreviation is on The Joint Commission "Do Not Use" list?
- **a.** U
- **b.** IU
- **c.** MS
- **d.** all of the above

Clinical Situations

1 The stat sample drawn by the phlebotomist was QNS to R/O a Dx of cardiac disease.
- *a.* What priority of sample is to be drawn?
- *b.* Why was the sample to be drawn?
- *c.* Was there a problem with the sample?
- *d.* What body system is being evaluated?
- *e.* Identify each word part in the medical term: phlebotomist.

2 A CBC was ordered on a patient in the ED with LRQ pain and a FUO. The lab result indicated leukocytosis with neutrophilia. The physician diagnosed appendicitis and stated the pre-op patient must be NPO.
- *a.* Define the abbreviations: CBC, ED, LRQ, FUO, and NPO.
- *b.* What is an appendicitis?
- *c.* What does leukocytosis with neutrophilia indicate?

CHAPTER 6

Basic Anatomy and Physiology

Learning Objectives

Upon completion of this unit, the reader will be able to:

1. Explain the levels of organization of the human body.
2. Use directional terms to describe the position and location of body structures.
3. List the body cavities and name the main organs contained in each cavity.
4. State the four quadrants of the abdominopelvic cavity.
5. List all the body systems and identify their functions and major components.
6. List the major disorders associated with each body system.
7. Relate the major diagnostic laboratory tests to their associated systems.

A basic knowledge of anatomy and physiology is essential for effective work in the health-care professions. Anatomy is the study of the structure of the body, whereas physiology is the study of how the body functions. Knowing the location and the function of each body part helps the phlebotomist to communicate effectively with coworkers in the medical setting. An understanding of normal physiology will make disorders and diseases easier to understand.

ORGANIZATIONAL LEVELS OF THE BODY

The human body develops into a complex organism through different levels of structure and function, from the simplest to the most complex. Each level includes the previous level to build on. These levels of organization, in ascending order, are cells, tissues, organs, body systems, and the organism.

Cells

The smallest functioning unit of the body is the cell. Over 30 trillion cells provide the basic building blocks for the various structures that make up the human body. The size, shape, and composition of the cell determine cell function. There are several different types of cells, each with a specialized function and the ability to carry out specialized chemical reactions to communicate with other cells throughout the body.

Tissues

Groups of specific cells with similar structure and function form the different types of body tissue and together perform specialized functions. There are four basic types of tissue:

- Epithelial tissue: flat cells in a sheet-like arrangement that cover and line body surfaces
- Connective tissue: blood, bone, cartilage, and adipose cells that support and connect tissues and organs and provide a support network for the organs
- Muscle tissue: long, slender cells that provide the contractile tissue for movement of the body
- Nerve tissue: cells capable of transmitting electrical impulses to regulate body functions

Organs

Organs are body structures formed by the combination of two or more different types of tissue. Each organ is a specialized component of the body (e.g., the heart, brain, skin, and kidneys) and accomplishes a specific function.

Body Systems

Groups of organs functioning together for a common purpose make up the body systems. The major body systems are the integumentary, skeletal, muscular, nervous, respiratory, digestive, urinary, endocrine, reproductive, circulatory, and lymphatic. Table 6-1 lists the organs and functions of each body system. The body systems are discussed separately in this chapter and in Chapter 7 that covers the circulatory system.

Organism

Several body systems make up a complete living entity called an organism. The human body has attained the highest level of organization. The ability of these body systems to work together to sustain life and keep the body functioning normally, in spite of constantly changing internal and external conditions, is an essential function referred to as homeostasis.

ANATOMIC DESCRIPTION OF THE BODY

Key Terms
Anatomic position
Frontal plane
Midsagittal plane
Sagittal plane
Transverse plane

Directional Terms

Health-care providers effectively communicate with one another and the patient through universally adopted reference systems for the anatomic description of the body. These reference systems include directional terms, body planes, and cavities. The *anatomic position* for the body is standing erect, the head facing forward, and the arms by the sides with the palms facing to the front.

TABLE 6-1 • Summary of Body Systems

SYSTEM	FUNCTION	ORGANS
Integumentary	Protects against harmful pathogens and chemicals and regulates temperature	Skin, hair, nails, and glands
Skeletal	Supports and protects internal organs, stores minerals, and is the location of blood cell formation	Bones, ligaments, joints, and cartilage
Muscular	Skeletal movement and heat production	Muscles and tendons
Nervous	Recognizes and interprets sensory stimuli and regulates responses to stimuli by coordinating other body systems	Brain, spinal cord, and nerves
Respiratory	Exchanges oxygen and carbon dioxide between the air and circulating blood	Nose, pharynx, larynx, trachea, bronchi, and lungs
Digestive	Breaks down food to usable molecules to be absorbed by the body and eliminates waste products	Mouth, pharynx, esophagus, stomach, small intestine, large intestine, and rectum
Urinary	Removes waste products and regulates water and salt balance	Kidneys, ureters, urinary bladder, and urethra
Endocrine	Produces and regulates hormones	Thyroid gland, parathyroid gland, adrenal gland, pancreas, pituitary gland, ovaries, testes, thymus, and pineal gland
Reproductive	Sexual reproduction and development of male and female sexual characteristics	Female: Ovaries, fallopian tubes, uterus, vagina, and breasts Male: Testes, epididymides, vas deferens, seminal vesicles, prostate gland, bulbourethral glands, and penis
Lymphatic	Returns excess tissue fluid to the blood stream and defends against disease	Lymph vessels, ducts, lymph nodes, spleen, tonsils, and thymus
Circulatory	Transports oxygen, nutrients, and waste products	Heart, arteries, veins, and capillaries

Directional terms indicate the location and position of an area or body part. Table 6-2 contains common directional terms.

 Technical Tip 6-1. When studying anatomic illustrations, note that the right and left sides are opposite your own.

Body Planes

An anatomic plane is an imaginary flat surface that divides portions of the body or an organ into front, back, right, left, upper, and lower sections. Figure 6-1 illustrates the body planes and directions.

- *Frontal* (coronal) *plane*—divides the body into the anterior (front or ventral) and posterior (back or dorsal) portions
- *Sagittal plane*—divides the body vertically into right and left portions
- *Midsagittal plane*—vertically divides the body into equal right and left portions
- *Transverse plane*—cross-sectional division separating the body horizontally into upper (superior) and lower (inferior) portions

Body Cavities

Body cavities are hollow spaces containing the internal organs. Classified into two major groups depending

TABLE 6-2 • Common Directional Terms		
TERM	**DEFINITION**	**EXAMPLE**
Anterior	In front of or before	The chest is anterior to the spine.
Posterior	Toward the back	The spine is posterior to the chest.
Superior	Above/in an upward direction	The head is superior to the chest.
Inferior	Below/in a downward direction	The chest is inferior to the head.
Proximal	Point of attachment near the body center	The knee is proximal to the foot.
Distal	Point of attachment further from center	The foot is distal to the knee.
Lateral	To the side	The shoulder is lateral to the chest.
Medial	Nearest the midline	The chest is medial to the shoulder.
Ventral	The front side	The chest is on the ventral side of the body.
Dorsal	The back side	The spine is on the dorsal side of the body.
Superficial	Toward the surface	The skin is a superficial organ.
Deep	Toward the interior	The femoral artery is deep in the body.

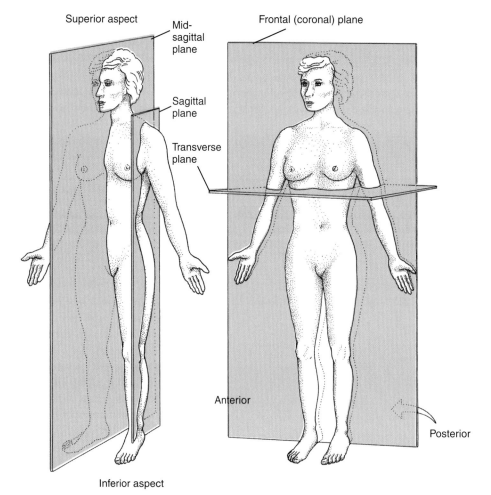

FIGURE 6-1 The planes of the body. *(Modified from Scanlon, VC, and Sanders, T: Essentials of Anatomy and Physiology, ed. 5. FA Davis, 2007, Philadelphia, with permission.)*

on their location, the anterior and posterior cavities enclose five subcavities (Fig. 6-2).

The ventral cavity (anterior) consists of the thoracic cavity, abdominal cavity, and pelvic cavity. Pleural membranes line the organs of the thoracic cavity. A muscular wall called the diaphragm separates the thoracic and abdominal cavities.

The dorsal cavity (posterior) contains the cranial cavity and spinal cavity. Table 6-3 lists the main organs contained in these cavities.

Abdominopelvic Cavity

The abdominopelvic cavity combines the abdominal and pelvic cavities. An imaginary cross formed by a transverse plane and a midsagittal plane that cross at the umbilicus divides the abdominopelvic cavity into four quadrants for clinical evaluation and diagnostic purposes. The four divisions are the right upper quadrant (RUQ), right lower quadrant (RLQ), left

TABLE 6-3 ● Body Cavities and Their Organs		
PLANE	**CAVITY**	**ORGANS**
Anterior	Thoracic	Lungs and heart
	Abdominal	Stomach, small and large intestines, spleen, liver, gallbladder, pancreas, and kidneys
	Pelvic	Bladder, ovaries, and testes
Posterior	Cranial	Brain
	Spinal	Spinal cord

upper quadrant (LUQ), and left lower quadrant (LLQ) (Fig. 6-3).

 Technical Tip 6-2. A patient with appendicitis might present with right lower quadrant pain.

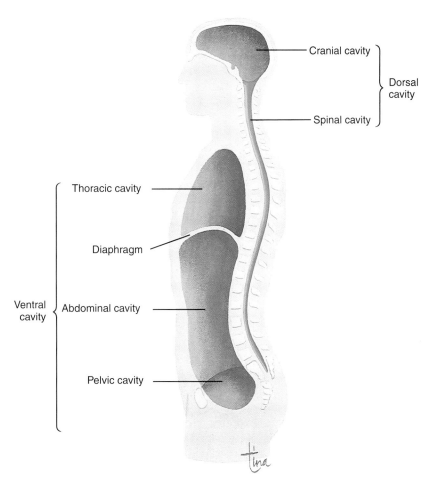

FIGURE 6-2 The cavities of the body. *(From Scanlon, VC, and Sanders, T: Essentials of Anatomy and Physiology, ed. 5. FA Davis, 2007, Philadelphia, with permission.)*

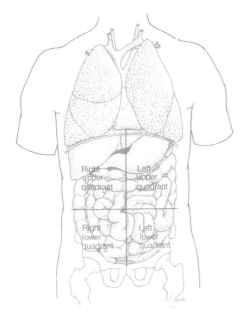

FIGURE 6-3 Four quadrants of the abdominopelvic cavity. *(From Scanlon, VC, and Sanders, T: Essentials of Anatomy and Physiology, ed. 5. FA Davis, 2007, Philadelphia, with permission.)*

INTEGUMENTARY SYSTEM

Key Terms

Dermis (DER mis)
Epidermis (EP i DER mis)
Erythema (ER i THE ma)
Keratin (KER a tin)
Melanin (MEL a nin)
Sebaceous gland (se BA shus)
Subcutaneous (SUB ku TA ne us)
Sudoriferous gland (su dor IF er us)

Function

The skin covers the outer surface of the body and provides the functions of protection, regulation, sensation, and secretion.

Skin protects the body against invasion by microorganisms and environmental chemicals, minimizes the loss or entry of water, helps block the harmful effects of sunlight, and helps produce vitamin D.

Skin regulates temperature by insulating the body and raising or lowering body temperature in response to environmental changes. Blood vessels in the skin dilate to bring blood to the surface when the body needs to lose heat and constrict to allow blood to flow to the muscles and organs when the body needs to conserve heat.

Embedded in the skin are sensory receptors to receive the sensations of heat, cold, pain, touch, and pressure that provide information about the external environment.

Millions of glands under the skin produce secretions to lubricate the skin and produce sweat to keep the body cool.

Components

The integumentary system consists of the skin, hair, nails, *sebaceous glands,* and *sudoriferous glands,* hair, and nails. The skin is the body's largest organ. On the average adult, it weighs about 7 pounds and, when stretched out, would cover about 18 square feet. The skin consists of three layers, the *epidermis, dermis,* and *subcutaneous* layer (Fig. 6-4).

- The epidermis is the thinnest layer of skin and contains no blood vessels or nerve endings. It depends on the blood supply in the capillaries of the dermis to provide oxygen and nutrients. Four or five layers of squamous epithelial cells make up the epidermis. The outer cells produce the hard protein *keratin* that prevents the loss or entry of water and resists the entry of pathogens and harmful chemicals. Melanocytes, the cells that produce the skin pigment *melanin,* are located in the epidermis. The amount of melanin produced by exposure to ultraviolet (UV) light determines the darkness of skin color.
- The dermis lies below the epidermis. The dermis is thicker than the epidermis, and this irregular fibrous connective tissue contains capillaries, lymph vessels, nerve fibers, sudoriferous glands, sebaceous glands, and hair follicles. A layer of dermal papillae acts as peg-like projections that help bind the dermis to the epidermis. The uneven ridges and grooves created by this junction form the fingerprints and footprints.
- A layer of subcutaneous tissue connects the skin to the underlying organs, protects and cushions the deep tissues of the body, stores fat for energy, and acts as a heat insulator.
- Sudoriferous glands are small, coiled glands with ducts extending up through the epidermis to small pores on almost all body surfaces. Activated by high external temperature and exercise, the perspiration (sweat) produced by these

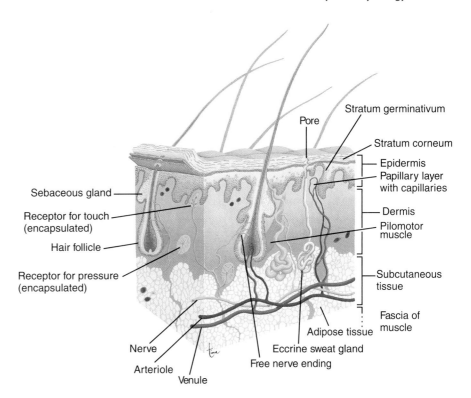

FIGURE 6-4 **Cross-section of the skin.** *(Adapted from Scanlon, VC, and Sanders, T: Essentials of Anatomy and Physiology, ed. 5. FA Davis, 2007, Philadelphia, with permission.)*

glands regulates body temperature by evaporation and eliminates waste products through the pores of the skin.

- Sebaceous glands are the oil-secreting glands of the skin. Secreted through tiny ducts into hair follicles or directly to the skin surface to prevent drying of the hair and skin is an oily substance called sebum.
- Hair consists of dead cells filled with keratin. Hair fibers grow in sheaths of epidermal tissue called hair follicles. Mitosis takes place in the hair root located at the base of the follicle. The new cells produce keratin, obtain their color from melanin, and grow into the visible portion of the follicle, called the hair shaft.
- Nails consist of hard keratin plates that cover and protect the fingers and toes. As with the hair fiber, new cells constantly form in the nail root of a nail follicle. The new cells produce keratin and then die to form the nail plate.

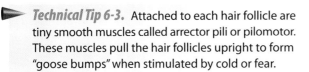 *Technical Tip 6-3.* Attached to each hair follicle are tiny smooth muscles called arrector pili or pilomotor. These muscles pull the hair follicles upright to form "goose bumps" when stimulated by cold or fear.

Disorders

Common disorders of the integumentary system are shown in Box 6-1.

Diagnostic Tests

The most frequently ordered diagnostic tests associated with the integumentary system and their clinical correlations are presented in Table 6-4.

BOX 6-1 Disorders of the Integumentary System

Acne (AK ne): An oversecretion of sebum by the sebaceous glands that causes blockage of ducts and formation of pustules.

Eczema (EK ze ma): An allergic reaction with an itchy rash that may blister and is aggravated by infection, emotional stress, food allergy, and sweating.

Fever blisters (cold sores): Caused by the herpes simplex virus, usually at the edge of the lip; may become dormant and are triggered by stress or illness.

Fungal infections: infections such as ringworm, athlete's foot, and jock itch; caused by the dermatophyte fungi that can produce itching, scaling, and *erythema*.

Continued

| BOX 6-1 | Disorders of the Integumentary System—cont'd |

Impetigo (im pe TI go): A highly contagious bacterial infection caused by *Staphylococcus* or *Streptococcus*, frequently seen in younger children; may present with erythema and progress into blisters that rupture, producing yellow crusts.

Keloid (KE loyd): Excess collagen scar formation in the area of surgical incisions or skin wounds.

Psoriasis (so RI a sis): A chronic inflammatory skin condition characterized by itchy, scaly, red patches; scales are on top of raised lesions called plaques.

Skin cancer: Squamous cell carcinoma, basal cell carcinoma, and malignant melanoma are the most common types of skin cancer.

TABLE 6-4 • **Diagnostic Laboratory Tests Associated with the Integumentary System**

TEST	CLINICAL CORRELATION
Culture and sensitivity (C & S)	Bacterial infection
Fungal culture	Fungal infection
Gram stain	Microbial infection
Potassium hydroxide (KOH) prep	Fungal infection
Skin biopsy (Bx)	Malignancy

SKELETAL SYSTEM

Key Terms

Articulation (ar TIK u LA shun)
Bursa (BUR sa)
Cartilage (KAR ti lij)
Hematopoiesis (hem a to poy E sis)
Ligament (LIG a ment)
Sarcoma (sar KO ma)
Synovial (Sin O ve al)
Tendon (TEN dun)

Function

The five main functions of the skeletal system are support, protection, movement, mineral storage, and

blood cell formation (*hematopoiesis*). As the framework of the body, the skeletal system provides support and protects vital organs. Movement is possible because bone is the anchor point for muscles, joints, *tendons*, and *ligaments*. Phosphorus and calcium are stored in the bones and are released to the blood as needed. The important function of hematopoiesis takes place in the center (marrow) of bones.

Components

The components of the skeletal system are the bones, joints, tendons, *cartilage*, and ligaments.

Bones

There are four types of bones that make up the skeleton of the body.

- Long bones—bones in the extremities (arms and legs): leg (femur, tibia, fibula), arm (humerus, radius, ulna), hand (metacarpals, phalanges)
- Short bones—bones in the wrists and ankles
- Flat bones—the ribs, shoulder blades, hips, and skull bones
- Irregular bones—the vertebrae and facial bones

The major bones of the body are shown in Figure 6-5.

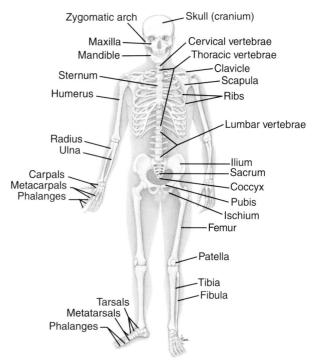

FIGURE 6-5 The major bones of the body. (*From Scanlon, VC, and Sanders, T: Essentials of Anatomy and Physiology, ed. 5. FA Davis, 2007, Philadelphia, with permission.*)

Connective Tissue

Cartilage fibers imbedded in a gel-like material coats the ends of the joint-forming bones. The remainder of the bone is covered by a fibrous tissue membrane that serves as an attachment for ligaments and tendons. Ligaments consisting of fibrous connective tissue attach bones not involved in joint formation to other bones.

Tendons attach muscles to bones to coordinate movement.

Joints

Joints are formed by the ***articulation*** of the ends of two long bones. They are classified by the amount of movement in the joint. Types of joints and examples are:

- Immovable: skull sutures
- Partially moveable: vertebrae
- Free moving: knees, hips, elbows, wrist, feet

Free-moving joints are ***synovial*** joints. The ends of the bones are connected by a joint capsule containing viscous synovial fluid that reduces friction between the two bones. Small sacs of synovial fluid called ***bursae*** located between the joint and tendons allow tendons to slide easily across joints (Fig. 6-6).

 Technical Tip 6-4. Samples of synovial fluid are frequently received in the laboratory to determine the cause of joint inflammation.

Disorders

Common disorders of the skeletal system are shown in Box 6-2.

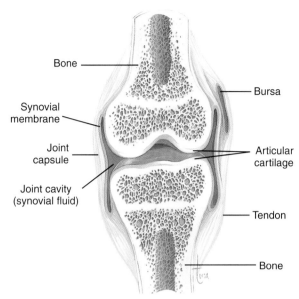

FIGURE 6-6 **Synovial joint.** *(From Scanlon, VC, and Sanders, T: Essentials of Anatomy and Physiology, ed. 5. FA Davis, 2007, Philadelphia, with permission.)*

 Technical Tip 6-5. Osteomyelitis can be caused by local trauma to the bone such as improper heel punctures in phlebotomy.

Diagnostic Tests

The most frequently ordered diagnostic tests associated with the skeletal system and their clinical correlations are presented in Table 6-5.

BOX 6-2 Disorders of the Skeletal System

Arthralgia (ar THRAL je a): Pain without swelling or redness in the joints; can be caused by tension, virus infections, unusual exertion, or accidents.

Arthritis (ar THRI tis): Inflammation of the joint, causing swelling, redness, warmth, and pain on movement. The most common types are osteoarthritis, rheumatoid arthritis, and gout.

Bursitis (bur SI tis): Inflammation of the bursae located between the joints and the tendons, commonly causing swelling and pain in the shoulder, elbow, and heel.

Fractures (Fx): Breaking of bone caused by stress, cancer, or metabolic disease.

Gout (gowt): Painful metabolic condition caused by uric acid crystals forming in the joints, frequently the big toe, the ankle, or the knee.

Osteoarthritis (OS te o ar THRI tis): Swelling and pain, primarily in weight-bearing joints caused by calcium deposits in the joint capsules.

Osteomalacia (OS te o mal A she a): Softening of the bones resulting from inability to absorb calcium, caused by a vitamin D deficiency; often called rickets.

Continued

BOX 6-2 • Disorders of the Skeletal System—cont'd

Osteomyelitis (OS te o MI el I tis): Inflammation of the bones and bone marrow caused by a bacterial infection.

Osteoporosis (OS te o por O sis): Bone disease involving decreased bone density, producing porous bones that can become brittle and easily broken.

Rheumatoid arthritis (RA) (ROO ma toyd): Chronic inflammation of the joints caused by an autoimmune reaction involving the joint connective tissue.

Sarcoma: A malignant bone tumor.

Scoliosis (SKO le O sis): Lateral curvature of the spine with deviation either to the right or left that gives the spine the shape of an "S."

Spina bifida (SPI na BI fid a): Congenital disorder characterized by an abnormal closure of the spinal canal resulting in the malformation of the spine.

TABLE 6-5 • Diagnostic Laboratory Tests Associated with the Skeletal System

TEST	CLINICAL CORRELATION
Alkaline phosphatase (ALP)	Bone disorders
Antinuclear antibody (ANA)	Systemic lupus erythematosus
Calcium (Ca)	Bone disorders
Erythrocyte sedimentation rate (ESR)	Inflammation
Fluorescent antinuclear antibody (FANA)	Systemic lupus erythematosus
Gram stain	Microbial infection
Phosphorus (P)	Skeletal disorders
Rheumatoid arthritis (RA)	Rheumatoid arthritis
Synovial fluid analysis	Arthritis
Uric acid	Gout
Vitamin D	Calcium absorption

MUSCULAR SYSTEM

Key Terms

Cardiac muscle (KAR de ak)
Insertion
Origin
Skeletal muscle
Smooth muscle
Striated

Function

The muscular system works in conjunction with the skeletal and nervous systems to provide body movement. Muscles are attached to the bones of the skeleton by tendons. The ability of the muscle to contract provides the body with movement and posture. Muscles not only provide skeletal movement but also pass food through the digestive system, propel blood through blood vessels, and contract the bladder to expel urine.

Muscle Movement

Tendons, cords of fibrous connective tissue, attach skeletal muscle to bones. A muscle attaches to a stationary bone, the *origin,* and to a movable bone, the *insertion.* As the muscle contracts and shortens, the insertion bone moves toward the stationary bone. A muscle pulls when it contracts, but it cannot push. An opposing muscle contracts to pull the bone in the other direction. A muscle that produces movement is the prime mover, and the opposing muscle is an antagonist. Table 6-6 lists the major muscle movements.

TABLE 6-6 • Major Muscle Movements*

MOTION	ACTION
Abduction	Moving away from the middle of the body
Adduction	Moving toward the middle of the body
Extension	Straightening of a limb
Flexion	Bending of a limb
Pronation	Turning the palm down
Supination	Turning the palm up
Dorsiflexion	Elevating the foot
Plantar flexion	Lowering the foot
Rotation	Moving a bone around its longitudinal axis

*Grouped in pairs of antagonistic function (except for rotation).

The concept of muscular movement is illustrated in Figure 6-7.

Components

The three types of muscle found in the body are skeletal, smooth, and cardiac. They are classified by their function and appearance. The three types of muscle are shown in Figure 6-8.

Skeletal muscle is a *striated* voluntary muscle that attaches to bones and is responsible for movement of the body. It is called a voluntary muscle because a person has control over its activity. It is a striated muscle because of its cross-striped appearance when examined microscopically.

Smooth muscle is an unstriated involuntary muscle that lacks the cross-striped appearance microscopically. It is controlled by the autonomic nervous system. Found in the walls of veins and arteries and in the internal organs of the digestive, respiratory, and urinary systems, smooth muscle functions without conscious control.

Cardiac muscle is the muscle of the heart wall. Like skeletal muscle, it is a striated muscle. However, it is also an involuntary muscle. Controlled by the autonomic nervous system, cardiac muscle rhythmically contracts without conscious control.

Disorders

The common disorders of the muscular system are shown in Box 6-3.

Diagnostic Tests

The most frequently ordered diagnostic tests associated with the muscular system and their clinical correlations are presented in Table 6-7.

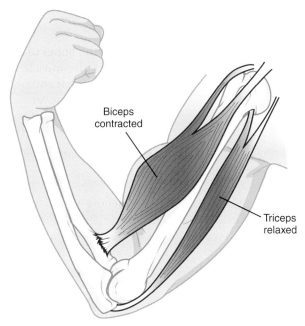

FIGURE 6-7 **An example of muscular movement.**

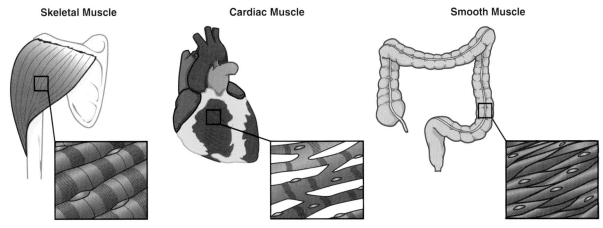

FIGURE 6-8 **The three types of muscle.**

BOX 6-3 Disorders of the Muscular System

Atrophy (AT ro fe): Wasting away of muscle caused by inactivity.

Fibromyalgia syndrome (FMS): A condition causing chronic muscle pain, fatigue, sleep problems, irritable bowel syndrome, morning stiffness, anxiety, and memory problems.

Muscular dystrophy (DIS tro fe) (MD): An inherited disorder in which the muscles are replaced by fat and fibrous tissue and progressively weaken.

Myalgia (mi AL je a): Muscle pain that can be caused by tension, viral infections, exertion, and accidents.

Myasthenia gravis (mI as THE ne a): A neuromuscular disorder of the skeletal muscle that affects the transmission of nerve impulses to the muscles of the eyes, face, and limbs.

Poliomyelitis (POL e o MI el I tis): Viral infection of the nerves controlling skeletal movement, resulting in muscle weakness and paralysis.

Tendinitis (TEN din I tis): Inflammation of the tendons caused by excess exertion.

TABLE 6-7 • Diagnostic Laboratory Tests Associated With the Muscular System

TEST	CLINICAL CORRELATION
Creatinine kinase (CK [CPK])	Muscle damage
Creatinine kinase isoenzymes (CK-MM, MB)	Muscle damage
Lactic acid	Muscle fatigue
Magnesium (Mg)	Musculoskeletal disorders
Myoglobin	Muscle damage
Potassium (K)	Muscle function

NERVOUS SYSTEM

Key Terms

Afferent neuron
Axon (AK son)
Central nervous system
Cerebrospinal fluid
Dendrite (DEN drit)

Efferent neuron
Meninges (men IN jez)
Myelin sheath (MI el in)
Neuroglia (nû ROG le a)
Neuron (NU ron)
Peripheral nervous system
Synapse (SIN aps)

Function

The primary functions of the nervous system are to recognize sensory stimuli, to interpret these sensations, and to initiate the appropriate response that provides the communication, integration, and control of all body functions.

Components

The nervous system is divided into the *central nervous system* (CNS) and the *peripheral nervous system* (PNS). The CNS lies in the center of the body and consists of the brain and the spinal cord. The PNS consists of nerves located outside the skull and spinal column that extend out into the body and connect the brain and spinal cord to all parts of the body. The main functioning cell that conducts nerve impulses is the *neuron.*

Neurons

Neurons are the main functional cells of the nervous system. A neuron consists of three main parts: *dendrites,* a cell body, and an *axon.* Several dendrites branch out to receive and carry impulses to the cell body. The axon, which is a single long projection, extends out and carries impulses away from the cell body. Neurons are held together by *neuroglia* cells that act as support for the neurons but do not conduct impulses.

The point at which the axon of one neuron and the dendrite of another neuron come together is called a *synapse.* Nerve impulses are transmitted at the synapse. The nerve impulse from an axon stops at the synapse, chemical signals are sent across the gap, and the impulse then continues along the dendrites, cell body, and the axon of the next neuron (Fig. 6-9).

Different types of neurons are classified by the way they transmit impulses.

- Sensory neurons, also called *afferent neurons,* transmit impulses from the sensory organs to the brain and spinal cord.
- Motor or *efferent neurons* transmit impulses away from the brain and spinal cord to the muscles

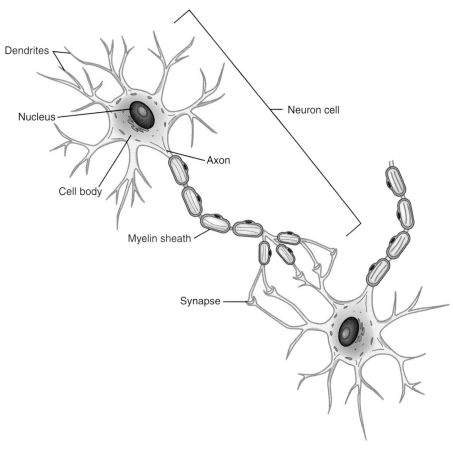

Dendrites

Nucleus

Cell body

Myelin sheath

Axon

Neuron cell

Synapse

FIGURE 6-9 **The neuron and its function.**

and glands to produce a response of either contraction or secretion.

Central Nervous System

The CNS, consisting of the brain and spinal cord, is the communication center of the nervous system. It receives impulses from all parts of the body, processes the information, and initiates a response. The brain is one of the largest organs in the body and is the center for regulating body functions. The spinal cord has an ascending nerve tract to carry sensory impulses to the brain. A descending nerve tract carries motor impulses away from the brain to the muscles and organs.

The brain and spinal cord are protected not only by the skull and vertebrae but also by three layers of tissue called the **meninges. Cerebrospinal fluid** (CSF) circulates between the layers of the meninges to cushion the brain and spinal cord from external shock (Fig. 6-10).

▶ **Technical Tip 6-6.** CSF obtained by puncture into the meninges between the vertebrae is frequently received in the laboratory for analysis. These samples must be processed with extreme care.

Peripheral Nervous System

The PNS is the nerve network branching throughout the body from the brain and spinal cord. The PNS includes the autonomic nervous system that consists of the motor neurons to control the involuntary bodily functions such as heartbeat, stomach contractions, respiration, and gland secretions and the sensory neurons to carry voluntary impulses to the musculoskeletal system.

The involuntary actions of the autonomic system are regulated by the sympathetic and parasympathetic divisions of the autonomic nervous system. The sympathetic division controls stress situations such as

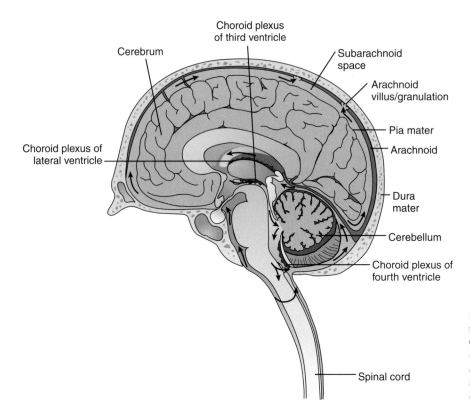

Choroid plexus of third ventricle

Cerebrum

Subarachnoid space

Arachnoid villus/granulation

Pia mater

Arachnoid

Choroid plexus of lateral ventricle

Dura mater

Cerebellum

Choroid plexus of fourth ventricle

Spinal cord

FIGURE 6-10 The brain and spinal cord showing circulation of CSF through the meninges. *(Adapted from Strasinger, SK, and Di Lorenzo, MS: Urinalysis and Body Fluids, ed. 5. FA Davis, 2008, Philadelphia.)*

anger or fear by increasing the heart rate and dilating vessels. The parasympathetic controls relaxed situations by decreasing the heart rate and the other body activities to normal levels.

Disorders

The common disorders of the nervous system are shown in Box 6-4.

Diagnostic Tests

The most frequently ordered diagnostic tests associated with the nervous system and their clinical correlations are presented in Table 6-8.

RESPIRATORY SYSTEM

Key Terms

Carbaminohemoglobin (kar bam i no he mo glo bin)
External respiration
Hemoglobin
Internal respiration
Oxyhemoglobin
Partial pressure of carbon dioxide
Partial pressure of oxygen
Surfactant

Function

The function of the respiratory system is to exchange the gases oxygen and carbon dioxide between the circulating blood and the air and tissues. This system is crucial to the survival of cells. Oxygen is a colorless, odorless, combustible gas found in the air; carbon dioxide is a colorless, odorless, incombustible gas that is a waste product of cell metabolism.

The exchange of gases involves two types of respiration processes: *external respiration* and *internal respiration.* External respiration is the exchange of gases between the blood and the lungs. Internal respiration is the exchange of gases between the blood and tissue cells.

Blood transports oxygen and carbon dioxide through the *hemoglobin* in red blood cells (RBCs). Hemoglobin with oxygen attached is called *oxyhemoglobin* and is carried to the tissues for use by the body cells. Twenty percent of the total carbon

BOX 6-4 Disorders of the Nervous System

Alzheimer's disease (ALTS hi merz): Characterized by diminished mental capabilities, including memory loss, anxiety, and confusion.

Amyotrophic lateral sclerosis (ALS) (a MI o TROF ik) (skle RO sis): A disorder of the motor neurons in the brain and spinal cord that causes skeletal and muscular weakness; also called Lou Gehrig's disease.

Bell's palsy (PAWL ze): Inflammation of a facial nerve that causes paralysis and numbness of the face.

Cerebral palsy: A condition associated with birth defects, marked by partial paralysis and poor muscle coordination.

Cerebrovascular accident (CVA): Stroke, which can be caused by a cerebral hemorrhage or arteriosclerosis (hardening of the arteries). A decrease in the flow of blood to the brain causes destruction of the brain tissue from lack of oxygen.

Encephalitis (en SEF a LI tis): Inflammation of the brain caused by a virus; symptoms are lethargy, stiff neck, or convulsions.

Epilepsy (EP i LEP se): Recurring seizure disorder resulting from abnormal electrical activity or malfunctioning of the chemical substances of the brain.

Meningitis (men in JI tis): Inflammation of the membranes of the brain or spinal cord caused by a variety of microorganisms.

Multiple neurofibromatosis (NU ro fi BRO ma TO sis): Fibrous tumors throughout the body causing crippling deformities.

Multiple sclerosis (MS): A chronic degenerative disease of the CNS that destroys the *myelin sheath* of the brain and spinal cord.

Myelitis (mi e LI tis): Inflammation of the spinal cord.

Neuralgia (nu RAL je a): Pain of the nerves.

Neuritis (nu RI tis): Inflammation of nerves associated with a degenerative process.

Parkinson's disease: Chronic disease of the nervous system characterized by muscle tremors, muscle weakness, and loss of equilibrium.

Reye's syndrome (riz): An acute disease that causes edema of the brain and fatty infiltration of the liver and other organs; viral in origin; seen in children after aspirin administration.

Shingles (herpes zoster): An acute viral disease caused by varicella zoster, the virus that causes chickenpox, which can remain dormant in the body and reappear in the form of shingles.

TABLE 6-8 • Diagnostic Laboratory Tests Associated With the Nervous System

TEST	CLINICAL CORRELATION
Cerebrospinal fluid (CSF) analysis	
Cell count/differential	Neurological disorders or meningitis
Culture and Gram stain	Meningitis
Glucose and protein	Neurological disorders or meningitis
Creatinine kinase isoenzymes (CK-BB)	Brain damage
Culture and sensitivity (C & S)	Microbial infection
Drug screening	Therapeutic drug monitoring or drug abuse
Lead	Neurological function
Lithium (Li)	Antidepressant drug monitoring
Lumbar puncture (LP)	Cerebrospinal fluid collection prodedure

dioxide attaches to hemoglobin to form *carbamino-hemoglobin,* which is carried to the lungs, where the carbon dioxide is expelled. The remaining carbon dioxide is carried as bicarbonate ion in the plasma. In the lungs, the bicarbonate ion enters the RBC, and carbon dioxide is re-formed and diffuses into the alveoli to be exhaled by the body (Fig. 6-11).

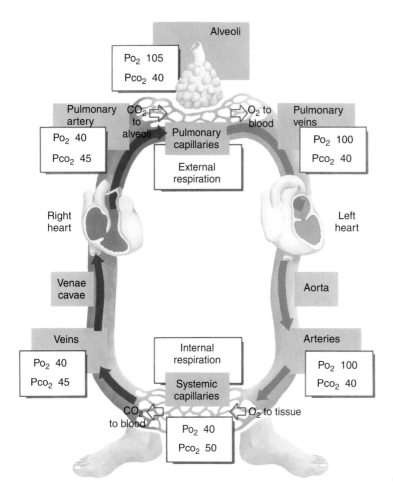

FIGURE 6-11 External and internal respiration.
(From Scanlon, VC, and Sanders, T: Essentials of Physiology, ed. 5. FA Davis, 2007, Philadelphia, with permission.)

The amount of oxygen and carbon dioxide in the blood is determined in the laboratory by measuring the ***partial pressure of oxygen*** and the ***partial pressure of carbon dioxide*** (Po_2 and Pco_2) of the two gases in arterial blood. Arterial blood should have a higher Po_2 than Pco_2 because it is delivering oxygen to the cells. Venous blood should have a higher Pco_2 than Po_2 because it has picked up carbon dioxide from the cells to be expelled by the lungs.

Components

The respiratory system consists of the upper respiratory tract, which includes the nose, pharynx, larynx, and upper trachea, and the lower respiratory tract, which includes lungs, lower trachea, bronchi, and alveoli (Fig. 6-12).

- The nose filters, moistens, and warms inhaled air.
- The pharynx serves as a pathway for air inhaled by the nose to reach the larynx.
- The larynx passes air through the trachea and contains the vocal chords.

- The trachea (windpipe) divides into two pathways called major bronchi to pass air to the right and left lungs.
- The lungs lie on either side of the heart and are enclosed in a serous membrane called pleura. The right lung is divided into three lobes and the left lung into two lobes. The lungs are where the oxygen and carbon dioxide exchange take place.
- The bronchi divide into tree-like branches called bronchioles that extend thoughout the lungs.
- The alveoli are miniature air sacs coated with a ***surfactant*** to prevent collapsing at the termination of the bronchioles. Exchanges of oxygen and carbon dioxide with the capillary blood take place in the alveoli. Oxygen attached to hemoglobin in the RBCs is passed to the body cells and carbon dioxide in the cells is then attached to the hemoglobin to be returned to the lungs.

Disorders

The common disorders of the respiratory system are shown in Box 6-5.

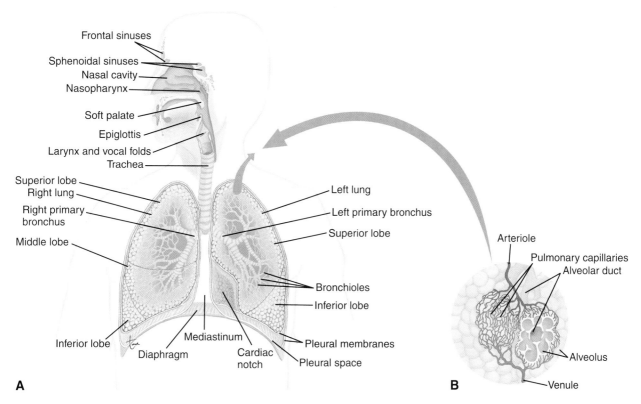

FIGURE 6-12 **The respiratory system. A, Anterior view of the upper and lower respiratory tracts.** *(From Scanlon, VC, and Sanders, T: Essentials of Anatomy and Physiology, ed. 5. FA Davis, 2007, Philadelphia, with permission.)* **B, Microscopic view of alveloi and pulmonary capillaries**

BOX 6-5 Disorders of the Respiratory System

Apnea (ap NE a): Cessation of breathing.

Asthma (AZ ma): Swelling or constriction of the bronchial tubes causing wheezing, a feeling of chest constriction, and difficulty in breathing.

Bronchitis (brong KI tis): Chronic inflammation of the bronchial tubes causing a deep cough that can produce sputum.

Chronic obstructive pulmonary disease (COPD): Inflammation or obstruction of the bronchi and/or alveoli over a long period.

Cystic fibrosis: A hereditary disorder causing production of viscous mucus that blocks the bronchioles.

Emphysema (EM fi SE ma): Chronic inflammation resulting in destruction of the bronchioles.

Infant respiratory distress syndrome (IRDS): A condition affecting prematurely born infants, caused by a lack of surfactant in the alveolar air sacs in the lungs.

Pleurisy (PLOO ris e): Inflammation of the pleural membrane covering the chest cavity and the outer surface of the lungs.

Pneumonia (nu MO ne a): Acute infection of the alveoli of the lungs in which the alveoli fill with fluid so that the air spaces are blocked and it is difficult to exchange oxygen and carbon dioxide.

Pulmonary edema (PUL mo ne re e DE ma): Accumulation of fluid in the lungs; frequently a complication of congestive heart failure.

Rhinitis (ri NI tis): Inflammation of the nasal mucous membranes resulting in a runny nose.

Strep throat: Inflammation of the pharynx caused by streptococcal group A bacteria.

Tuberculosis (TB): Infectious disease decreasing respiratory function, caused by *Mycobacterium tuberculosis*.

Upper respiratory infection (URI): Infection of the nose, pharynx, or larynx, including the common cold.

TABLE 6-9 • Diagnostic Tests Associated With the Respiratory System	
TEST	**CLINICAL CORRELATION**
Arterial blood gases (ABGs)	Acid-base balance
Bronchoalveolar lavage	Microbial infection
Cold agglutinins	Atypical pneumonia
Complete blood count (CBC)	Pneumonia
Electrolytes (Lytes)	Acid-base balance
Gram stain	Microbial infection
Pleural fluid analysis	Infection, malignancy, or organ failure
Sweat chloride test	Cystic fibrosis
Thoracentesis	Obtain pleural fluid analysis
Throat and sputum cultures	Bacterial infection/ tuberculosis

Diagnostic Tests

The most frequently ordered diagnostic tests associated with the respiratory system and their clinical correlations are presented in Table 6-9.

DIGESTIVE SYSTEM

Key Terms

Alimentary tract (AL i MEN tar e)
Bile
Bilirubin (bil i ROO bin)
Diarrhea (di a RE a)
Digestion
Feces
Insulin
Peristalsis

Function

The digestive system performs three major functions: *digestion*, absorption of nutrients, and elimination of waste products.

- Digestion occurs by both mechanical and chemical processes. The mechanical breakdown begins in the mouth, where the teeth and tongue physically alter the food into smaller pieces. Saliva moistens and lubricates the food to facilitate swallowing. Chemical digestion is performed by digestive enzymes and acids contributed by the primary and accessory organs of the digestive system.
- Absorption of the digested products of food occurs through the walls of the small intestine into the blood and lymph, which transport the nutrients to the other parts of the body to produce energy and nourish body cells.
- Elimination of waste products is the third function of the digestive system. Unusable products of digestion are concentrated as *feces* in the large intestine, from which they pass out of the body through the anus.

Components

Alimentary Tract/Gastrointestinal (GI) Tract

The GI tract forms a 30-foot continuous tube in adults that begins with the mouth and ends at the anus. The organs of the gastrointestinal tract include the mouth, pharynx, esophagus, stomach, small intestine, large intestine, rectum, and anus (Fig. 6-13).

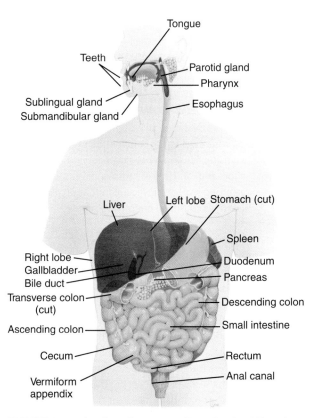

FIGURE 6-13 **The digestive system.** *(From Scanlon, VC, and Sanders, T: Essentials of Anatomy and Physiology, ed. 5. FA Davis, 2007, Philadelphia, with permission.)*

- The pharynx and esophagus propel food from the mouth to the stomach by muscular contractions called *peristalsis.*
- The stomach stores food for chemical digestion and produces hydrochloric acid (HCl) for further degradation of food and maintains a low pH to destroy ingested pathogens.
- The small intestine completes the digestive process and permits nutrients to be reabsorbed into the blood and lymph fluid.
- The large intestine (colon) absorbs water, minerals, and vitamins and propels undigested food material to the rectum by peristalsis.
- The rectum eliminates undigested food material in the form of feces by reflux action through the anus.

Accessory organs and structures that assist in the breakdown of food include the teeth, tongue, salivary glands, liver, gallbladder, and pancreas (Fig. 6-14).

- Teeth and tongue break food into small pieces.
- The salivary glands produce amylase to digest fats.
- The liver forms *bilirubin* and secretes it in the form of *bile* for fat digestion and absorption.
- The gallbladder concentrates and stores excess bile.
- The pancreas secretes the digestive enzymes lipase, amylase, and trypsin and produces *insulin* that regulates the carbohydrate glucose by converting excess glucose to glycogen.

Disorders

The common disorders of the digestive system are shown in Box 6-6.

Diagnostic Tests

The most frequently ordered diagnostic tests associated with the digestive system and their clinical correlations are presented in Table 6-10.

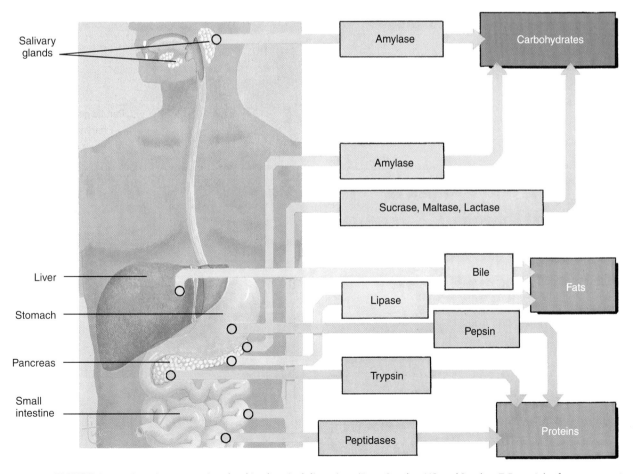

FIGURE 6-14 **Digestive organs involved in chemical digestion.** *(From Scanlon, VC, and Sanders, T: Essentials of Anatomy and Physiology, ed. 5. FA Davis, 2007, Philadelphia, with permission.)*

BOX 6-6 Disorders of the Digestive System

Appendicitis (a PEN di SI tis): Inflammation of the appendix requiring surgical removal.

Cholecystitis (KO le sis TI tis): Inflammation of the gallbladder caused by gallstones made up of precipitated bile blocking the bile duct.

Cirrhosis (si RO sis): Chronic inflammation of the liver caused by alcoholism, hepatitis, or malnutrition, resulting in degeneration of liver cells.

Colitis (ko LI tis): Acute or chronic inflammation of the colon.

Crohn's disease (kronz): Autoimmune disorder producing chronic inflammation of the intestinal tract accompanied by *diarrhea* and malabsorption.

Diverticulosis (DI ver TIK u LO sis): Inflammation of the pouches in the walls of the colon.

Gastritis (gas TRI tis): Inflammation of the stomach lining.

Gastroenteritis (GAS tro en ter I tis): Inflammation of the stomach and intestinal tracts.

Hemorrhoids (HEM o royds): Enlargement of the veins in the anorectum.

Hernia (HER ne a): Protrusion of an organ or structure through the wall of the body cavity in which it is contained.

Hepatitis: Acute inflammation of the liver caused by exposure to toxins or the hepatitis viruses.

Pancreatitis (PAN kre a TI tis): Inflammation of the pancreas.

Peritonitis (PER i to NI tis): Inflammation of the lining of the abdominal cavity (the peritoneum).

Ulcer: Open lesion in the lining of the stomach, caused by increased acid secretion or bacterial infection.

TABLE 6-10 • Diagnostic Tests Associated With the Digestive System

TEST	CLINICAL CORRELATION
Alanine aminotransferase (ALT)	Liver disorders
Albumin	Malnutrition or liver disorders
Alcohol	Intoxication
Alkaline phosphatase (ALP)	Liver disorders
Ammonia	Severe liver disorders
Amylase	Pancreatitis
Aspartate aminotransferase (AST)	Liver disorders
Bilirubin	Liver disorders
Carcinoembryonic antigen (CEA)	Carcinoma detection and monitoring
Complete blood count (CBC)	Appendicitis or other infection
Fecal fat	Fat absorption
Gamma-glutamyl transferase (GGT)	Early liver disorders
Gastrin	Gastric malignancy
Hepatitis A, B, and C immunoassays	Hepatitis A, B, and C screening
Lactic dehydrogenase (LD)	Liver disorders
Lipase	Pancreatitis
Occult blood	Gastrointestinal bleeding or intestinal malignancy
Ova and parasites (O & P)	Parasitic infection
Peritoneal fluid analysis	Bacterial infection
Stool culture	Pathogenic bacteria
Total protein (TP)	Liver disorders

URINARY SYSTEM

Key Terms

Nephron (NEF ron)
Renal (RE nal)
Renal dialysis (di AL i sis)
Uremia (u RE me a)

Function

The urinary system removes metabolic waste products, and excess water from the body in the form of urine and maintains the body's essential water and electrolyte balance.

Urine is formed in the *nephrons* of the kidney by a process of filtration and reabsorption. Blood enters the kidney through the *renal* artery, which branches into arterioles leading to the nephrons and then into a collection of capillaries called the glomerulus. The nonselective filtration process takes place in the glomerulus, where all small molecular weight substances are filtered out of the blood. Large proteins and cells remain in the blood.

Reabsorption of water, glucose, sodium, and other essential nutrients required by the body begins as the glomerular filtrate passes through the tubules of the nephron. Substances not filtered by the glomerulus are secreted by the tubules into the urinary filtrate. The actual amount of urine produced depends on the body's state of hydration and normally averages about 1000 mL (1 liter) per 24 hours. The kidneys also produce hormones, such as renin to control blood pressure, and erythropoietin to regulate the production of RBCs (Fig. 6-15).

Components

The urinary system consists of two kidneys, two ureters, the urinary bladder, and the urethra.

- The kidneys are bean-shaped organs containing an outer cortex region and an inner medulla region. The functioning unit of the kidney is the nephron, which consists of the Bowman's capsule, the glomerulus, the proximal convoluted tubule, the loop of Henle, the distal convoluted tubule, and collecting duct. Each kidney contains approximately one million nephrons.

- The two ureters are muscular tubes that conduct urine from the kidney to the bladder.
- The urinary bladder is an expandable sac located in the anterior portion of the pelvic cavity. The bladder stores the urine formed by the nephron. When the bladder becomes full, muscles in the bladder walls squeeze urine into the urethra for elimination.
- The urethra is a tube extending from the bladder to an external opening, called the urinary meatus. The male urethra transports urine and semen. The female urethra carries only urine.

Disorders

The common disorders of the urinary system are shown in Box 6-7.

Diagnostic Tests

The most frequently ordered diagnostic tests associated with the urinary system and their clinical correlations are presented in Table 6-11.

ENDOCRINE SYSTEM

Key Terms

Endocrine (EN do krin)
Gland
Hormone (HOR mon)
Hyperglycemia (HI per gli SE me a)

Function

The *endocrine* system produces and regulates *hormones.* Hormones regulate activities such as metabolism, growth and development, reproduction, and responses to stress. The system interacts with the nervous system to communicate, regulate, and control body functions. Unlike the nervous system, which commands and controls with nerve impulses, the *glands* of the endocrine system direct long-term changes in body activities by secreting chemical substances called hormones. Endocrine glands are ductless glands that secrete hormones directly into the bloodstream to circulate throughout the body until they reach a target organ. Hormones bind to a specific receptor site located on the cell membrane of a target organ and cause specific

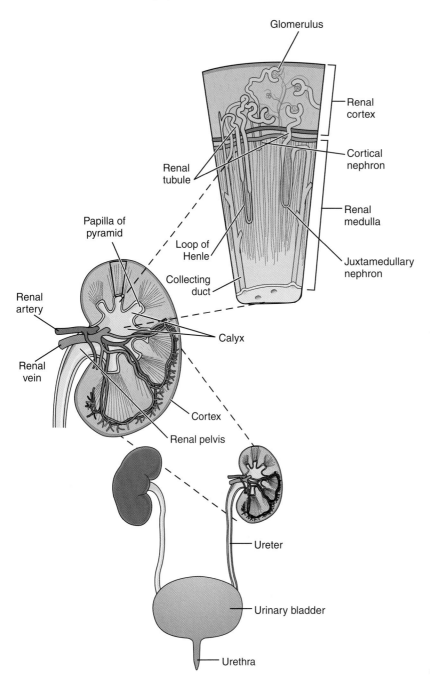

FIGURE 6-15 **The relationship of the nephron to the kidney and excretory system.** *(From Strasinger, SK, and Di Lorenzo, MS: Urinalysis and Body Fluids, ed. 5. FA Davis, 2008, Philadelphia, with permission.)*

chemical reactions to occur. A feedback system regulated by supply and demand stimulates or decreases the release of hormones.

Components

The endocrine glands include the pituitary gland, thyroid gland, four parathyroid glands, two adrenal glands, pancreas, two female ovaries, two male testes, thymus, and pineal gland (Fig. 6-16). Each gland produces hormones that perform a specific function as listed in Table 6-12.

 Technical Tip 6-7. Notice in Table 6-12 the large number of hormones secreted by the pituitary gland. The pituitary gland is commonly called the master gland because many of its hormones target other hormone-producing organs and stimulate them to produce their hormones.

BOX 6-7 Disorders of the Urinary System

Cystitis (sis TI tis): Inflammation of the urinary bladder, usually caused by a bacterial infection.

Glomerulonephritis (glo MER u lo ne FRI tis): Inflammation of the glomerulus of the kidney caused by an immune disorder or infection.

Pyelonephritis (PI e lo ne FRI tis): Inflammation of the renal pelvis and connective tissue of the kidney, usually caused by a bacterial infection.

Renal calculi (KAL ku li): Stones composed of calcium, phosphate, uric acid, oxalate, or other chemicals that crystallize within the kidney.

Renal failure: Complete cessation of renal function resulting in the need for *renal dialysis* and kidney transplantation.

Uremia (u RE me a): Excess urea, creatinine, uric acid, and other metabolic waste products in the blood.

Urinary tract infection (UTI): Bacterial infection involving any of the organs of the urinary system; includes urethritis, cystitis, and pyelonephritis.

TABLE 6-11 ● Diagnostic Tests Associated With the Urinary System

TEST	CLINICAL CORRELATION
Albumin	Kidney disorders
Ammonia	Kidney function
Blood urea nitrogen (BUN)	Kidney function
Serum creatinine	Kidney function
Creatinine clearance	Glomerular filtration
Electrolytes (Lytes)	Fluid balance
Osmolality	Fluid and electrolyte balance
Routine urinalysis (UA)	Renal or metabolic disorders
Total protein (TP)	Kidney disorders
Uric acid	Kidney function
Urine culture	Bacterial infection

TABLE 6-12 ● Summary of Endocrine Hormones

GLAND	HORMONE	FUNCTION
Anterior pituitary	Growth hormone (GH) (Somatropin)	Stimulates bone and body growth
	Thyroid-stimulating hormone (TSH)	Stimulates the thyroid gland hormones thyroxine (T_4) and triiodothyronine (T_3)
	Adrenocorticotropic hormone (ACTH)	Stimulates adrenal cortex to secrete cortisol
	Follicle-stimulating hormone (FSH)	Stimulates growth of ovarian follicles in females and sperm production in males
	Luteinizing hormone (LH)	Stimulates ovulation in females and produces testosterone in males
	Prolactin (PRL)	Stimulates milk production by mammary glands and promotes growth of breast tissue
	Melanocyte-stimulating hormone (MSH)	Regulates melanin deposits that influence skin pigmentation
Posterior pituitary	Antidiuretic hormone (ADH)	Stimulates water reabsorption by the kidney to maintain body hydration
	Oxytocin	Stimulates uterine contraction and milk secretion by the mammary gland
Thyroid	Triiodothyronine (T_3) and thyroxine (T_4)	Regulate cell metabolism and increase energy production
	Calcitonin	Decreases the reabsorption of calcium and phosphate from bones into the blood

Continued

TABLE 6-12 • Summary of Endocrine Hormones—cont'd

Parathyroid	Parathyroid hormone (PTH)	Increases the reabsorption of calcium and phosphate from the bones into the blood
Adrenal cortex	Aldosterone	Regulates sodium and potassium levels in the blood
	Cortisol	Regulates metabolism of proteins, carbohydrates, and fats and suppresses inflammation
	Androgens and estrogens	Maintain secondary sex characteristics
Adrenal medulla	Epinephrine (adrenaline)	Increases cardiac activity
	Norepinephrine (noradrenalin)	Constricts blood vessels and increases blood pressure
Pancreas	Insulin	Lowers blood sugar by transporting glucose from blood to the cells
	Glucagon	Increases blood sugar levels by converting glycogen to glucose
Ovaries	Estrogen and progesterone	Maintain female reproductive system and develop secondary female sex characteristics
Testes	Testosterone	Promotes maturation of spermatozoa and development of male secondary sex characteristics
Thymus	Thymosin	Promotes maturation of T lymphocytes and development of the immune system
Pineal	Melatonin	Regulates the body's internal clock

Disorders

Common disorders of the endocrine system are shown in Box 6-8.

Diagnostic Tests

The most frequently ordered diagnostic tests associated with the endocrine system and their clinical correlations are presented in Table 6-13.

REPRODUCTIVE SYSTEM

Key Terms

Gamete (GAM et)
Menopause (MEN o pawz)
Menstruation (men stroo A shun)
Ova
Ovulation (OV u LA shun)
Semen (SE men)
Spermatozoa (SPER mat o ZO a)

Function

The function of the reproductive system is the perpetuation of future generations of the human species. The organs and hormones specific to the male and female reproductive systems ensure sexual reproduction and the development of male and female secondary sex characteristics. The vital functions of the male and female reproduction systems are to produce *gametes,* to enable fertilization, and to provide a nourishing environment for the developing embryo/fetus.

Components

Female Reproductive System (Fig. 6-17)

- The ovaries produce the gametes called *ova.* Production (*ovulation)* begins at puberty and ends at *menopause.*
- The fallopian tubes transport unfertilized ova or a fertilized embryo to the uterus.
- The uterus is the organ for embryo development.

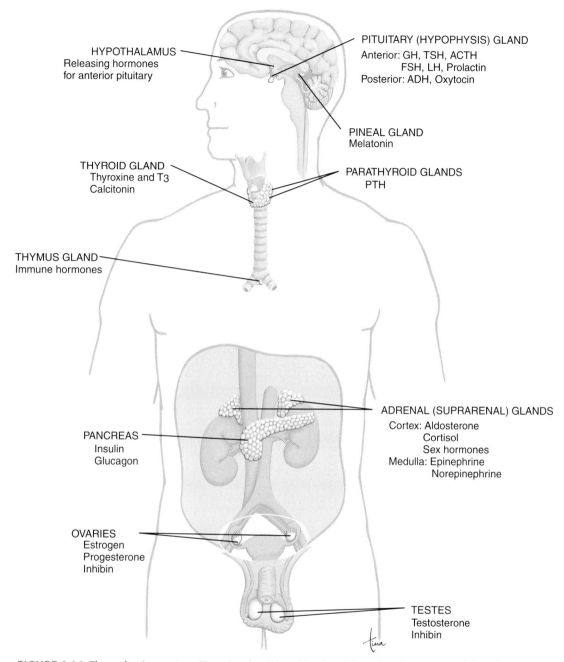

HYPOTHALAMUS
Releasing hormones
for anterior pituitary

PITUITARY (HYPOPHYSIS) GLAND
Anterior: GH, TSH, ACTH
FSH, LH, Prolactin
Posterior: ADH, Oxytocin

PINEAL GLAND
Melatonin

THYROID GLAND
Thyroxine and T3
Calcitonin

PARATHYROID GLANDS
PTH

THYMUS GLAND
Immune hormones

ADRENAL (SUPRARENAL) GLANDS
Cortex: Aldosterone
Cortisol
Sex hormones
Medulla: Epinephrine
Norepinephrine

PANCREAS
Insulin
Glucagon

OVARIES
Estrogen
Progesterone
Inhibin

TESTES
Testosterone
Inhibin

FIGURE 6-16 **The endocrine system.** *(From Scanlon, VC, and Sanders, T: Essentials of Anatomy and Physiology, ed. 5. FA Davis, 2007, Philadelphia, with permission.)*

- The vagina receives sperm during intercourse, discharges menstrual blood, and acts as the birth canal during delivery of a fetus.
- The mammary glands (breasts) produce milk for newborn nourishment.

Male Reproductive System (Fig. 6-18)

- The testes, enclosed in the scrotum, produce *spermatozoa* (sperm).
- The epididymis is an organ for storage and maturation of sperm.

BOX 6-8 Common Disorders of the Endocrine System

Pituitary

Acromegaly: Marked enlargement of the bones in the hands, feet, and face caused by hypersecretion of growth hormone (GH) in adulthood.

Diabetes insipidus (DI): Hyposecretion of antidiuretic hormone (ADH), causing a failure of the kidneys to reabsorb water and resulting in excessive urination (polyuria) and thirst (polydipsia).

Dwarfism: Abnormally small body size caused by hyposecretion of GH in childhood. Bones are underdeveloped but well proportioned to the body.

Gigantism: Marked increase in body size caused by hypersecretion of GH in childhood.

Thyroid

Cretinism: Congenital deficiency in the secretion of the thyroid hormones (hypothyroidism) resulting in mental retardation, impaired growth, and abnormal bone formation.

Goiter: An enlargement of the thyroid gland caused by hyperthyroidism.

Graves' disease: Increased cellular metabolism caused by excessive production of thyroid hormones (hyperthyroidism).

Myxedema: A condition of subcutaneous tissue swelling caused by hypothyroidism that develops in adulthood.

Parathyroid

Hyperparathyroidism: Excessive parathyroid hormone (PTH) secretion, often caused by a benign tumor.

Hypoparathyroidism: Deficient PTH secretion caused by injury or surgical removal of the gland.

Adrenal

Addison's disease: Caused by hyposecretion of cortisol.

Cushing's disease: Hypersecretion of cortisol as a result of increased adrenal cortex stimulation by adrenocorticotropic hormone (ACTH) from the pituitary gland, caused by a tumor of the pituitary gland or adrenal cortex gland.

Pancreas

Diabetes mellitus (DM): Insulin deficiency that prevents sugar from leaving the blood and entering the body cells, resulting in **hyperglycemia**.

Hypoglycemia: Abnormally decreased blood sugar level associated with increased insulin production.

TABLE 6-13 • Diagnostic Laboratory Tests Associated With the Endocrine System

TEST	CLINICAL CORRELATION
Adrenocorticotropic hormone (ACTH)	Adrenal and pituitary gland function
Aldosterone	Regulation of sodium blood levels
Antidiuretic hormone (ADH)	Water reabsorption in the nephron
Calcium (Ca)	Parathyroid function
Catecholamines	Adrenal function
Cortisol	Adrenal cortex function
Glucose	Hypoglycemia or diabetes mellitus
Glucose tolerance test (GTT)	Hypoglycemia or diabetes mellitus
Growth hormone (GH)	Pituitary gland function
Insulin level	Glucose metabolism and pancreatic function
Parathyroid hormone (PTH)	Parathyroid function
Phosphorus (P)	Endocrine disorders
Testosterone	Testicular function
Thyroid function (T_3, T_4, TSH) studies	Thyroid function

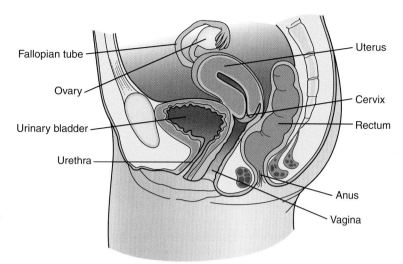

FIGURE 6-17 **The female reproductive system.** *(Adapted from Scanlon, VC, and Sanders, T: Essentials of Anatomy and Physiology, ed. 5. FA Davis, 2007, Philadelphia.)*

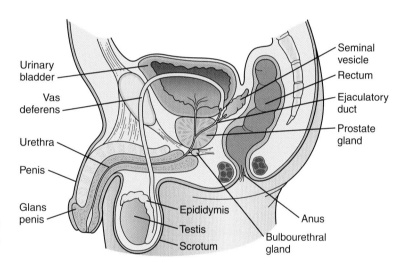

FIGURE 6-18 **The male reproductive system.** *(From Strasinger, SK, and Di Lorenzo, MS: Urinalysis and Body Fluids, ed. 5. FA Davis, 2008, Philadelphia, with permission.)*

- The vas deferens is a tube that propels mature sperm from the epididymis to the ejaculatory duct.
- The seminal vesicles produce fluid for sperm nourishment and motility. The fluid mixes with the sperm in the ejaculatory duct.
- The prostate gland propels *semen* through the urethra for ejaculation and contributes additional chemicals for sperm nourishment and acid for semen liquifaction after ejacualation.
- The bulbourethral glands contribute additional chemicals for sperm viability just before the semen is propelled to the urethra.
- The urethra is a tube running through the penis to expel the semen.

Disorders

Common disorders of the male and female reproductive systems are shown in Box 6-9.

Diagnostic Tests

The most frequently ordered diagnostic tests associated with the reproductive system and their clinical correlations are presented in Table 6-14.

LYMPHATIC SYSTEM

Key Terms

B lymphocytes
Cell-mediated immunity
Humoral immunity (HU mor al)
Lymph (limf)
Lymph nodes
T lymphocytes

BOX 6-9 Disorders of the Reproductive System

Carcinoma: Malignant tumors of the cervix (Cx), ovary, prostate, or testes.

Endometriosis: Increased endometrial (uterine lining) tissue that migrates outside the uterus.

Fibroids: Benign uterine tumors that may cause excessive uterine bleeding.

Pelvic inflammatory disease (PID): Inflammation of the ovaries, cervix, uterus, or fallopian tubes, caused by infection that may result in infertility or septicemia.

Premenstrual syndrome (PMS): Characterized by symptoms including depression, irritability, mood swings, weight gain, breast tenderness, water retention, and nervousness occurring 7 to 14 days before *menstruation.*

Sexually transmitted diseases (STDs): Diseases transmitted by sexual contact such as chlamydiosis, gonorrhea, herpes genitalis, syphilis, trichomoniasis, and AIDS.

TABLE 6-14 • Diagnostic Tests Associated With the Reproductive System

TEST	CLINICAL CORRELATION
Amniocentesis	Fetal maturity or genetic defects
Chorionic villus sampling (CVS)	Genetic defects
Estradiol, estriol, and estrogen	Ovarian or placental function
Fluorescent treponemal antibody-absorbed (FTA-ABS)	Syphilis
Genital culture	Bacterial infection
Gram stain	Microbial infection
Human chorionic gonadotropin (HCG)	Pregnancy
Pap smear (Pap)	Cervical or vaginal carcinoma
Prostate-specific antigen (PSA)	Prostatic cancer
Prostatic acid phosphatase (PAP)	Prostatic cancer
Rapid plasma reagin (RPR)	Syphilis
Rubella titer	Immunity to German measles
Semen analysis	Fertility or effectiveness of a vasectomy
Toxoplasma antibody screening	*Toxoplasma* infection
Vaginal wet prep	Microbial infection
Venereal Disease Research Laboratory (VDRL)	Syphilis

Function

The lymphatic system drains excess fluid from the tissue spaces and transports the nutrients and waste products back to the bloodstream. It provides a defense mechanism against disease by storing lymphocytes and monocytes that protect the body from foreign substances through phagocytosis and the immune response. It acts as the passageway for the absorption of fats from the small intestine into the bloodstream.

The lymphatic system is the body's "other" vessel system and connects to the circulatory system. Lymphatic vessels extend throughout the body to propel *lymph* fluid back to the circulatory system.

Components

- The parts of the lymphatic system are the lymph, lymph vessels, right lymphatic duct, thoracic duct, *lymph nodes,* tonsils, thymus, and spleen. Lymph forms from interstitial fluid, the tissue fluid that leaks from blood capillaries and surrounds the body cells. It is a clear, colorless fluid consisting of 95 percent water, proteins, salts, sugar, lymphocytes, monocytes, and waste products of metabolism. It does not contain platelets or RBCs. Lymph flows through the lymphatic vessels, entering the bloodstream through ducts that connect to veins in the upper chest.

- Lymph vessels consist of capillaries, venules, and veins. The capillaries collect lymph from the interstitial space and move it to the larger venules and veins that move it to the lymphatic ducts. Valves in the lymph vessels allow the lymph to flow in only one direction toward the chest cavity by skeletal muscle contraction.
- The right lymphatic duct receives lymph from the upper right quadrant of the body and empties into the right subclavian vein.
- The thoracic duct receives lymph from the left upper quadrant of the body and lower body and returns it to the blood in the left subclavian vein.

Figure 6-19 displays the relationship between the lymphatic and circulatory systems.
- Lymph nodes (masses of lymphatic tissue) located along the lymphatic pathway filter the lymph as it flows through the lymphatic vessels. Lymph nodes store lymphocytes and monocytes needed to phagocytize bacteria and foreign substances, stimulate the immune response, and recognize and destroy cancer cells.
- The tonsils, thymus gland, and spleen also contain lymphoid tissue to store lymphocytes and monocytes.

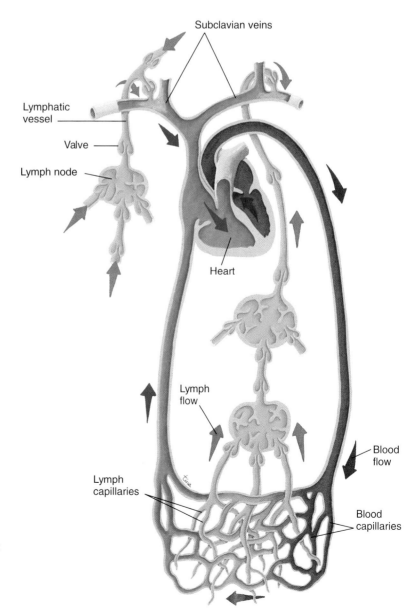

FIGURE 6-19 **The relationship of lymphatic vessels to the cardiovascular system.** *(From Scanlon, VC, and Sanders, T: Essentials of Anatomy and Physiology, ed. 5. FA Davis, 2007, Philadelphia, with permission.)*

- The tonsils (located in the pharynx) filter bacteria at the entrance of the respiratory and digestive tracts.
- The thymus gland, located between the lungs, controls the immune system. It produces T cells to provide cellular immunity.
- The spleen, located in the upper left quadrant of the abdomen, filters cell debris, bacteria, parasites, and old RBCs.

Immune System

The lymphatic system controls the body's immune system by the recognition of foreign antigens filtered through the lymph nodes and spleen, and the maintenance of a high concentration of B and T lymphocytes. An antigen is a large molecule located on cells that stimulates the formation of antibodies. Cells are recognized as "self" or foreign by the antigens present on the cell membrane.

An antibody (immunoglobulin) is a protein that is produced by exposure to antigens. *Humoral immunity* or antibody-mediated immunity involves the production of antibodies to specific antigens by *B lymphocytes* in the spleen and lymph nodes. Humoral immunity is the major immune response against bacterial infections.

T lymphocytes produce chemical substances (lymphokines) rather than antibodies for the destruction of foreign antigens in cellular or *cell-mediated immunity.* T cells also differentiate into helper T cells to aid in the humoral immune response to produce antibodies. Cell-mediated immunity is the major protection against intracellular microorganisms, such as viruses, and tumor cells. It also can cause rejection of transplanted tissue.

 Technical Tip 6-8. In AIDS, it is the helper T cells that are infected by HIV. Without the helper T cells, the immune system is severely compromised.

Disorders

The common disorders of the lymphatic system are shown in Box 6-10.

Diagnostic Tests

The most frequently ordered diagnostic tests associated with the lymphatic system and their clinical correlations are presented in Table 6-15.

BOX 6-10 Disorders of the Lymphatic System

AIDS: A suppressed immune system caused by the pathogen HIV, transmitted through sexual contact, blood products, and needles, or from mother to infant perinatally.

Hodgkin's disease: A malignant tumor of the lymphatic tissue that produces painless enlarged lymph nodes.

Infectious mononucleosis (IM): Infectious disease caused by the Epstein-Barr virus characterized by enlarged lymph nodes, increased lymphocytes, weakness, fatigue, fever, and sore throat.

Lymphoma: A solid tumor, frequently malignant, of the lymphatic tissue such as Burkitt's lymphoma and non-Hodgkin's lymphoma.

Lymphosarcoma: A diffuse malignant tumor of the lymphatic tissue.

Multiple myeloma: Malignant proliferation of plasma cells in the bone marrow.

TABLE 6-15 ● Diagnostic Laboratory Tests Associated With the Lymphatic System

TEST	CLINICAL CORRELATION
Anti-HIV	HIV screening test
Antinuclear antibody (ANA)	Systemic lupus erythematosus
Complete blood count (CBC)	Infectious mononucleosis
Fluorescent antinuclear antibody (FANA)	Systemic lupus erythematosus
Immunoglobin (Ig) levels	Immune system function
Monospot	Infectious mononucleosis
Protein electrophoresis	Multiple myeloma
T-cell count	HIV/AIDS monitoring
Viral load	HIV/AIDS monitoring
Western blot	HIV confirmation test

BIBLIOGRAPHY

Scanlon, VC, and Sanders, T: Essentials of Anatomy and Physiology, ed. 5. FA Davis, 2007, Philadelphia.

Strasinger, SK, and Di Lorenzo, MS: Urinalysis and Body Fluids, ed. 5. FA Davis, 2008, Philadelphia.

Key Points

✦ The organizational levels of the body are cells (smallest functional units), tissues (epithelial, connective, muscle, and nerve), organs (two or more tissues performing a specific function), and body systems (groups of organs working together with a common purpose).

✦ Directional terms refer to areas of the body when viewed in anatomic position. They include the terms shown in Table 6-2.

✦ Body cavities contain the internal organs. Thoracic (lungs and heart), abdominal (liver, stomach, intestines, kidneys), pelvic (uterus, testes, bladder), cranial (brain), and spinal (spinal cord). Refer to Table 6-3.

✦ The abdominopelvic cavity contains four quadrants. When the cavity is divided at the umbilicus, they are the right and left upper quadrants and the right and left lower quadrants.

✦ Body systems and organs include integumentary (skin), skeletal (bone), muscular (muscles), nervous (brain, nerves), respiratory (lungs), digestive (stomach, intestines), urinary (kidneys, bladder), endocrine (glands), reproductive (ovaries, testes, uterus), and lymphatic (vessels, nodes, B and T cells). Refer to Table 6-1.

✦ Primary functions of the body systems are integumentary (protection and temperature regulation), skeletal (support, organ protection, blood cell formation), muscular (body movement), nervous (communication among systems), respiratory (external and internal exchange of O_2 and CO_2), digestive (breakdown and absorption of nutrients, elimination of waste products), urinary (produce urine to remove metabolic wastes, maintain body hydration and electrolyte balance), endocrine (production and regulation of hormones), reproductive (production of gametes, fertilization, and maintenance of embryos), and lymphatic (removal of cellular waste and production of B and T cells).

✦ Each body system is subject to a variety of disorders that affect its function and can then lead to the malfunction of additional systems. (Refer to Boxes 6-1, 6-2, 6-3, 6-4, 6-5, 6-6, 6-7, 6-8, 6-9, and 6-10.)

✦ Many laboratory tests can be of diagnostic value for several body systems as shown in Tables 6-4, 6-5, 6-7, 6-8, 6-9, 6-10, 6-11, 6-13, 6-14, and 6-15. Primary tests for systems include integumentary (Gram stains and cultures), skeletal (calcium, phosphorus, synovial fluid analysis), muscular (creatine kinase), nervous (CSF analysis), respiratory (arterial blood gases, pleural fluid analysis), digestive (amylase, bilirubin, occult blood), urinary (routine urinalysis and culture, blood urea nitrogen), endocrine (glucose, thyroid-stimulating hormone), reproductive (beta human chorionic gonadotropin, prostate-specific antigen, Pap smear), and lymphatic (antinuclear antibody, monospot, T cell count).

Study Questions

1. Match the following disorders with the body system that they affect.
   _____ Nervous
   _____ Skeletal
   _____ Integumentary
   _____ Digestive
   _____ Reproductive
   a. appendicitis
   b. fibroids
   c. meningitis
   d. acne
   e. arthritis

2. The nephron is part of which body system?
   a. nervous
   b. endocrine
   c. urinary
   d. reproductive

3. Synovial fluid is found in the:
   a. joints
   b. testes
   c. lymph nodes
   d. spinal cord

4. All of the following are types of muscle **EXCEPT:**
   a. connective
   b. smooth
   c. cardiac
   d. skeletal

Continued

Study Questions—cont'd

5. A synapse is part of which body system?
   a. endocrine
   b. nervous
   c. skeletal
   d. reproductive

6. The type of hemoglobin found in the alveoli is:
   a. methemoglobin
   b. carbaminohemoglobin
   c. oxyhemoglobin
   d. both B and C

7. Digestive enzymes are secreted by all of the following **EXCEPT:**
   a. large intestine
   b. pancreas
   c. liver
   d. salivary glands

8. The master gland of the endocrine system is the:
   a. thyroid
   b. pituitary
   c. parathyroid
   d. adrenal

9. Which of the following body planes divides the body into superior and inferior portions?
   a. sagittal
   b. midsagittal
   c. frontal
   d. transverse

10. Keratin is found in all of the following **EXCEPT:**
    a. skin
    b. dermis
    c. nails
    d. hair

11. The lungs and heart are located in the:
    a. cranial cavity
    b. abdominal cavity
    c. pelvic cavity
    d. thoracic cavity

12. The basic structure of the body is the:
    a. cell
    b. tissue
    c. skeleton
    d. organ

13. The body system that produces B cells and T cells is the:
    a. nervous
    b. reproductive
    c. lymphatic
    d. integumentary

14. Match the following laboratory tests with the body system they are primarily evaluating.
    _____ Muscular   a. blood urea nitrogen (BUN)
    _____ Respiratory   b. cortisol level
    _____ Urinary   c. monospot
    _____ Lymphatic   d. myoglobin
    _____ Endocrine   e. arterial blood gases

Clinical Situations

1 When blood is collected for each of the following tests on the same patient, what is the primary body system being evaluated?

a. Calcium, phosphorous, and vitamin D
b. HCG, PSA, RPR
c. Serum creatinine and serum osmolarity
d. Western blot

2 What body system are the following laboratory tests evaluating?

a. Fecal sample for ova and parasites
b. KOH preparation
c. Sputum culture
d. Occult blood

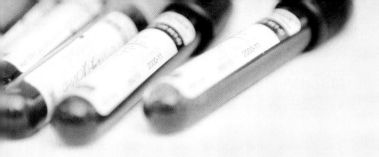

CHAPTER 7

Circulatory System

Learning Objectives

Upon completion of this chapter, the reader will be able to:

1. Briefly describe the functions of the blood vessels, heart, and blood.
2. Differentiate between arteries, veins, and capillaries by structure and function.
3. Locate the femoral, radial, brachial, and ulnar arteries.
4. Locate the basilic, cephalic, median cubital, radial, and saphenous veins.
5. Trace the pathway of blood through the heart and define the function of each chamber.
6. Identify the components of blood.
7. State the major function of red blood cells, white blood cells, and platelets.
8. Briefly explain the coagulation process.
9. Describe the major disorders associated with the circulatory system.
10. State the clinical correlations of laboratory tests associated with the circulatory system.

Key Terms

Arteriole (ar TE re ol)
Artery
Atrium (A tre um)
Capillary (KAP I LAR e)
Cardiovascular
Erythrocyte (e RITH ro sight)
Leukocyte (LOO ko sight)
Lumen (LU men)
Thrombocyte (THROM bo sight)
Vascular (VAS ku lar)
Vein
Vena cava (VE na KA va)
Ventricle (VEN trik l)
Venule (VEN ul)

The circulatory (*cardiovascular*) system consists of the heart, blood vessels, and the blood. Blood is circulated through the blood vessels by the heart to deliver oxygen and nutrients to the cells and transport waste products to the organs that remove them from the body.

BLOOD VESSELS

The three types of blood vessels that transport blood throughout the body are *arteries, veins,* and *capillaries.*

Blood Vessel Structure (Fig. 7-1)

The walls of the arteries and veins consist of three layers.

- Tunica externa: the outer layer composed of connective tissue.
- Tunica media: the middle layer composed of smooth muscle and elastic tissue.
- Tunica intima: the inner layer composed of a lining of epithelial cells.

The space within a blood vessel through which the blood flows is called a *lumen.*

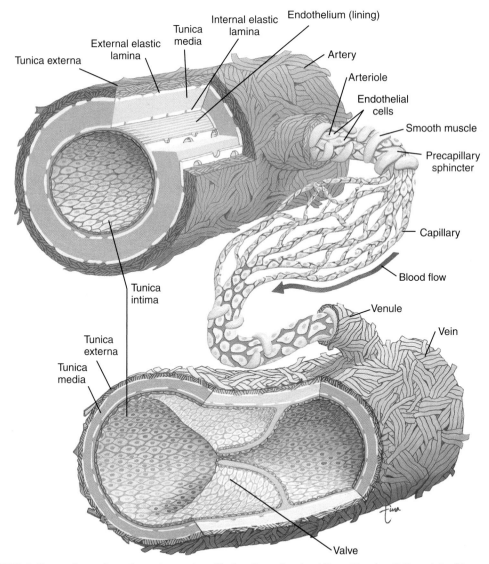

FIGURE 7-1 **Comparison of arteries, veins, and capillaries.** *(From Scanlon, VC, and Sanders, T: Essentials of Anatomy and Physiology, ed. 5. FA Davis, 2007, Philadelphia.)*

Arteries

Arteries are large thick-walled blood vessels that propel oxygen-rich blood away from the heart to the capillaries. Arteries branch into smaller thinner vessels called **arterioles** that connect to capillaries. Notice the increased thickness of the arterial walls versus the venous walls in Figure 7-1. The thicker walls aid in the pumping of blood, maintain normal blood pressure (BP), and give arteries the strength to resist the high pressure caused by the contraction of the heart ventricles. The elastic walls expand as the heart pushes blood through the arteries. Also notice in Figure 7-1 the smooth muscle surrounding the arterioles as they branch off from the artery. This is necessary to maintain the pumping pressure to distribute the blood from the artery through the arterioles to the capillaries.

The major arteries of the body are shown in Figure 7-2. Common arteries encountered in health care are described in Table 7-1.

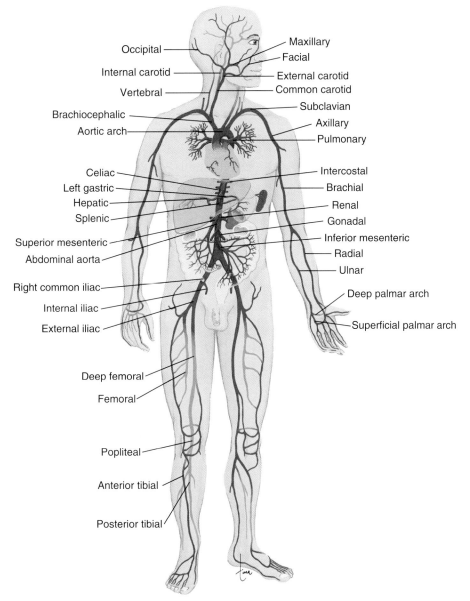

FIGURE 7-2 **The major arteries.** *(From Scanlon, VC, and Sanders, T: Essentials of Anatomy and Physiology, ed. 5. FA Davis, 2007, Philadelphia, with permission.)*

TABLE 7-1 ● Major Arteries Associated with Health Care	
ARTERY	**FUNCTION**
Aorta	The largest artery, branches into smaller arteries to distribute oxygen-rich blood throughout the body
Radial	Located near the thumb side of the wrist, the most common site for obtaining a pulse rate
Carotid	Located near the side of the neck, the most accessible site in an emergency, such as cardiac arrest, to check for a pulse rate
Brachial	Located in the antecubital space of the elbow, the most common site to obtain a BP
Femoral	Located in the groin area, may be used for arterial punctures by specially trained personnel
Pulmonary	The only artery that does not carry oxygenated blood

Veins

Veins have thinner walls than arteries and carry oxygen-poor blood, carbon dioxide, and other waste products back to the heart. No gaseous exchange takes place in the veins, only in the capillaries. The thinner walls of veins have less elastic tissue and less connective tissue than arteries because the BP in the veins is very low. Veins have one-way valves to keep blood flowing in one direction as the blood flows through the veins by skeletal muscle contraction. The leg veins have numerous valves to return the blood to the heart against the force of gravity. Figure 7-3 shows the principal veins of the body.

Most blood tests are performed on venous blood. Venipuncture is the procedure for removing blood from a vein for analysis. The veins of choice for venipuncture are the basilic, cephalic, and median cubital veins located in the antecubital area of the elbow, as shown in Figure 7-4. Common veins encountered in health care that are not associated with venipuncture are described in Table 7-2.

Venules

Venules are small veins that connect capillaries to larger veins.

Capillaries

Capillaries are the smallest blood vessels. They consist of a single layer of epithelial cells to allow exchanges of oxygen, carbon dioxide, nutrients, and waste products between the blood and tissue cells. The blood in capillaries is a mixture of arterial and venous blood.

HEART

The heart is a hollow muscular organ located in the thoracic cavity between the lungs and slightly to the left of the body midline that consists of two pumps to circulate blood throughout the circulatory system. It is enclosed in a membranous sac called the pericardium (Fig. 7-5).

The heart has four chambers and is divided into right and left halves by a partition called the septum. Each side has an upper chamber called an **atrium** to collect blood and a lower chamber called a **ventricle** to pump blood from the heart. The right side is the "pump" for the pulmonary circulation, and the left side is the "pump" for the systemic circulation. The heart contracts and relaxes to pump oxygen-poor blood through the heart to the lungs and return oxygenated blood to the heart for distribution throughout the body. Refer to Figure 7-6 to follow the circulation of blood through the heart.

Valves located at the entrance and exit of each ventricle prevent a backflow of blood and keep it flowing in one direction. Table 7-3 describes the heart valves. They are listed in order of blood flow through the heart as shown in Figures 7-6 and 7-7.

 Technical Tip 7-1. Both veins and ventricles have valves.

 Technical Tip 7-2. Heart sounds created by the opening and closing of the valves are the "lub-dup" sounds heard with a stethoscope. The first sound, the "lub," is the closure of the entrance valves as the ventricles contract. The second sound, the "dup," is the closure of the exit valves.

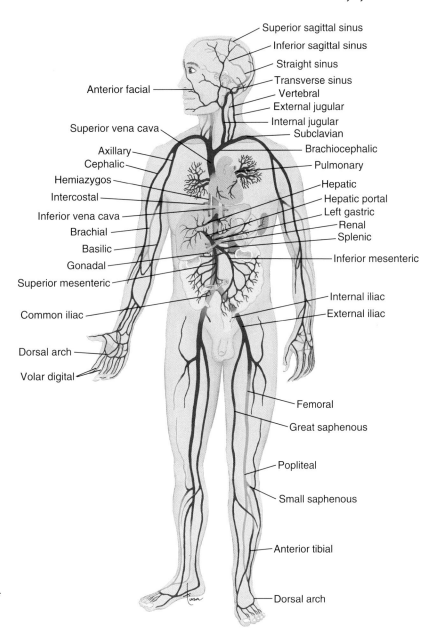

Superior sagittal sinus
Inferior sagittal sinus
Straight sinus
Transverse sinus
Vertebral
External jugular
Internal jugular
Subclavian
Brachiocephalic
Pulmonary
Hepatic
Hepatic portal
Left gastric
Renal
Splenic
Inferior mesenteric
Internal iliac
External iliac
Femoral
Great saphenous
Popliteal
Small saphenous
Anterior tibial
Dorsal arch

Anterior facial
Superior vena cava
Axillary
Cephalic
Hemiazygos
Intercostal
Inferior vena cava
Brachial
Basilic
Gonadal
Superior mesenteric
Common iliac
Dorsal arch
Volar digital

FIGURE 7-3 **The major veins.** *(From Scanlon, VC, and Sanders, T: Essentials of Anatomy and Physiology, ed. 5. FA Davis, 2007, Philadelphia, with permission.)*

 Technical Tip 7-3. A heart murmur is an abnormal heart sound that occurs when the valves close incorrectly.

Pathway of Blood Through the Heart

Two large veins, the superior *vena cava* and the inferior vena cava, transport oxygen-poor blood to the right atrium of the heart. The superior vena cava collects blood from the upper portion of the body, and the inferior vena cava collects blood from the lower portion of the body. The blood passes through the tricuspid valve to the right ventricle. The right ventricle contracts to pump the blood through the pulmonary semilunar valve into the right and left pulmonary arteries that carry it to each lung. In the lung capillaries, blood releases carbon dioxide and acquires oxygen. The right and left pulmonary veins carry the oxygenated blood from the lungs to the left atrium of the heart. The blood flows through the mitral valve into the left ventricle that contracts to pump blood through the aortic semilunar valve into

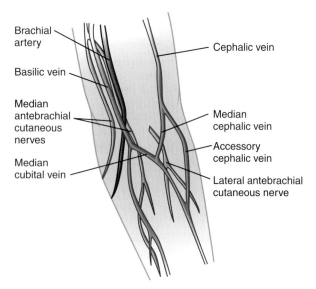

FIGURE 7-4 Veins in the arm used for venipuncture.

TABLE 7-2 • Common Veins Not Associated With Venipuncture	
VEIN	**FUNCTION**
Superior vena cava	Carries oxygen-poor blood from the upper body to the heart
Inferior vena cava	Carries oxygen-poor blood from the lower body to the heart
Great saphenous	The principal vein in the leg and the longest in the body
Pulmonary	The only vein carrying oxygenated blood

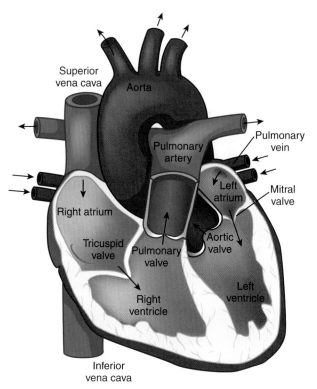

FIGURE 7-6 Chambers of the heart.

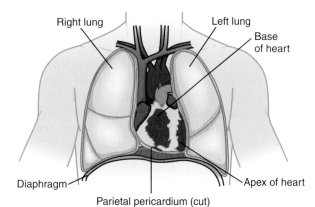

FIGURE 7-5 Body location of the heart.

TABLE 7-3 • Heart Valves Listed in Order of Blood Flow Through the Heart		
NAME	**LOCATION**	**FUNCTION**
Tricuspid	Entrance to the right ventricle	Prevents back-flow into the right atrium
Pulmonary semilunar	Exit of the right ventricle	Allows blood flow into the pulmonary artery
Mitral/ bicuspid	Entrance to the left ventricle	Prevents back-flow into the left atrium
Aortic semilunar	Exit of the left ventricle	Allows blood flow into the aorta

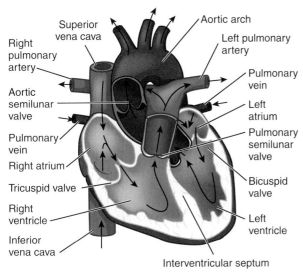

FIGURE 7-7 **Circulation of blood through the heart.**

the aorta. Blood travels throughout the body to the capillaries from arteries that branch off the aorta. Refer to Figures 7-7 and 7-8 to follow the circulation of blood thoughout the heart.

As the major player to circulate nourishment to the body, the heart has its own *vascular* system to sustain it (Fig. 7-9). The right and left coronary arteries are the first blood vessels branching off the aorta. They branch into smaller arteries, arterioles, and capillaries to nourish the heart muscle. The capillaries merge to form venules and then veins to return the blood to the coronary sinus and then back to the right atrium.

▶ *Technical Tip 7-4.* When the coronary arteries become obstructed, heart muscle dies because of lack of oxygen, and a heart attack can occur.

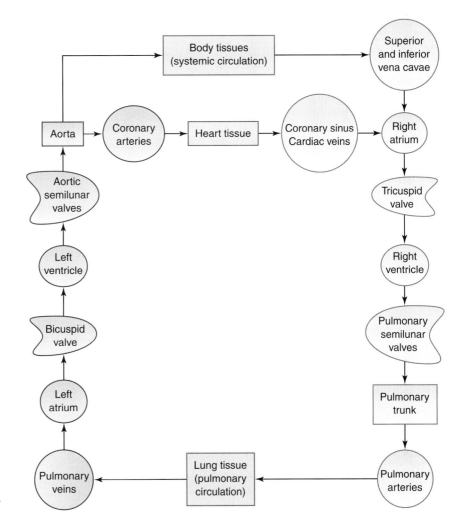

FIGURE 7-8 **Diagram of the pathway of blood through the heart.**

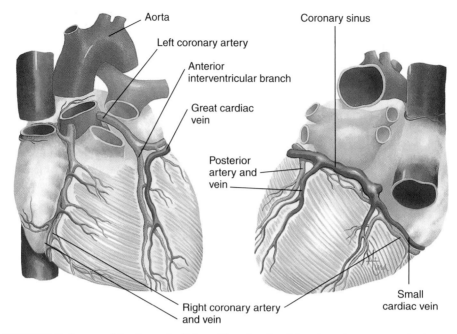

FIGURE 7-9 **Coronary blood vessels.** *(Adapted from Scanlon, VC, and Sanders, T: Essentials of Anatomy and Physiology, ed. 5. FA Davis, 2007, Philadelphia.)*

Cardiac Cycle

The cardiac cycle is the contraction phase (systole) and the relaxation phase (diastole) of the cardiac muscle that occurs in one heartbeat. Cardiac muscle is under involuntary control; therefore, the electrical impulses of the cardiac cycle are essential to produce rhythmic contraction and relaxation of the heart muscle.

The following steps in the cardiac cycle are illustrated in Figure 7-10:

1. The sinoatrial (SA) node, located in the upper right atrium, is the pacemaker of the heart and initiates the heartbeat.
2. The atrioventricular (AV) node located in the lower interatrial septum receives the electrical impulse and both the right and left atria contract forcing blood to the ventricles.
3. The impulse passes to the AV bundle that separates into right and left bundle branches.
4. In the right and left bundle branches the impulse travels to the Purkinje fibers covering the ventricles, causing them to contract, forcing blood into the aorta and pulmonary artery.
5. The cycle starts again.

Electrocardiogram (ECG)

The cardiac cycle is measured with an ECG by placing electrodes connected to a recorder on the patient's arms, legs, and chest. As shown in Figure 7-11, the

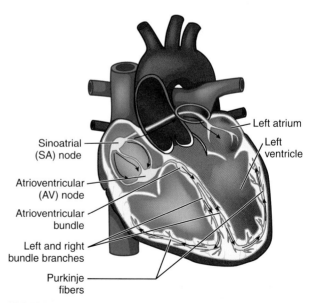

FIGURE 7-10 **Conduction pathway of the heart.**

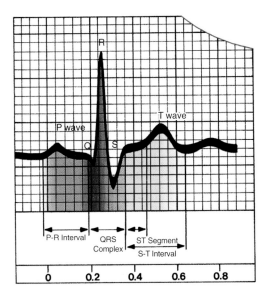

FIGURE 7-11 **Electrocardiogram tracing.** *(From Scanlon, VC, and Sanders, T: Essentials of Anatomy and Physiology, ed. 5. FA Davis, 2007, Philadelphia.)*

ECG measures the total time of one cardiac cycle and the timing of the atrial and ventricular contractions and relaxations.

Heart Rate/Pulse Rate

The heart contracts approximately 60 to 80 times per minute, which represents the heart rate or pulse rate. The arterial pulse is a rhythmic recurring wave that occurs through the arteries during normal pumping action of the heart. The pulse is most easily detected by palpation where an artery crosses over a bone or firm tissue. Common pulse sites are the temporal, carotid, brachial, and radial arteries.

In adults and children older than 3 years, the radial artery is usually the easiest to locate. Two fingers are pressed against the radius just above the wrist on the thumb side (Fig. 7-12). When taking the pulse, the rate (number of beats per minute), the rhythm (pattern of beats or regularity), and strength of the beat are determined. (The normal count is taken for 30 seconds and multiplied by two.) If the patient's pulse is irregular, it should always be counted for a full 60 seconds.

Blood Pressure

BP is the pressure exerted by the blood on the walls of blood vessels during contraction and relaxation of the ventricles. Systolic and diastolic readings

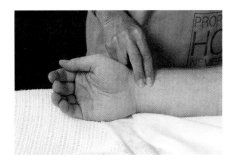

FIGURE 7-12 **Proper placement of fingers along the radial artery.** *(From Wilkinson, JM, and Van Leuven, K: Fundamentals of Nursing, Vol 2. FA Davis, 2008, Philadelphia, with permission.)*

are taken and reported in millimeters of mercury (mm Hg). The systolic pressure is the higher of the two numbers and indicates the BP during contraction of the ventricles. The diastolic pressure is the lower number and is the BP when the ventricles are relaxed.

To measure the BP, a BP cuff called a sphygmomanometer is placed over the upper arm and a stethoscope is placed over the brachial artery to listen for heart sounds (Fig. 7-13). The BP cuff is inflated to restrict the blood flow in the brachial artery and then slowly deflated until loud heart sounds are heard with the stethoscope. The first heart sounds

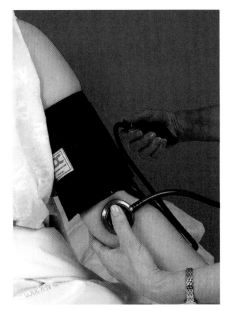

FIGURE 7-13 **Taking a blood pressure from the brachial artery.** *(From Wilkinson, JM, and Van Leuven, K: Fundamentals of Nursing, Vol 2. FA Davis, 2008, Philadelphia, with permission.)*

heard represent the systolic pressure during contraction of the ventricles and is the top number of a BP reading. The cuff continues to be deflated until the sound is no longer heard. This represents the diastolic pressure during the relaxation of the ventricles and is the bottom number of a BP reading. An average BP for an adult is 120/80, representing a systolic pressure of 120 mm Hg and a diastolic pressure of 80 mm Hg.

 Technical Tip 7-5. The pulse rate and blood pressure measure heart function, are considered vital signs, and are routinely tested.

BLOOD

Blood is the body's main fluid for transporting nutrients, waste products, gases, and hormones through the circulatory system. An average adult has a blood volume of 5 to 6 liters. Blood consists of two parts: a liquid portion called plasma, and a cellular portion called the formed elements (Fig. 7-14).

Plasma comprises approximately 55% of the total blood volume. It is a clear, straw-colored fluid that is about 91% water and 9% dissolved substances. It is the transporting medium for the plasma proteins, nutrients, minerals, gases, vitamins, hormones, and blood cells, as well as waste products of metabolism. The formed elements constitute approximately 45% of the total blood volume and include the *erythrocytes* (red blood cells [RBCs]), *leukocytes* (white

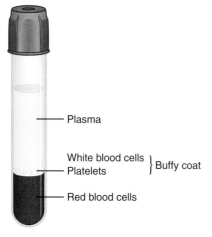

Plasma

White blood cells ⎫
Platelets   ⎬ Buffy coat

Red blood cells

FIGURE 7-14 Tube of centrifuged blood showing plasma and formed elements.

blood cells [WBCs]), and *thrombocytes* (platelets). Blood cells are produced in the bone marrow, which is the spongy material that fills the inside of the major bones of the body. Cells originate from stem cells in the bone marrow, differentiate, and mature through several stages in the bone marrow and lymphatic tissue until they are released to the circulating blood (Fig. 7-15).

 Technical Tip 7-6. Examination of the bone marrow is used to diagnose many blood disorders.

Erythrocytes

Erythrocytes (RBCs) are anuclear biconcave disks that are approximately 7.2 microns in diameter. Erythrocytes contain the protein hemoglobin to transport oxygen and carbon dioxide. Hemoglobin consists of two parts, heme and globin. The heme portion requires iron for its synthesis.

Erythrocytes mature through several stages in the bone marrow and enter the circulating blood as reticulocytes that contain fragments of nuclear material. There are approximately 4.5 to 6.0 million erythrocytes per microliter (µL) of blood, with men having slightly higher values than women. The normal life span for an erythrocyte is 120 days. Macrophages in the liver and spleen remove the old erythrocytes from the bloodstream and destroy them. The iron is reused in new cells.

Blood Group and Type

The surface of erythrocytes contains antigens that determine the blood group and type of an individual, frequently referred to as the person's ABO group and Rh type. As shown in Figure 7-16A, four blood groups exist based on the antigens present on the erythrocyte membrane. Group A blood has the "A" antigen (Ag), and group B blood has the "B" antigen. Group AB blood has both the "A" and "B" antigens, and group O blood has neither the "A" nor the "B" antigens. Groups O and A are the most common, and group AB is the least common.

The plasma of an individual contains naturally occurring antibodies (Abs) for those antigens not present on the erythrocytes. Group A blood has anti-B antibodies in the plasma, and group B blood has anti-A antibodies. Group O blood has both the anti-A and anti-B antibodies, and group AB blood has neither anti-A nor anti-B antibodies. The naturally

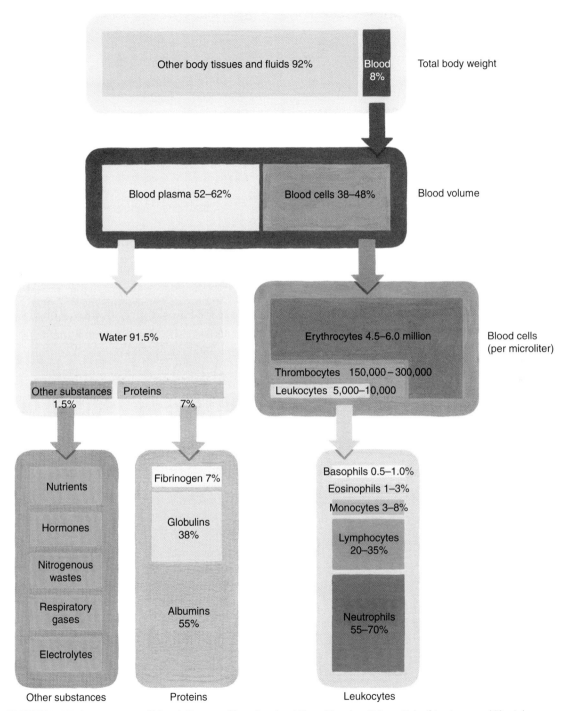

FIGURE 7-15 **Components of blood diagram.** *(From Scanlon, VC, and Sanders, T: Essentials of Anatomy and Physiology, ed. 5. FA Davis, 2007, Philadelphia.)*

A   ABO blood types
B   Typing and cross-matching

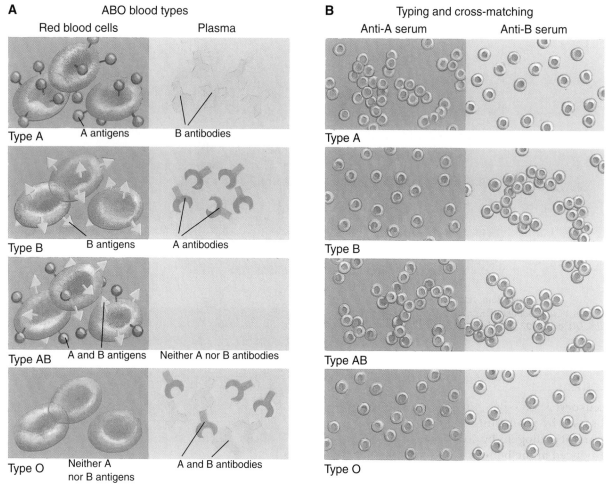

FIGURE 7-16   **ABO blood groups.** *(From Scanlon, VC, and Sanders, T: Essentials of Anatomy and Physiology, ed. 5. FA Davis, 2007, Philadelphia.)*

occurring antibodies react with erythrocytes carrying antigens that are not present on the individual's own erythrocytes (Fig. 7-16B).

A transfusion reaction may occur when a person receives a different group of blood because a person's natural antibodies will destroy the donor RBCs that contain the antigen specific for the antibodies. Patients receive group-specific blood to avoid this type of transfusion reaction (Fig. 7-17).

Rh Type

The presence or absence of the RBC antigen called the Rh factor or D antigen determines whether a person is type Rh-positive or Rh-negative. Rh-negative people do not have natural antibodies to the Rh factor but will form antibodies if they receive Rh-positive blood. A second transfusion of Rh-positive blood will cause a transfusion reaction.

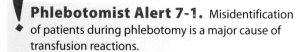

Phlebotomist Alert 7-1. Misidentification of patients during phlebotomy is a major cause of transfusion reactions.

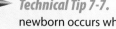

Technical Tip 7-7. Hemolytic disease of the newborn occurs when an incompatibility is present between maternal and fetal blood Rh antigens.

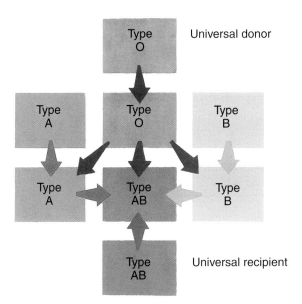

FIGURE 7-17 **Compatibility of ABO blood groups.** *(From Scanlon, VC, and Sanders, T: Essentials of Anatomy and Physiology, ed. 5. FA Davis, 2007, Philadelphia.)*

Leukocytes

Leukocytes, or WBCs, provide immunity to certain diseases by producing antibodies and destroying harmful pathogens by phagocytosis. Leukocytes are produced in the bone marrow from a stem cell and develop in the thymus and bone marrow. They differentiate and mature through several stages before being released into the bloodstream. Leukocytes circulate in the peripheral blood for several hours and then migrate to the tissues through the capillary walls. The normal number of leukocytes for an adult is 4,500 to 11,000 per μL of blood.

Five types of leukocytes are present in the blood, each with a specific function. They are distinguished by their morphology, as shown later. When stained with Wright's stain, the cells are examined microscopically for granules in the cytoplasm, the shape of the nucleus, and the size of the cell. The five normal types of leukocytes are neutrophils, lymphocytes, monocytes, eosinophils, and basophils.

▶ *Technical Tip 7-8.* A differential cell count determines the percentage of each type of leukocyte.

Neutrophils (40% to 60%)

Neutrophils, the most numerous leukocytes, provide protection against infection through phagocytosis. Neutrophils are called segmented or polymorphonuclear cells because the nucleus has several lobes. The number of neutrophils increases in bacterial infections (Fig. 7-18).

Lymphocytes (20% to 40%)

Lymphocytes, the second most numerous leukocytes, provide the body with immune capability by means of B and T lymphocytes. The lymphocyte has a large round purple nucleus with a rim of sky blue cytoplasm. The number of lymphocytes increases in viral infections (Fig. 7-19).

Monocytes (3% to 8%)

Monocytes are the largest circulating leukocytes and act as powerful phagocytes to digest foreign material. The cytoplasm has a fine blue-gray appearance with vacuoles and a large, irregular nucleus. A tissue monocyte is known as a macrophage. The number of monocytes increases in intracellular infections and tuberculosis (Fig. 7-20).

Neutrophil

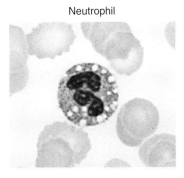

FIGURE 7-18 **Neutrophil.** *(From Harmening, DM: Clinical Hematology and Fundamentals of Hemostasis, ed. 5. FA Davis, 2009, Philadelphia, with permission.)*

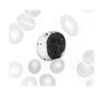

FIGURE 7-19 **Lymphocyte.** *(From Harmening, DM: Clinical Hematology and Fundamentals of Hemostasis, ed. 5. FA Davis, 2009, Philadelphia, with permission.)*

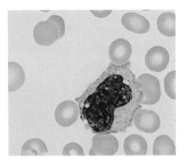

FIGURE 7-20 **Monocyte.** *(From Harmening, DM: Clinical Hematology and Fundamentals of Hemostasis, ed. 5. FA Davis, 2009, Philadelphia, with permission.)*

Eosinophils (1% to 3%)

The granules in cytoplasm of eosinophils stain red-orange, and the nucleus has only two lobes. Eosinophils detoxify foreign proteins and increase in allergies, skin infections, and parasitic infections (Fig. 7-21).

Basophils (0% to 1%)

Basophils are the least common of the leukocytes. The cytoplasm contains large granules that stain purple-black and release histamine in the inflammation process and heparin to prevent abnormal blood clotting (Fig. 7-22).

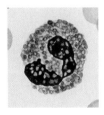

FIGURE 7-21 **Eosinophil.** *(From Harmening, DM: Clinical Hematology and Fundamentals of Hemostasis, ed. 5. FA Davis, 2009, Philadelphia, with permission.)*

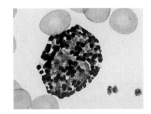

FIGURE 7-22 **Basophil.** *(From Harmening, DM: Clinical Hematology and Fundamentals of Hemostasis, ed. 5. FA Davis, 2009, Philadelphia, with permission.)*

Thrombocytes

Thrombocytes or platelets are small, irregularly shaped disks formed from the cytoplasm of very large cells in the bone marrow called the megakaryocytes. Platelets have a life span of 9 to 12 days. The average number of platelets is between 140,000 and 440,000 per μL of blood. Platelets play a vital role in blood clotting in all stages of the coagulation mechanism (Fig. 7-23).

COAGULATION/HEMOSTASIS

A complex coagulation mechanism that involves blood vessels, platelets, and the coagulation factors maintains hemostasis. Hemostasis is the process of forming a blood clot to stop the leakage of blood when injury to a blood vessel occurs and lysing the clot when the injury has been repaired. A basic understanding of coagulation can be obtained by dividing the process into four stages.

Stage 1

In Stage 1, also called primary hemostasis, blood vessels and platelets respond to an injury to a blood vessel. Blood vessels constrict to slow the flow of blood to the injured area. Platelets become sticky, clump together (platelet aggregation), and adhere to the injured blood vessel wall (platelet adhesion) to form a temporary platelet plug to stop the bleeding (Fig. 7- 24).

 Technical Tip 7-9. The bleeding time test evaluates formation of the platelet plug.

Stage 2

In stage 2, often called secondary hemostasis, the coagulation cascade shown in Figure 7-25 initiates the

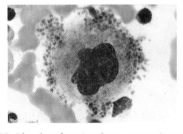

FIGURE 7-23 **Platelets forming from a megakaryocyte.** *(From Harmening, DM. Clinical Hematology and Fundamentals of Hemostasis, ed. 5. FA Davis, 2009, Philadelphia, with permission.)*

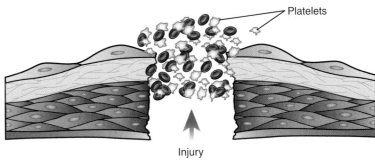

FIGURE 7-24 **Stage 1 of the coagulation cascade.**

1. Primary Coagulation

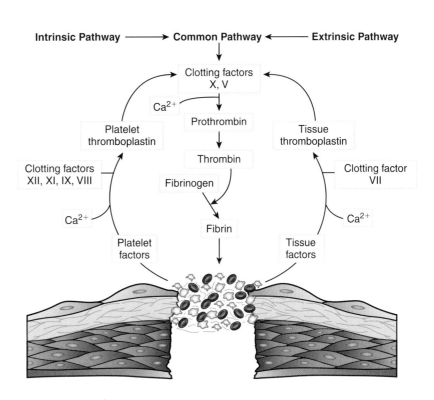

FIGURE 7-25 **Stage 2 of the coagulation cascade.**

2. Coagulation Cascade

formation of fibrin strands to strengthen the platelet plug by forming a fibrin clot. In the coagulation cascade, one factor becomes activated, which activates the next factor in a specific sequence. Notice in Figure 7-25 two pathways, extrinsic and intrinsic come together, called the common pathway, to complete the cascade.

 Technical Tip 7-10. The activated partial thromboplastin time and the activated clotting time tests evaluate the intrinsic pathway and monitor heparin therapy. The prothrombin time test evaluates the extrinsic pathway and monitors warfarin (Coumadin) therapy.

Stage 3

The last factor in the coagulation cascade (Factor XIII) stabilizes the fibrin clot.

This produces retraction (tightening) of the clot (Fig. 7-26).

 Technical Tip 7-11. The thrombin time and the fibrinogen level evaluate this end stage of fibrin clot production.

Stage 4

After the injury to the blood vessel has healed the process of fibrinolysis degrades (breaks down) the fibrin clot into fibrin degradation products (FDPs) (Fig. 7-27).

 Technical Tip 7-12. The measurement of FDPs or D-dimers monitors fibrinolysis.

DISORDERS OF THE CIRCULATORY SYSTEM

Disorders of the circulatory system are shown in Boxes 7-1 through 7-4.

DIAGNOSTIC TESTS

The most frequently ordered diagnostic tests associated with the circulatory system and their clinical correlations are presented in Table 7-4.

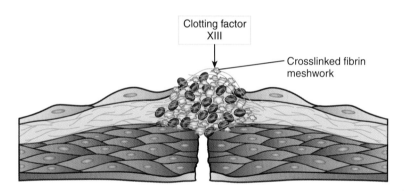

3. Fibrin Stabilizing, and Clot Retraction

FIGURE 7-26 Stage 3 of the coagulation cascade.

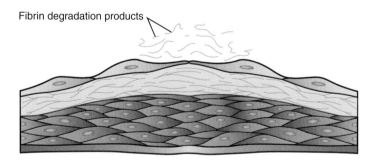

4. Fibrinolysis

FIGURE 7-27 Stage 4 of the coagulation cascade.

BOX 7-1 Disorders of the Blood Vessels

Aneurysm (AN u rizm): A bulge formed by a weakness in the wall of a blood vessel, usually an artery, that can burst and cause severe hemorrhaging.

Arteriosclerosis (ar TE re o skle RO sis): Hardening of the artery walls contributing to aneurysm or stroke.

Atherosclerosis (ATH er O skle RO sis): A form of arteriosclerosis characterized by the accumulation of lipids and other materials in the walls of arteries causing the lumen of the vessel to narrow and stimulate clot formation.

Embolism (EM bo lizm): A moving clot that can obstruct a blood vessel.

Phlebitis (fle BI tis): Inflammation of the vein wall causing pain and tenderness.

Thrombosis (throm BO sis): Obstruction of a blood vessel by a stationary blood clot.

Varicose veins: Swollen peripheral veins caused by damaged valves, allowing backflow of blood that causes swelling (edema) in the tissues.

BOX 7-2 Disorders of the Heart

Angina pectoris (an JI na): Sharp chest pain caused by deceased blood flow to the heart, usually because of an obstruction in the coronary arteries.

Bacterial endocarditis (EN do kar DI tis): Inflammation of the inner lining of the heart caused by a bacterial infection.

Congestive heart failure: Congestive heart failure impairs the ability of the heart to pump blood efficiently, causing fluid accumulation in the lungs and other tissues.

Myocardial infarction (mi o KAR de al): Death (necrosis) of the heart muscle caused by a lack of oxygen to the

myocardium because of an occluded coronary artery, commonly known as a heart attack.

Pericarditis (per I kar DI tis): Inflammation of the membrane surrounding the heart, the pericardium, induced by bacteria, viruses, trauma, or malignancy.

Rheumatic heart disease (roo MAT ik): An autoimmune disorder affecting heart tissue following a streptococcal infection.

BOX 7-3 Disorders of the Blood

Anemia (a NE me a): A decrease in the number of erythrocytes or the amount of hemoglobin in the circulating blood.

Leukemia (loo KE me a): A marked increase in the number of WBCs in the bone marrow and circulating blood; leukemias are named for the particular type of leukocyte that is increased.

Leukocytosis (LOO ko si TO sis): An abnormal increase in the number of normal leukocytes in the circulating blood, as seen in infections.

Leukopenia (LOO ko PE ne a): A decrease below normal values in the number of leukocytes, often caused by exposure to radiation or chemotherapy.

Polycythemia (POL e si THE me a): A consistent increase in the number of erythrocytes and other formed elements causing blood to have a viscous consistency.

Thrombocytopenia (THROM bo SI to PE ne a): A decrease in the number of circulating platelets, frequently seen in patients receiving chemotherapy; spontaneous bleeding can result.

Thrombocytosis (THROM bo si TO sis): An increase in the number of circulating platelets.

BOX 7-4 Disorders of the Coagulation System

Disseminated intravascular coagulation: Spontaneous activation of the coagulation system by certain foreign substances entering the circulatory system.

Hemophilia (HEM o FIL e a): A hereditary disorder characterized by excessive bleeding because of the lack of a coagulation cascade factor.

TABLE 7-4 • Diagnostic Tests Associated With the Circulatory System

TEST	CLINICAL CORRELATION
Activated clotting time (ACT)	Heparin therapy
APTT/PTT	Heparin therapy or coagulation disorders
Antibody (Ab) screen	Blood transfusion
Anti-Xa Heparin Assay	Heparin therapy
Antithrombin III	Coagulation disorders
Apo-A, Apo-B lipoprotein	Cardiac risk
Aspartate aminotransferase (AST)	Cardiac muscle damage
Bilirubin	Hemolytic disorders
Bleeding time (BT)	Platelet function
Blood culture	Microbial infection
Blood group and type	ABO group and Rh factor
Bone marrow aspiration	Blood cell disorders
Brain natriuretic peptide (BNP)	Congestive heart failure
C-reactive protein (CRP)	Inflammatory disorders
Cholesterol	Coronary artery disease
Complete blood count (CBC)	Bleeding disorders, anemia, or leukemia
Creatine kinase (CK)	Myocardial infarction
Creatine kinase isoenzymes (CK-MB)	Myocardial infarction
Direct antihuman globulin test (DAT)	Anemia or hemolytic disease of the newborn
Erythrocyte sedimentation rate (ESR)	Inflammatory disorders
Fibrin degradation products (FDP)	Disseminated intravascular coagulation
Fibrinogen	Coagulation disorders
Hematocrit (Hct)	Anemia
Hemoglobin (Hgb)	Anemia
Hemoglobin (Hgb) electrophoresis	Hemoglobin abnormalities
High-density lipoprotein (HDL)	Coronary risk
Iron	Anemia
Lactic dehydrogenase (LD)	Myocardial infarction
Low-density lipoprotein (LDL)	Coronary risk
Myoglobin	Myocardial infarction
Platelet (plt) count	Bleeding tendencies
Prothrombin time (PT)	Coumadin therapy and coagulation disorders

TABLE 7-4 ● Diagnostic Tests Associated With the Circulatory System—cont'd	
Reticulocyte (retic) count	Bone marrow function
Sickle cell screening	Sickle cell anemia
Total iron binding capacity (TIBC)	Anemia
Triglycerides	Coronary artery disease
Troponin I and T	Myocardial infarction
Type and crossmatch (T & C)	Blood transfusion
Type and screen	Blood transfusion
White blood cell (WBC) count	Infections or leukemia

APTT, Activated partial thromboplastin time; PTT, partial thromboplastin time.

Key Points

✦ The three types of blood vessels that transport blood throughout the body are arteries, veins, and capillaries. The heart circulates blood through the pulmonary and systemic circulations. Blood transports nutrients, waste products, gases, and hormones through the circulatory system.

✦ Arteries are large thick-walled blood vessels that propel oxygen-rich blood away from the heart. Veins are thinner-walled vessels that carry deoxygenated blood back to the heart. Capillaries are the smallest blood vessels (one cell thick) that connect arteries and veins and provide exchanges of gases, nutrients, and waste products between the blood and body cells.

✦ The radial artery (site for taking a pulse) is located on the thumb side of the wrist and the ulnar artery is on the opposite side of the wrist. The brachial artery (site for taking a BP) is located in the antecubital fossa area of the elbow. Carotid arteries in the neck area are another area for obtaining a pulse. The femoral artery is located in the groin area. The pulmonary artery is the only artery to carry deoxygenated blood.

✦ The primary veins used for venipuncture are the median cubital, cephalic, and basilic located in the elbow area of the arm. The longest vein in the body is the saphenous vein located in the leg. The superior and inferior vena cavae carry oxygen-poor blood back to the heart. The pulmonary vein is the only vein to carry oxygenated blood.

✦ Blood from the vena cavae enters the right atrium, flows to the right ventricle to the pulmonary arteries through the lungs to the pulmonary veins to the left atrium then to the left ventricle, and leaves the heart through the aorta. The heart has two circulation systems: the pulmonary and the systemic.

✦ The coronary arteries branch off the aorta to nourish the heart muscle.

✦ The cardiac cycle initiates an impulse from the SA node continuing to the AV node, the AV bundle, the right and left bundle branches, and the Purkinje fibers.

✦ The electrical impulses of the heart are monitored by an ECG.

✦ Blood consists of approximately 55% plasma and 45% formed elements. Plasma contains water and dissolved nutrients and wastes. Formed elements include erythrocytes, leukocytes, and thrombocytes.

✦ Erythrocytes transport oxygen and carbon dioxide attached to hemoglobin throughout the body. The surface of the erythrocytes contains the antigens to determine the ABO group of the blood and the Rh type. Leukocytes consist of neutrophils, lymphocytes, monocytes, eosinophils,

Continued

Key Points—cont'd

and basophils. Leukocytes protect the body from infection. Platelets participate in coagulation by forming platelet plugs at the site of an injury and contributing to the coagulation cascade.

✦ Hemostasis consists of four stages: (1) vasoconstriction and platelet aggregation and adhesion,

(2) coagulation cascade formation of the initial fibrin clot, (3) retraction and tightening of the fibrin clot, and (4) degradation of the fibrin clot.

✦ Review Boxes 7-1 through 7-4 and Table 7-4 for disorders and tests of the circulatory system.

BIBLIOGRAPHY

Scanlon, VC, and Sanders, T: Essentials of Anatomy and Physiology, ed. 5. FA Davis, 2007, Philadelphia.

Tamparo, CD, and Lewis, MA: Diseases of the Human Body, ed. 4. FA Davis, 2005, Philadelphia.

 ## Study Questions

1. The smallest blood vessel is a/an:
   a. arteriole
   b. venule
   c. capillary
   d. vein

2. Valves are found in all of the following **EXCEPT** the:
   a. capillaries
   b. left ventricle
   c. right ventricle
   d. saphenous vein

3. All of the following carry oxygenated blood **EXCEPT** the:
   a. pulmonary vein
   b. aorta
   c. radial artery
   d. pulmonary artery

4. When checking a person's pulse rate, you could use the:
   a. carotid artery
   b. aorta
   c. radial artery
   d. both A and C

5. Deoxygenated blood enters the heart in which chamber?
   a. right atrium
   b. left atrium
   c. right ventricle
   d. left ventricle

6. Blood is pumped into the aorta from the:
   a. right atrium
   b. left atrium
   c. right ventricle
   d. left ventricle

7. The pacemaker of the heart is the:
   a. AV node
   b. AV bundle
   c. Purkinje fibers
   d. SA node

8. A person's blood group is determined by testing:
   a. erythrocytes
   b. leukocytes
   c. plasma
   d. both A and C

Study Questions—cont'd

9. Which stage of coagulation does a blood test for fibrin degradation products evaluate?
   a. Stage 1
   b. Stage 2
   c. Stage 3
   d. Stage 4

10. Match the following leukocytes with their function.
    ____ Basophil   a. increased in allergies
    ____ Neutrophil   b. becomes a macrophage
    ____ Monocyte   c. releases histamine
    ____ Lymphocyte   d. phagocytizes bacteria
    ____ Eosinophil   e. recognizes foreign antigens

11. Match the following disorders with the components of the circulatory system they affect.
    ____ Leukemia   a. blood vessels
    ____ Hemophilia   b. heart
    ____ Aneurysm   c. blood
    ____ Embolism   d. coagulation
    ____ Endocarditis
    ____ Anemia

12. Match the following laboratory tests with the component of the circulatory system that each evaluates.
    ____ Reticulocyte count   a. blood vessels
    ____ Group and type   b. heart
    ____ Bleeding time   c. blood
    ____ Creatine kinase   d. coagulation
    ____ Prothrombin time
    ____ Triglycerides

Clinical Situations

1 John has A antigens on his RBCs.
   a. What antibody (s) will be in his plasma?
   b. With what blood group(s) can he be transfused?
   c. To what blood group(s) can he donate blood?

2 Name two vital signs that might be evaluated on a patient who faints while having blood collected.
   1.
   2.

3 A patient is being evaluated for a bleeding disorder. The physician must determine which stage of the coagulation system is affected. Name a laboratory test that evaluates each stage of the coagulation system.
   Stage 1
   Stage 2
   Stage 3
   Stage 4

Phlebotomy Techniques

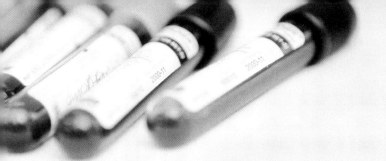

CHAPTER 8

Venipuncture Equipment

Learning Objectives

Upon completion of this chapter, the reader will be able to:

1. Discuss the use of a blood collection tray, transport carriers, and drawing stations.
2. List the items that may be carried on a phlebotomist's tray.
3. Differentiate among the various needle sizes as to gauge, length, and purpose.
4. Describe the OSHA-required safety needles and equipment.
5. Discuss methods to dispose of contaminated needles safely.
6. Differentiate among an evacuated tube system, a syringe, and a winged blood collection set, and state the advantages and disadvantages of each.
7. Identify the types of evacuated tubes by color code, and state the anticoagulants and additives present, any special characteristics, and the purpose of each.
8. State the mechanism of action, advantages, and disadvantages of the anticoagulants EDTA, sodium citrate, potassium oxalate, and heparin.
9. List the correct order of draw when collecting multiple tubes of blood.
10. Describe the purpose and types of tourniquets.
11. Name the substances used to cleanse the skin before venipuncture.
12. Discuss the use of gauze, bandages, gloves, and slides when performing venipuncture.
13. Describe the quality control of venipuncture equipment.
14. Correctly select and assemble venipuncture equipment when presented with a clinical situation.

Key Terms

Acid citrate dextrose (ACD)
Anticoagulant
Antiseptic
Antiglycolytic agent
Bevel
Clot activator
Ethylenediamine-
   tetraacetic acid (EDTA)
Evacuated tube
Gauge
Heparin
Holder
Hub
Hypodermic needle
Lumen
Multisample needle
Plasma separator tube
   (PST)
Polymer barrier gel
Potassium oxalate
Serum separator tubes
   (SST)
Shaft
Sodium citrate
Sodium fluoride
Sodium polyanethol
   sulfonate (SPS)
Winged blood
   collection set

The first step in learning to perform a venipuncture is knowledge of the needed equipment. Considering the many types of blood samples that may be required for laboratory testing and the risks to both patients and health-care personnel associated with blood collection, it is understandable that a considerable amount of equipment is required for the procedure. This chapter covers the latest types of equipment used when performing venipunctures with evacuated tube systems (ETS), syringes, and *winged blood collection sets.* Discussion includes the advantages and disadvantages of the various pieces of equipment, the situations in which they are used, and when appropriate, the mechanisms by which the equipment works.

Equipment necessary to perform venipunctures includes needles, sharps disposal containers, *holders,* evacuated blood collection tubes, syringes, winged blood collection sets, tourniquets, *antiseptic* cleansing solutions, gauze pads, bandages, and gloves. Box 8-1 lists routine venipuncture equipment.

ORGANIZATION OF EQUIPMENT

An important key to successful blood collection is making sure that all the required equipment is conveniently present in the collection area. Maintaining a well-equipped blood collection tray that the phlebotomist carries into the patient's room is the ideal way to prevent unnecessary errors during blood collection. Trays designed to organize and transport collection equipment are available from several manufacturers (Fig. 8-1). The phlebotomy tray provides a convenient way for the phlebotomist to carry equipment to the patients' rooms. Except in isolation situations, the tray is carried into the patient's room. It should be placed on a solid surface, such as a nightstand, and not on the patient's bed, where it could be knocked off. Only the needed equipment should be brought directly to the patient's bed.

 Technical Tip 8-1. A well-organized tray instills patient confidence.

Mobile phlebotomy workstations with swivel caster wheels have replaced the traditional phlebotomy tray in some institutions. With the increased amounts of required equipment necessary for safe phlebotomy, these versatile mobile workstations can be configured to accommodate phlebotomy trays, hazardous waste containers, sharps containers, and storage drawers and shelves. The cart is designed to be wheeled around the hospital and up to the patient's bedside to eliminate placing equipment or a phlebotomy tray on the patient's bed (Fig. 8-2).

In outpatient settings, a more permanent arrangement can be located at the drawing station (Fig. 8-3). A blood drawing chair has an attached or adjacently

---

BOX 8-1 Routine Venipuncture Equipment

Phlebotomy collection tray
Evacuated tube system holders
Syringes
Winged blood collection sets
Needles
Needle disposal sharps containers
Evacuated collection tubes
Transfer devices
Tourniquets
Gloves
70 percent isopropyl alcohol, iodine swabs,
   chlorhexidine gluconate swabs
2 × 2-inch gauze pads
Bandages
Slides
Antimicrobial hand gel
Marking pen

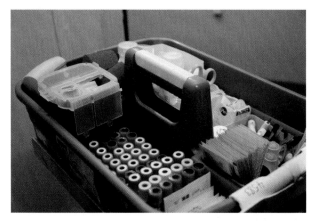

FIGURE 8-1 Phlebotomy collection tray.

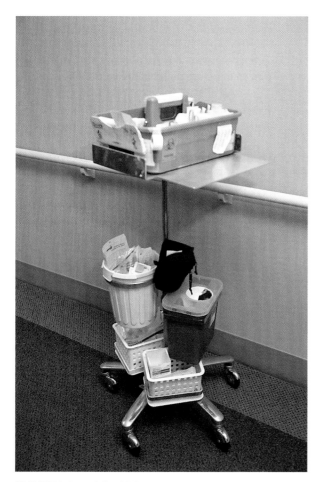

FIGURE 8-2 **Mobile phlebotomy workstation.**

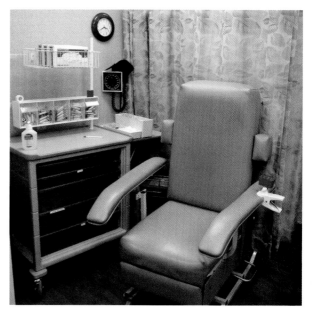

FIGURE 8-3 **Phlebotomy drawing station, including a reclining chair.**

placed stand to hold equipment. Drawing chairs have an armrest that locks in place in front of the patient to provide arm support and protect the patient from falling out of the chair if he or she faints. A reclining chair or bed should be available for special procedures or for patients who feel faint or ill. Infant cradle pads or portable infant phlebotomy stations are available for collection of blood from an infant (Fig. 8-4).

The duties of a phlebotomist include the cleaning, disinfecting, and restocking of the phlebotomy trays, workstations, and outpatient drawing stations. Trays should be totally emptied and disinfected on a weekly basis. Trays also contain equipment for performing the microcollection techniques to be discussed in Chapter 12, arterial puncture equipment discussed in Chapter 14, and point-of-care equipment discussed in Chapter 15.

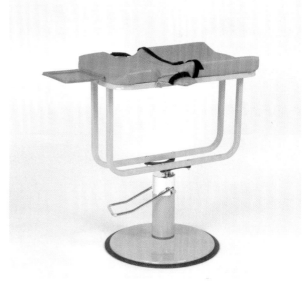

FIGURE 8-4 **Portable infant phlebotomy station.** *(Courtesy of Custom Medtek, Winter Park, FL.)*

EVACUATED TUBE SYSTEM

The evacuated tube system (ETS) (Fig. 8-5) is the most frequently used method for performing venipuncture. Blood is collected directly into the

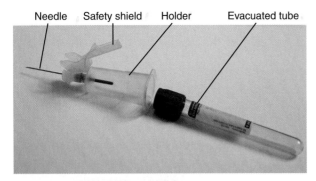

Needle   Safety shield   Holder   Evacuated tube

FIGURE 8-5 Evacuated tube system.

evacuated tube, eliminating the need for transfer of specimens and minimizing the risk of biohazard exposure. The evacuated tube system consists of a double-pointed needle to puncture the stopper of the collection tube, a holder to hold the needle and blood collection tube, and color-coded evacuated tubes.

NEEDLES

Venipuncture needles include **multisample needles,** hypodermic needles, and winged blood collection needles. All needles used in venipuncture are sterile, disposable, and are used only once. Needle size varies by both length and gauge (diameter). For routine venipuncture, 1-inch and 1.5-inch lengths are used.

> **Technical Tip 8-2.** Many phlebotomists believe that using a 1-inch needle gives better control and is less frightening to the patient.

Needle **gauge** refers to the diameter of the needle bore. Needles vary from large (16-gauge) needles used to collect units of blood for transfusion to much smaller (23-gauge) needles used for very small veins. Notice that the smaller the gauge number the bigger the diameter of the needle. Needles with gauges smaller than 23 are available, but they can cause hemolysis when used for drawing blood samples. They are most frequently used for injections and intravenous (IV) infusions.

> **Technical Tip 8-3.** Although a 20-gauge needle will allow blood to flow more quickly into the tube, it is not recommended for routine blood collection. Many patients are on blood thinners and the use of a 20-gauge needle can result in postpuncture bleeding and hematomas because of the larger opening in the vein.

> **Technical Tip 8-4.** Using 25-gauge needles is not recommended because of the longer time the needle is in the vein causing the tube to fill more slowly, the formation of microclots, and increased frequency of hemolysis.

Manufacturers package needles individually in sterile twist-apart sealed shields that are color coded by gauge for easy identification. Needles must not be used if the seal is broken (Fig. 8-6).

As shown in Figure 8-7, needle structure varies to adapt to the type of collection equipment being used. All needles consist of a **bevel** (angled point), **shaft, lumen,** and **hub.** Needles should be visually examined before use to determine if any structural defects, such as nonbeveled points or bent shafts, are present. Defective needles should not be used. Needles should never be recapped once the shield is removed regardless of whether they have or have not been used.

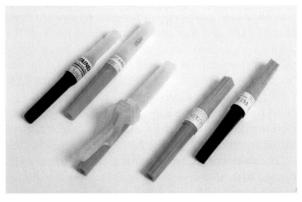

FIGURE 8-6 Multisample needles with color-coded caps, both traditional and BD Eclipse safety needle with the safety shield attached, Greiner Bio-One black 22 gauge, green 21 gauge.

[handwritten annotation: × Never ever recap a needle]

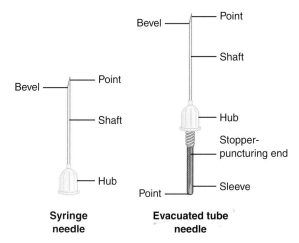

FIGURE 8-7 **Needle structure.**

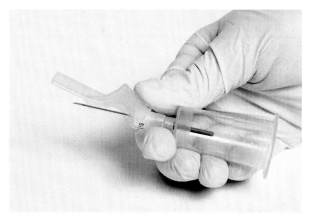

FIGURE 8-8 **Eclipse blood collection needle.**

Evacuated tube system needles are threaded in the middle and have a beveled point at each end designed so that one end is for venipuncture and the other end punctures the rubber stopper of the evacuated blood collection tube. Evacuated tube system needles are designated as multisample needles. Multisample needles have the stopper puncturing needle covered by a rubber sheath that is pushed back when a tube is attached and returns to full needle coverage when the tube is removed. This prevents leakage of blood when tubes are being changed.

 Safety Tip 8-1. The Needlestick Prevention and Safety Act mandates the evaluation and use of safety needle devices. State mandates also have been issued.

Various safety shields and blunting devices are available from different manufacturers. The BD Vacutainer Eclipse blood collection needle (Becton, Dickinson, Franklin Lakes, NJ) uses a shield that the phlebotomist locks over the needle tip after completion of the venipuncture (Fig. 8-8).

Self-blunting needles (PUNCTUR-GUARD, Gaven Medical LLC, Vernon, CT) are available to provide additional protection against needlestick injuries by making the needles blunt before removal from the patient. A hollow, blunt inner needle is contained inside the standard needle. Before removing the needle from the patient's vein, an additional push on the final tube in the holder advances the internal blunt cannula past the sharp tip of the outer needle. The blunt cannula is hollow, allowing blood to continue to flow into the tube (Fig. 8-9).

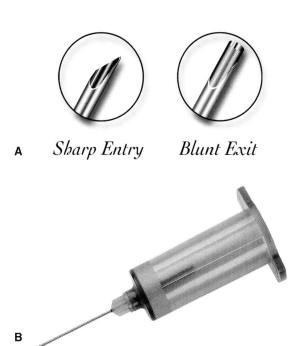

FIGURE 8-9 **A, Blunting needle principle. B, Puncture-Guard Self-blunting needle.** *(Courtesy of Gaven Medical LLC, Vernon, CT.)*

NEEDLE HOLDERS

Needles used in the evacuated tube collection systems attach to a holder that holds the collection tube. Holders are made of rigid plastic and may be designed to act as a safety shield for the used needle. Complete units are available that include the holder and a sterile preattached multisample needle with safety shield. Various types of holders are shown in Figure 8-10. As discussed in Chapter 4, the Occupational Safety and Health Administration (OSHA) directs that holders must be discarded with the used needle.

The One-Use Holder by Becton, Dickinson is available with a different threading to allow a needle to be threaded into the holder only one time (Fig. 8-11). The entire needle/holder assembly is discarded in a sharps container after use.

Another type of holder that includes the safety device is the Venipuncture Needle-Pro (Smith Medical, Weston, MA) that consists of a plastic sheath attached by a hinge to the end of the evacuated tube holder. The shield hangs free during the venipuncture and is engaged over the needle using a single-handed technique against a flat surface after the puncture is performed. The plastic shield can be rotated to provide the phlebotomist a better view of the venipuncture site and needle placement. The entire device is discarded in the sharps container (Fig. 8-12A).

Holders that retract the needle include The ProGuard II and the VanishPoint tube holder. The ProGuard II safety needle holder (Coviden, Mansfield, MA) uses

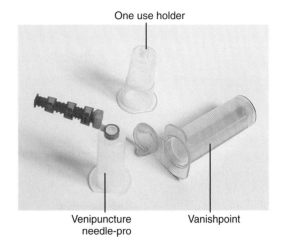

One use holder

Venipuncture needle-pro   Vanishpoint

FIGURE 8-11 **One-Use Holder (Becton Dickinson), Venipuncture Needle-Pro (Smith Medical) and VanishPoint (Retractible Technologies) holders.**

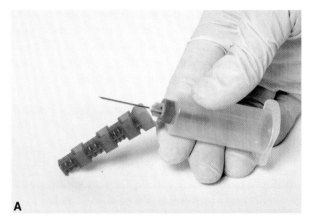

A

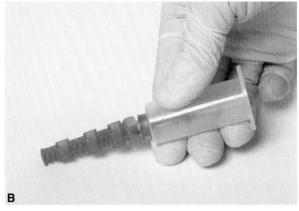

B

FIGURE 8-12 **A, Venipuncture Needle-Pro Holder with safety shield. B, Venipuncture Needle-Pro with safety shield activated.**

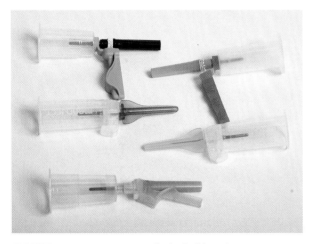

FIGURE 8-10 **Various types of tube holders.** *(Vacuette, Venipuncture Needle Pro, Monoject, and Becton Dickinson.)*

a one-handed method to retract the needle into the holder and a cover for the end that is open to the stopper- puncturing needle. The VanishPoint tube holder (Retractible Technologies, Little Elm, TX) automatically retracts the needle by securely closing the end cap while the needle is still in the patient's vein (Fig. 8-13A).

The VACUETTE QuickShield Safety Tube Holder comes with a protective cap and is designed to use with Vacuette multisample needles. The VACUETTE Quickshield Complete style includes both the holder and a sterile preattached needle. After completion of blood collection, the needle is removed from the patient's vein and the protective cap is pressed over the needle against a hard surface using a one-handed technique. The VACUETTE QuickShield Complete Plus system includes a holder and Vacuette Visio Plus

multisample needle. In this combination, a "flash" is observed that confirms penetration of the vein.

The BD Vacutainer Passive Shielding Blood Collection Needle (Becton, Dickinson) and the VACUETTE Premium Safety Needle System (Greiner Bio-One) are the new generation of safety devices. The systems include a preassembled multisample needle with safety device and holder. In both systems, the insertion of the first tube into the holder releases the safety shield, which then rests against the patient's skin. As the needle is removed from the vein after blood collection, a spring in the holder causes the safety shield to automatically move forward to cover the needle. An advantage to these systems is that the needle is immediately covered when the needle moves out of the vein due to an unexpected move by the patient. The BD Vacutainer Passive Shielding Blood Collection Needle (Fig. 8-14) has a safety shield indicator arrow that judges the depth of needle insertion. The holders have a flat side to lay against the skin for shallow angle of needle entry.

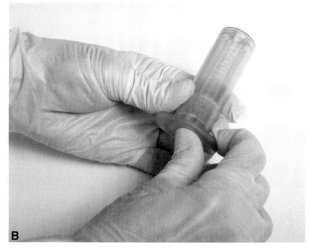

FIGURE 8-13 VanishPoint Tube Holder. A, Tube in holder. B, Tube removed, needle retracted and sealed.

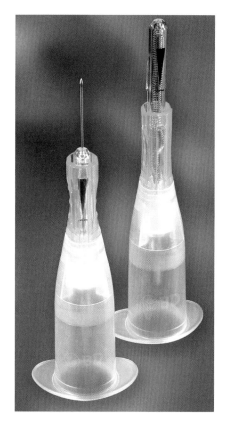

FIGURE 8-14 BD Vacutainer Passive Shielding Blood Collection Needle. *(Courtesy of Becton, Dickinson and Company.)*

Holders are available to accommodate collection tubes of different sizes. To provide proper puncturing of the rubber stopper and maximum control, tubes should fit securely in the holder. Ribbed pediatric holder inserts can be inserted into the regular size holder for pediatric tubes.

The rubber-sheathed puncturing end of an evacuated tube system needle screws securely into the small opening at one end of the holder, and the evacuated blood collection tube is placed into the large opening at the opposite end of the holder. The first tube can be partially advanced onto the stopper-puncturing needle in the holder. A marking near the top of the holder indicates the distance an evacuated tube may be advanced into the stopper-puncturing needle without entering the tube and losing the vacuum (Fig. 8-15). The tube is fully advanced to the end of the holder when the needle is in the vein. Blood will flow into the tube once the needle penetrates the stopper. The flared ends of the needle holder aid the phlebotomist during the changing of tubes in multiple-sample situations. Tubes are removed with a slight twist to help disengage them from the needle.

Safety Tip 8-2. If the evacuated tube needle does not have a safety device, the tube holder must have one.

Technical Tip 8-5. Loss of tube vacuum is a primary cause of failure to obtain blood. The venipuncture can be performed before placing the tube on the needle. Practice both methods, and choose the one with which you are most comfortable.

NEEDLE DISPOSAL SYSTEMS

To protect phlebotomists from accidental needlesticks by contaminated needles, a means of safe disposal must be available whenever phlebotomy is performed. In recent years, because of the increased concern over exposure to bloodborne pathogens and mandates by the OSHA, many disposal systems have been developed.

Needles with safety devices activated must always be placed in rigid, puncture-resistant, leak-proof disposable "sharps" containers labeled BIOHAZARD that are easily sealed and locked when full. Syringes with the needles attached, winged blood collection sets, and

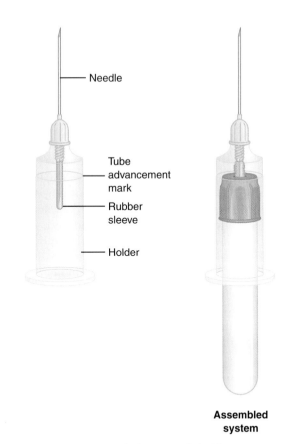

Assembled system

FIGURE 8-15 Diagram of a basic needle holder.

holders with needles attached are disposed of directly into puncture-resistant containers (Fig. 8-16). *Under no circumstances should a needle be recapped.*

Safety Tip 8-3. Sharps containers should be filled only to the designated mark and never overfilled.

Safety Tip 8-4. To prevent accidental punctures from contaminated needles, become thoroughly familiar with the operation of your needle safety system before performing blood collection.

COLLECTION TUBES

Tubes used for blood collection are called *evacuated tubes* because they contain a premeasured amount of vacuum. The collection tubes used with the evacuated

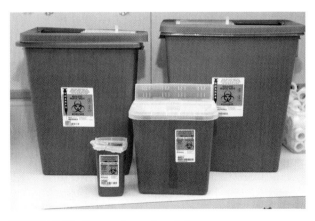

FIGURE 8-16 **Sharps disposal containers.**

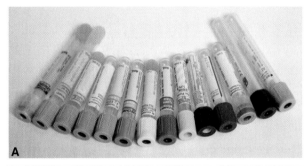

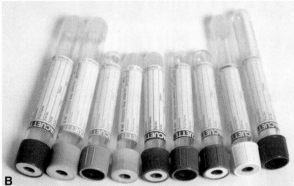

FIGURE 8-17 **Examples of evacuated tubes. A, BD Vacutainer tubes (Becton, Dickinson, Franklin Lakes, NJ). B, Vacuette evacuated tubes (Greiner Bio-One, Monroe, NC).**

tube system are often referred to as Vacutainers (Becton, Dickinson, Franklin Lakes, NJ), although they are also available from other manufacturers. Use of evacuated tubes with their corresponding needles and holders provides a means of collecting blood directly into the tube. Laboratory instrumentation is also available for direct sampling from the evacuated tubes, providing additional protection for laboratory workers.

The amount of blood collected in an evacuated tube ranges from 1.8 to 15 mL and is determined by the size of the tube and the amount of vacuum present. As shown in Figure 8-17, a wide variety of sizes is available to accommodate adult, pediatric, and geriatric patients. When selecting the appropriate size tube, the phlebotomist must consider the amount of blood needed, the age of the patient, and the size and condition of the patient's veins. Using a 23-gauge needle with a large evacuated tube can produce hemolysis, because red blood cells are damaged when the large amount of vacuum causes them to be rapidly pulled through the small lumen of the needle. Therefore, if it is necessary to use a small-gauge needle, the phlebotomist should collect two small tubes instead of one large tube.

Evacuated tubes are available in glass and plastic.

> ▌ **Safety Tip 8-5.** For safety reasons glass tubes
> ▲ are less routinely used.

Tubes are sterile and many are silicone coated to prevent cells from adhering to the tube, or to prevent the activation of clotting factors in coagulation studies. Information about the characteristics of a tube is

contained on the write-on label attached to the tube and should be verified by the phlebotomist when special collection procedures are needed. Tubes may also contain *anticoagulants* and additives. The tubes are labeled with the type of anticoagulant or additive, the draw volume, and the expiration date. The manufacturer guarantees the integrity of the anticoagulant and vacuum in the tube until the expiration date (Fig. 8-18).

As shown in Figure 8-19, evacuated tubes have thick rubber stoppers with a thinner central area to allow puncture by the needle. To aid the phlebotomist in identifying the many types of evacuated tubes, the stoppers are color-coded. Color coding for

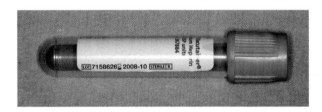

FIGURE 8-18 **Collection tube label.**

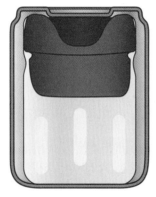

FIGURE 8-19 Cut-away view of a vacuum tube stopper (Hemogard closure). *(Adapted from product literature, Becton, Dickinson, Franklin Lakes, NJ.)*

routinely used tubes is generally universal; however, it may vary slightly by manufacturers, and instructions for sample collection usually refer to the tube color. This reference to tube color is found on most computer-generated forms (Example 8-1). Each laboratory department has specified sample requirements for the analysis of particular blood constituents. Phlebotomists and phlebotomy students should also understand that testing methodologies and types of instrumentation vary among laboratories. Therefore, the type of tube collected for a particular test may not be the same in all facilities. Direct sampling instrumentation may also be designed to only accept a specific type of tube, such as a rubber stopper and not a Hemogard closure or vice versa.

EXAMPLE 8-1

Draw one red top, one light blue top, and one lavender top tube.

Two types of color-coded tops are available. Rubber stoppers may be colored, or a color-coded plastic shield may cover the stopper, as with the Hemogard Vacutainer System. Many instruments in the laboratory are designed to identify a blood tube by its barcoded label and will directly pierce the stopper to aspirate blood into the instrument for testing.

❗ Safety Tip 8-6. Removing the rubber stoppers from evacuated tubes can be hazardous to laboratory personnel because an aerosol of blood can be produced if the stopper is quickly "popped off." Stoppers should be covered with a gauze pad and slowly loosened with the opening facing away from the body.

Hemogard closures provide additional protection against blood splatter by allowing the stoppers to be easily twisted and pulled off and have a shield over the stopper. The plastic shield protects the phlebotomist from blood that remains on the stopper after the tubes are removed from the needle. The color of the Hemogard closures varies slightly from that of rubber stoppers. Refer to the front and back inside covers of this book for two manufacturer's tube guides. Evacuated tubes fill automatically because a premeasured vacuum is present in the tube. This causes some tubes to fill almost to the top, whereas other tubes only partially fill. BD partial-fill tubes are distinguished from regular-fill tubes by translucent colored Hemogard closures in the same color as regular-fill tubes. When a tube has lost its vacuum, it cannot fill to the correct level. Loss of vacuum can be caused by dropping the tube, opening the tube, improper storage, manufacturer error, using the tube past its expiration date, prematurely advancing the tube onto the stopper-puncturing needle in the holder, or pulling the needle bevel out of the skin during venipuncture.

Principles and Use of Color-Coded Tubes

Color coding indicates the type of sample that will be obtained when a particular tube is used. As discussed in Chapter 2, tests may be run on plasma, serum, or whole blood. Tests may also require the presence of preservatives, inhibitors, ***clot activators,*** or barrier gels. To produce these necessary conditions, some tubes contain anticoagulants or additives, and others do not. Phlebotomists must be able to relate the color of the collection tubes to the types of samples needed and to any special techniques, such as tube inversion, that may be required. This section discusses the routinely used tubes with regard to anticoagulants, additives, types of tests for which they are used, and special handling required.

Tests requiring whole blood or plasma are collected in tubes containing an anticoagulant to prevent clotting of the sample. Anticoagulants prevent clotting by binding calcium or inhibiting thrombin in the coagulation cascade (Fig. 8-20). ***Ethylenediaminetetraacetic acid (EDTA)***, citrates, and oxalates are the most common anticoagulants that work by binding calcium. ***Heparin*** prevents clotting by inhibiting the formation of thrombin necessary to convert fibrinogen to fibrin

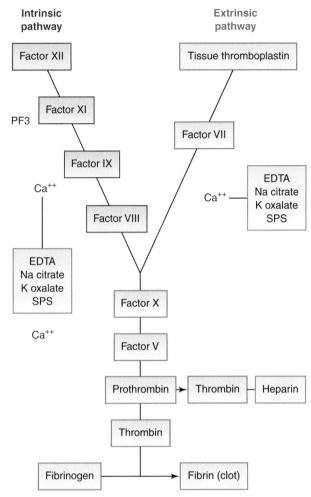

Intrinsic pathway

Extrinsic pathway

FIGURE 8-20 **The role of anticoagulants in the coagulation cascade.** *(Ca⁺⁺ = calcium; PF3 = platelet factor 3.)*

in the coagulation process. All tubes containing an anticoagulant must be gently inverted three to eight times immediately after collection to mix the contents and to avoid microclot formation.

 Technical Tip 8-6. Observing an air bubble moving through the tube from top to bottom during inversion ensures proper mixing.

Before use, tubes with powdered anticoagulant should be gently tapped to loosen the powder from the tube for better mixing with the blood. Tubes containing an anticoagulant must be filled to the designated volume draw to ensure the correct

blood-to-anticoagulant ratio and accurate test results. If a short draw is anticipated, a partial collection tube should be used. Tubes containing additives also must be gently mixed to ensure effectiveness. Blood collected in a tube containing an anticoagulant or additive cannot be transferred into a tube containing a different anticoagulant or additive.

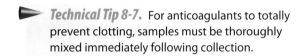 *Technical Tip 8-7.* For anticoagulants to totally prevent clotting, samples must be thoroughly mixed immediately following collection.

Technical Tip 8-8. Shaking an anticoagulated tube rather than gently inverting the tube may cause hemolysis and sample rejection.

Lavender (Purple) Top

Lavender stopper tubes and Hemogard closures contain the anticoagulant ethylenediaminetetraacetic acid (EDTA) in the form of liquid tripotassium or spray-coated dipotassium ethylenediaminetetraacetic acid (K_3EDTA or K_2EDTA). Coagulation is prevented by the binding of calcium in the sample to sites on the large EDTA molecule, thereby preventing the participation of the calcium in the coagulation cascade (see Fig. 8-20). Lavender stopper tubes should be gently inverted eight times.

For hematology procedures that require whole blood, such as the complete blood count (CBC), K_2EDTA is the anticoagulant of choice because it maintains cellular integrity better than other anticoagulants, inhibits platelet clumping, and does not interfere with routine staining procedures.

 Preexamination Consideration 8-1.

The Clinical and Laboratory Standards Institute (CLSI) recommends spray-coated K_2EDTA for hematology tests because liquid K_3 EDTA dilutes the sample and can result in lower results.

K_2EDTA tubes are also used for immunohematology testing and blood donor screening. The lavender stopper tube should be completely filled to avoid excess EDTA that may shrink the red blood cells and decrease the hematocrit level, red blood cell indices, and erythrocyte sedimentation rate (ESR) results.

Lavender stopper tubes cannot be used for coagulation studies because EDTA interferes with factor V and the thrombin-fibrinogen reaction.

Pink Top

Pink stopper tubes and Hemogard closure tubes also contain a spray-coated K_2EDTA anticoagulant and are used specifically for blood bank in some facilities.

Preexamination Consideration 8-2.

Using a designated tube for blood bank is believed to help prevent testing of samples from the wrong patient.

The tubes are designed with special labels for patient information required by the American Association of Blood Banks (AABB). Tubes should be inverted eight times.

White Top

White Hemogard closure tubes containing a spray-coated K_2EDTA anticoagulant and a separation gel are called plasma preparation tubes (PPTs). This differentiates them from *plasma separator tubes* that contain heparin as the anticoagulant. White Hemogard closure tubes are primarily used for molecular diagnostics but can be used for myocardial infarction (MI) panels and ammonia levels, depending on the test methodology and instrumentation. Tubes should be inverted eight times. Greiner Bio-One EDTA gel tubes have purple plastic stoppers with yellow tops.

Light Blue Top

Light blue stopper tubes and Hemogard closures contain the anticoagulant **sodium citrate,** which also prevents coagulation by binding calcium. Centrifugation of the anticoagulated light blue stopper tubes provides the plasma used for coagulation tests. Sodium citrate (3.2% or 3.8%) is the required anticoagulant for coagulation studies because it preserves the labile coagulation factors. Tubes should be inverted three to four times. The ratio of blood to the liquid sodium citrate is critical and should be 9 to 1 (e.g., 4.5 mL blood and 0.5 mL sodium citrate). Therefore, light blue stopper tubes must be completely filled to ensure accurate results.

When collecting coagulation tests on patients with polycythemia or hematocrit readings greater than 55 percent, the amount of citrate anticoagulant should be decreased to prevent an increased amount of citrate in the plasma. The increased citrate in the sample will interfere with the coagulation tests. The Clinical and Laboratory Standards Institute (CLSI) recommends the use of tubes containing 3.2 percent sodium citrate to prevent this problem. If necessary, tubes can also be specially prepared as described in the CLSI guideline.

The glass CTAD tube with a light blue Hemogard closure is designed for specialized platelet testing of citrated plasma and contains a solution of sodium citrate, theophylline, adenosine, and dipyridamole. The purpose of this tube is to minimize in vitro platelet activation and the artificial entry of platelet factors into the plasma. Greiner Bio-One CTAD tubes have blue stoppers with yellow tops.

A special blue stopper tube containing thrombin and a soybean trypsin inhibitor is used when drawing blood and providing serum for determinations of certain fibrin degradation products.

Technical Tip 8-9. The laboratory always rejects incompletely filled light blue stopper tubes.

Technical Tip 8-10. Overmixing a light blue stopper tube can activate platelets and cause erroneous coagulation test results.

Black Top

Black stopper tubes containing buffered sodium citrate are used for Westergren sedimentation rates. They differ from light blue top tubes in that they provide a ratio of blood to liquid anticoagulant of 4 to 1. Specially designed tubes for Westergren sedimentation rates are available.

Green Top

Green stopper tubes and Hemogard closures contain the anticoagulant heparin combined with sodium, lithium, or ammonium ion. Heparin prevents clotting by inhibiting thrombin in the coagulation cascade (see Fig. 8-20). Green stopper tubes are primarily used for chemistry tests performed on whole blood or plasma, particularly stat tests or tests that require a fast turn around time (TAT). Interference by sodium and lithium heparin with their corresponding chemical tests and by ammonium heparin in blood urea nitrogen (BUN) determinations must be avoided. In general, lithium heparin has been shown to produce the least interference. Tubes should be inverted eight times. Green stopper tubes are not used for hematology because heparin interferes with the Wright's stained blood smear. Heparin causes the stain to have a blue background on the blood smear, making it difficult to interpret the differential cell identification.

Light Green Top

Light green Hemogard closure tubes and green/black stopper tubes containing lithium heparin and a separation gel are called plasma separator tubes (PSTs). PSTs are used for plasma determinations in chemistry. They are well suited for potassium determinations because heparin prevents the release of potassium by platelets during clotting, and the gel prevents contamination by red blood cell potassium. Tubes should be inverted eight times. Greiner Bio-One heparin gel tubes have green plastic stoppers with yellow tops.

 Technical Tip 8-11. Tubes containing a gel barrier may be referred to as PST and SST tubes or as gel barrier tubes depending on the manufacturer.

Gray Top

Gray stopper tubes and Hemogard closures are available with a variety of anticoagulants and additives for the primary purpose of preserving glucose. All gray stopper tubes contain the glucose preservative (*antiglycolytic agent*) *sodium fluoride*. Sodium fluoride maintains glucose stability for 3 days. Sodium fluoride is not an anticoagulant; therefore, if plasma is needed for analysis, an anticoagulant must also be present and the tubes must be inverted eight times. In gray stopper tubes the anticoagulant is *potassium oxalate* or Na_2EDTA, which prevents clotting by binding calcium. Gray tubes with only sodium fluoride for serum testing are available.

 Preexamination Consideration 8-3.
When monitoring patient glucose levels, tubes for the collection of plasma and serum should not be interchanged.

Sodium fluoride will interfere with some enzyme analyses; therefore, gray stopper tubes should not be used for other chemistry analyses. Gray stopper tubes

are not used in hematology because oxalate distorts cellular morphology.

Blood alcohol levels are drawn in gray stopper tubes containing sodium fluoride to inhibit microbial growth, which could produce alcohol as a metabolic end product. Tubes with or without potassium oxalate can be used, depending on the need for plasma or serum in the test procedure.

Royal Blue Top

Royal blue Hemogard closure tubes are used for toxicology, trace metal, and nutritional analyses. Because many of the elements analyzed in these studies are significant at very low levels, the tubes must be chemically clean and the rubber stoppers are specially formulated to contain the lowest possible levels of metal. Royal blue stopper tubes are available with a spray-coated silica clot activator for serum or with K_2EDTA or sodium heparin (Greiner Bio-One) for plasma to conform to a variety of testing requirements. Tubes with an anticoagulant present must be inverted eight times.

Tan Top

Tan Hemogard closure tubes are available for lead determinations. They are certified to contain less than 0.1 µg/mL of lead. The tubes contain the anticoagulant K_2EDTA and must be inverted eight times.

Yellow Top

Yellow stopper tubes are available for two different purposes and contain different additives. Yellow stopper tubes containing the red blood cell preservative *acid citrate dextrose (ACD)* are used for cellular studies in blood bank, human leukocyte antigen (HLA) phenotyping, and DNA and paternity testing. The acid citrate prevents clotting by binding calcium and dextrose preserves the red blood cells.

Sterile yellow stopper tubes containing the anticoagulant *sodium polyanethol sulfonate (SPS)* are used to collect samples to be cultured for the presence of microorganisms. SPS also prevents coagulation by binding calcium (Fig. 8-20). SPS aids in the recovery of microorganisms by inhibiting the actions of complement, phagocytes, and certain antibiotics. Yellow stopper tubes should be inverted eight times.

Light Blue/Black Top

Light blue/black rubber stopper glass tubes contain the anticoagulant sodium citrate and a polyester gel and a density gradient liquid and are called cell preparation tubes (CPTs). CPTs are specialty single tube systems used for whole blood molecular diagnostic testing so that mononuclear cells can be separated from whole blood and transported without removing them from the tube. The mononuclear cells and platelets are separated from the granulocytes and red bloods cells by the polyester gel and dense gradient liquid when centrifuged. The tube should be inverted eight times (Fig. 8-21).

Red/Green Top

Red/green rubber stopper glass tubes contain the anticoagulant sodium heparin and a polyester gel and density gradient liquid and are also CPTs. This tube is used for whole blood molecular diagnostic testing when the testing methodology requires heparinized blood. The tube is mixed by inverting eight times.

Yellow/Gray and Orange Top

Yellow/gray stopper tubes and orange Hemogard closures are found on tubes containing the clot activator thrombin. Notice in Figure 8-20 that thrombin is generated near the end of the coagulation cascade; addition of thrombin to the tube results in faster clot formation, usually within 5 minutes. Tubes should be inverted eight times. Tubes containing thrombin are used for stat serum chemistry determinations and on samples from patients receiving anticoagulant therapy.

Orange Top

Orange stopper tubes containing a thrombin-based medical clotting agent and separation gel are called rapid serum tubes (RST) (Becton, Dickinson). RST

tubes clot within 5 minutes and are centrifuged for 10 minutes at a high speed yielding serum in a short period of time, which is ideal for stat serum chemistry testing. Tubes should be inverted five times.

Red/Gray and Gold Top

Red/gray stopper tubes and gold Hemogard closures are found on tubes containing a clot activator and a separation gel. They are frequently referred to as ***serum separator tubes (SSTs)*** (Becton, Dickinson). The tubes are spray coated with the clot activator silica to increase platelet activation, thereby shortening the time required for clot formation. Tubes should be inverted five times to expose the blood to the clot activator. A ***polymer barrier gel*** that undergoes a temporary change in viscosity during centrifugation is located at the bottom of the tube. As shown in Figure 8-22, when the tube is centrifuged, the gel forms a barrier between the cells and serum to prevent contamination of the serum with cellular materials. To produce a solid separation barrier, samples must be allowed to clot completely before centrifuging. Clotting time is approximately 30 minutes. Samples should be centrifuged as soon as clot formation is complete. Greiner Bio-One serum gel tubes have red plastic stoppers with yellow tops.

 Preexamination Consideration 8-4.
Centrifugation of incompletely clotted SSTs can produce a nonintact gel barrier and possible cellular contamination of the serum.

 Technical Tip 8-12. Fibrin fibers in the serum of incompletely clotted centrifuged SSTs may cause blockages in the tubing of analyzers.

SSTs are used for most chemistry tests and prevent contamination of the serum by cellular chemicals and products of cellular metabolism. They are not suitable for use in the blood bank and for certain immunology and serology tests because the gel may interfere with the immunological reactions. SSTs are also not recommended for certain therapeutic drug testing.

Red Top

Red stopper plastic tubes and Hemogard closures contain silica as a clot activator. They are used for serum chemistry tests and serology tests and in blood

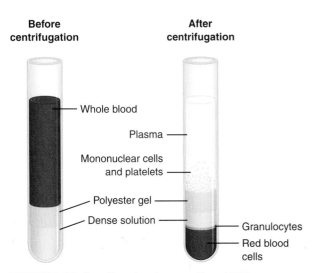
FIGURE 8-21 Centrifuged and uncentrifuged CPTs.

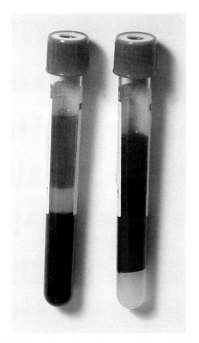

FIGURE 8-22 **Centrifuged and uncentrifuged SSTs.**

bank, where both serum and red blood cells may be used. The tubes are inverted five times to initiate the clotting process.

Red stopper glass tubes and Hemogard closures are often referred to as clot or plain tubes because they contain no anticoagulants or additives. Blood

collected in red stopper glass tubes clots by the normal coagulation process in about 60 minutes. Centrifugation of the sample then yields serum as the liquid portion. Red stopper tubes are used for the same purpose as the red plastic tubes. There is no need to invert glass red stopper tubes.

Red/Light Gray and Clear Top

Red/light gray stopper and clear Hemogard closures are plastic "discard tubes" because they contain no anticoagulants, additives, or gel. They are used as a discard tube for coagulation studies, when using a winged blood collection set, or as a secondary sample collection tube. No inverting of the tube is required.

 Technical Tip 8-13. Serum tubes with clot activator can not be used as a discard tube for coagulation studies.

Evacuated tubes are summarized in Table 8-1. Appendix I lists laboratory tests and the required types of anticoagulants and volume of blood required.

Order of Draw

When collecting multiple samples and samples for coagulation tests, the order in which tubes are drawn can affect some test results. Tubes must be collected in a specific order to prevent invalid test results

TABLE 8-1 • Summary of Evacuated Tubes			
STOPPER COLOR	**ANTICOAGULANT/ADDITIVE**	**SAMPLE TYPE**	**LABORATORY USE**
Lavender	Ethylenediaminetetraacetic acid (EDTA)	Whole blood/ plasma	Hematology
Pink	EDTA	Whole blood/ plasma	Blood bank
White	EDTA and gel	Plasma	Molecular diagnostics
Light blue	Sodium citrate	Plasma	Coagulation
Red/gray, gold	Clot activator and gel	Serum	Chemistry
Green	Ammonium heparin	Whole blood/ plasma	Chemistry
	Lithium heparin		
	Sodium heparin		
Light green, green/black	Lithium heparin and gel	Plasma	Chemistry

Continued

TABLE 8-1 • Summary of Evacuated Tubes—cont'd			
STOPPER COLOR	**ANTICOAGULANT/ADDITIVE**	**SAMPLE TYPE**	**LABORATORY USE**
Red (glass)	None	Serum	Blood bank, chemistry, serology
Red (plastic)	Clot activator	Serum	Chemistry, serology
Yellow/gray, orange	Thrombin	Serum	Chemistry
Gray	Potassium oxalate/sodium fluoride	Plasma	Chemistry glucose tests, alcohol
	Sodium fluoride	Serum	
	Sodium fluoride/Na_2EDTA	Plasma	
Tan	K_2EDTA	Plasma	Chemistry lead tests
Royal blue	Sodium heparin	Plasma	Chemistry trace elements, toxicology, and nutrient analyses
	K_2EDTA	Plasma	
	Clot activator	Serum	
Yellow	Sodium polyanethol sulfonate (SPS)	Whole blood	Microbiology blood cultures
	Acid citrate dextrose (ACD)	Whole blood	Blood bank
Black	Sodium citrate	Whole blood	Hematology sedimentation rates
Red/light gray, clear	None		Discard tube
Light blue/black	Sodium citrate, gel	Plasma	Molecular diagnostics
Red/green	Sodium heparin, gel	Plasma	Molecular diagnostics
Orange	Thrombin, gel	Serum	Chemistry, serology

caused by bacterial contamination, tissue fluid contamination, or carryover of additives or anticoagulants between tubes.

Preexamination Consideration 8-5.
Following the correct order of draw is essential to ensure accurate test results.

Technical Tip 8-14. CLSI standards state that a discard tube is not required for routine coagulation tests (activated partial thromboplastin time [APTT] and prothrombin time [PT]) unless special factor assays are being collected or when using a winged blood collection set.

Transfer of anticoagulants among tubes because of possible contamination of the stopper-puncturing needle must be avoided (Box 8-2). This is why tubes containing other anticoagulants or clot activators are drawn after the light blue stopper tube. EDTA and heparin can cause falsely increased PT and APTT time results that might cause a health-care provider to change the dosage of medication or misdiagnose a patient with a coagulation disorder. Tubes containing EDTA, which can bind calcium and iron, should not be drawn before a tube for chemistry tests on these substances. Contamination of a green, gold, or red stopper tube designated for sodium, potassium, and calcium determinations with EDTA, sodium citrate, or potassium oxalate would falsely decrease the calcium and elevate the sodium or potassium results. Tubes containing heparin should not be drawn before a tube for serum specimens. Holding blood collection tubes in a downward position so that the tube fills from the bottom up helps avoid the transfer of anticoagulants from tube to tube.

When sterile samples, such as blood cultures, are to be collected, they must be considered in the order of draw. Such samples are always drawn first in a sterile bottle or tube to prevent microbial contamination

BOX 8-2 Tests Affected by Anticoagulant/Additive Contamination

EDTA
- Alkaline phosphatase
- Calcium
- Activated partial thromboplastin time
- Creatine kinase-MB (CK-MB)
- Potassium
- Prothrombin time
- Iron
- Iron-binding capacity
- Sodium
- Amylase
- Alpha-1-antitrypsin
- Cholinesterase
- Ceruloplasmin
- Uric acid
- Creatinine
- Copper
- Lipase
- Lipids
- Acid phosphatase

Heparin
- Activated clotting time
- Activated partial thromboplastin time
- Acid phosphatase
- Erythrocyte sedimentation rate (ESR)
- Prothrombin time
- Sodium (sodium heparin)
- Lithium (lithium heparin)
- Blood urea nitrogen (BUN) (ammonium heparin)
- Ammonia (ammonium heparin)
- Albumin
- Cholinesterase
- CK-MB
- Iron
- Gamma-glutamyl transferase (Gamma-GT)

Potassium oxalate
- Potassium
- Red blood cell morphology
- Acid phosphatase
- Amylase
- Calcium
- Lactate dehydrogenase
- Prothrombin time
- Activated partial thromboplastin time
- Alkaline phosphatase
- Bilirubin
- Creatine kinase

- CK-MB
- Insulin
- Copper
- Low-density lipoprotein (LDL)-cholesterol
- Lipid electrophoresis
- Lithium
- Sodium
- Protein electrophoresis
- T_3 (triiodothyronine)
- Triglycerides
- Vitamin B_{12}
- Iron
- Gamma-GT

Sodium citrate
- Alkaline phosphatase
- Calcium
- Phosphorus
- Amylase
- Alpha-1-antitrypsin
- Bilirubin
- Cholesterol
- Creatine kinase
- CK-MB
- Iron
- Gamma-GT
- Glucose
- Uric acid
- High-density lipoprotein (HDL)-cholesterol
- Creatinine
- Copper
- Sodium
- Acid phosphatase
- Triglycerides

Sodium fluoride
- Alanine aminotransferase (ALT)
- Aspartate aminotransferase (AST)
- BUN
- Bilirubin
- Sodium
- Alkaline phosphatase
- Amylase
- Cholesterol
- Cholinesterase
- Creatine kinase
- CK-MB
- Gamma-GT
- Uric acid

Continued

BOX 8-2 Tests Affected by Anticoagulant/Additive Contamination—cont'd

HDL-cholesterol	Clot activator (silica)
Creatinine	Partial thromboplastin time
Copper	Prothrombin time
Lactate dehydrogenase (LDH)	
Acid phosphatase	
Triglycerides	

---

of the stopper puncturing needle from the unsterile stoppers of tubes used for the collection of other tests. The order of draw as recommended by the CLSI for both the evacuated tube system and when filling tubes from a syringe is: *need to know*

1. • Blood cultures (yellow stopper tubes, culture bottles)
2. • Light blue stopper tubes (sodium citrate)
3. • Red/gray, gold stopper tubes (serum separator tubes), red stopper plastic tubes (clot activator), and red stopper glass tubes
4. • Green stopper tubes and light green (plasma separator tubes) (heparin)
5. • Lavender stopper tubes (EDTA)
6. • Gray stopper tubes (potassium oxalate/sodium fluoride)
7. • Yellow/gray or orange stopper tubes (thrombin clot activator)

Other colored stopper tubes that contain EDTA such as the pink, white, royal blue, and tan should be drawn in the same order as the lavender stopper tube. If the royal blue stopper tube contains the anticoagulant sodium heparin, it should be drawn in the same order as the green stopper tubes. When the royal blue stopper tube does not contain an anticoagulant, it should be drawn in the same order as serum tubes.

SYRINGES

Syringes are often preferred over an evacuated tube system when drawing blood from patients with small or fragile veins. The advantage of this system is that the phlebotomist is able to control the suction pressure on the vein by slowly withdrawing the syringe plunger.

Syringes consist of a barrel graduated in milliliters (mL) or cubic centimeters (cc) and a plunger that fits tightly within the barrel, creating a vacuum when retracted (Fig. 8-23). Syringes routinely used for venipuncture range from 2 to 20 mL, and a size

corresponding to the amount of blood needed should be used.

Needles used with syringes are attached to a plastic hub designed to fit onto the barrel of the syringe. They are also individually packaged, sterile, and color coded as to gauge size. Routinely used syringe needles range from 21 to 23 gauge with 1-inch and 1.5-inch lengths.

▶ *Technical Tip 8-15.* An advantage when using syringe needles is that blood will appear in the hub of the needle when the vein has been successfully entered.

Needle protection devices are available for *hypodermic* syringe needles similar to evacuated tube needles. The Hypodermic Needle-Pro (Smiths Medical, Westin, MA) is a syringe needle with a disposable plastic sheath attached by a hinge (Fig. 8-24). The sheath hangs free during the venipuncture and is engaged over the needle by pressing the sheath against a flat surface after the procedure is complete. The SafetyGlide hypodermic needle by Becton, Dickinson (Fig. 8-25) has a movable shield that the phlebotomist pushes along the cannula with the thumb to enclose the needle tip after the venipuncture. Becton, Dickinson also has an Eclipse hypodermic needle that

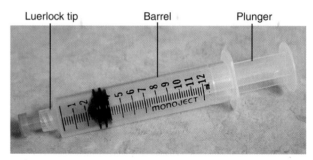

FIGURE 8-23 Diagram of a syringe.

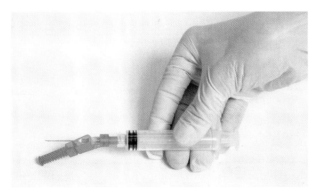

FIGURE 8-24 **Portex Blood Draw Hypodermic Needle-Pro.**

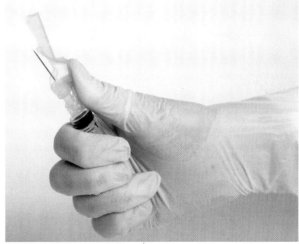

FIGURE 8-26 **BD Eclipse hypodermic needle.**

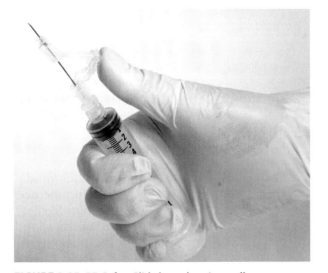

FIGURE 8-25 **BD SafetyGlide hypodermic needle.**

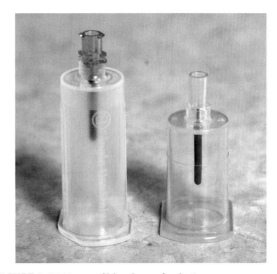

FIGURE 8-27 **Types of blood transfer devices.**

employs a shield that the phlebotomist locks over the needle tip after completion of the venipuncture procedure (Fig. 8-26). The entire needle and syringe assembly is discarded in the designated sharps container. The technique for use of syringes is discussed in Chapter 10.

Blood drawn in a syringe is immediately transferred to appropriate evacuated tubes to prevent the formation of clots. It is not acceptable to puncture the rubber stopper with the syringe needle and allow the blood to be drawn into the tube. A blood transfer device provides a safe means for blood transfer without using the syringe needle or removing the tube stopper (Fig. 8-27). It is an evacuated tube holder with a rubber-sheathed needle inside. After blood collection, the syringe tip is inserted

into the hub of the device and evacuated tubes are filled by pushing them onto the rubber-sheathed needle in the holder as in an evacuated tube system as shown in Figure 8-28.

 Technical Tip 8-16. It is important that the syringe and tube be held in a vertical position when using the blood transfer device to prevent carryover of anticoagulants or additives from previously filled tubes.

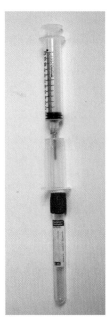

FIGURE 8-28 BD blood transfer device with syringe and evacuated tube.

The entire syringe/holder assembly is discarded in the sharps container after use. Only syringes with built-in needle protection shields should be used with this system. The shield must be activated immediately when the needle is removed from the vein to avoid accidental needle sticks.

▶ *Technical Tip 8-17.* Let the vacuum in the evacuated tube draw the appropriate amount of blood into the tube. Discard any extra blood left in the syringe; do not force it into the tube.

 Safety Tip 8-7. Do not unthread the syringe from the blood transfer device. Place the entire assembly in a sharps container. Use a safety needle device with this system.

When tubes are filled from a syringe, CLSI recommends the tubes be filled in the same order as recommended for the order of draw for the evacuated tube system. However, the personnel in some institutions believe that, because the portion of blood possibly contaminated by tissue thromboplastin is the first portion to enter the syringe, it is the last to be expelled. To avoid microclot formation in anticoagulated tubes, the order for tube fill from a syringe in these institutions would be:

- Sterile samples (blood cultures)
- Light blue stopper tubes
- Lavender stopper tubes
- Green stopper tubes
- Gray stopper tubes
- Red, SST, or orange stopper tubes

At the same time, the possible transfer of anticoagulants and additives among tubes must also be considered and will be minimized by using the CLSI protocol. Institutional protocol should be followed.

WINGED BLOOD COLLECTION SETS

Winged blood collection sets (or "butterflies" as they are routinely called) are used for the infusion of IV fluids and for performing venipuncture from very small or very fragile veins often seen in children and in the geriatric population. Winged blood collection needles used for phlebotomy are usually 21 or 23 gauge with lengths of 1/2 to 3/4 inch. Plastic attachments to the needle that resemble butterfly wings are used for holding the needle during insertion and to secure the apparatus during IV therapy. They also provide the ability to lower the needle insertion angle when working with very small veins. To accommodate the dual purpose of venipuncture and infusion, the needle is attached to flexible plastic tubing that can then be attached to an IV setup, syringe, or specially designed evacuated tube holders (Fig. 8-29).

 Safety Tip 8-8. Extreme care must be taken when working with winged blood collection needles to avoid accidental needle punctures. Always hold the apparatus by the needle wings and not by the tubing.

▶ *Technical Tip 8-18.* In the interest of cost containment, phlebotomists should not become dependent on the use of winged blood collection sets for patients with veins than can be accessed with a standard evacuated tube system.

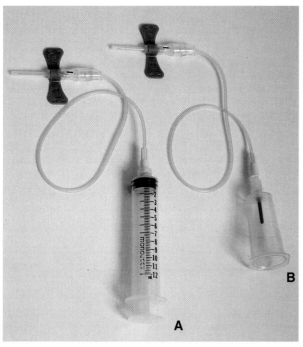

FIGURE 8-29 Winged blood collection sets. A, Syringe. B, Holder.

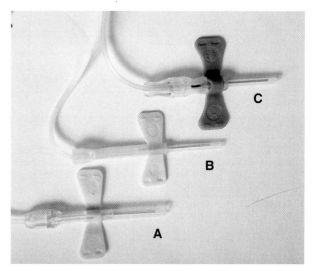

FIGURE 8-30 Examples of winged blood collection needles. A, Vacuette safety blood collection set (Greiner Bio-One, Kremsmuster, Austria). B, BD Vacutainer Safety-Lok blood collection set (Becton, Dickinson, Franklin Lakes, NJ). C, BD Vacutainer Push Button blood collection set (Becton, Dickinson, Franklin Lakes, NJ).

The flexible tubing can make the winged blood collection set more difficult to manage. The length of the tubing also results in approximately 0.5 mL less blood entering the first collection tube, which could interfere with coagulation tests. It is more expensive to use the winged blood collection set than the standard evacuated tube system, and phlebotomists should avoid becoming overly dependent on the winged blood collection set for sample collection.

 Technical Tip 8-19. A clear "discard" tube or another tube with the same additive should be drawn before tubes that are affected by an incorrect blood-to-anticoagulant ratio. Air in the winged blood collection set tubing will cause the first tube collected to underfill.

There are several winged blood collection sets with safety devices built into the system (Fig. 8-30). The BD Vacutainer Safety-Lok blood collection set (Becton, Dickinson, Franklin Lakes, NJ) uses a translucent protective shield that covers the needle immediately after removal from the vein. After use, the needle is completely retracted into the shield and locked in place by pushing the shield forward (Fig. 8-30B). The BD Vacutainer Push Button blood collection set uses in-vein activation of the needle. The needle is automatically retracted into the device when the phlebotomist pushes the activation button with the index finger while the needle is still in the vein. (Fig. 8-30C) The safety device for the Vacuette safety blood collection set (Greiner Bio-One, Kermsmuster, Austria) is activated by depressing both sides of the stopper and sliding it until the tip of the needle is retracted and covered by the protective shield (Fig. 8-30A). The Puncture Guard winged blood collection (Gaven Medical, Vernon, CT) produces a safety device that blunts the needle before withdrawal from the vein (Fig. 8-31). Another needle set is the Monoject Angel Wing safety needle (Kendall, Mansfield, MA). When the needle is withdrawn from the vein, a stainless steel safety shield is activated and locks in place to cover the needle.

The technique for use of winged blood collection sets is covered in Chapter 10.

COMBINATION SYSTEMS

The S-Monovette Blood Collection System (Sarstedt, Inc., Newton, NC) is an enclosed multisampling blood collection system that includes the blood

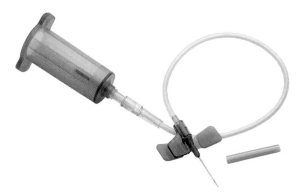

FIGURE 8-31 **Puncture Guard Winged Blood Collection Set.** *(With permission from Gaven Medical, Vernon, CT.)*

collection tube and collection device. Blood is collected using either an aspiration or vacuum principle of collection with multisampling needles with pre-assembled holders, needle protection devices, and a safety winged blood collection set (Fig. 8-32).

TOURNIQUETS

Tourniquets are used during venipuncture to make it easier to locate patients' veins. They do this by impeding venous but not arterial blood flow in the area just below where the tourniquet is applied. The distended vein then becomes more visible or palpable. Tourniquets are available in both adult and pediatric sizes.

The most frequently used tourniquets are flat latex or vinyl strips (Fig. 8-33). They are inexpensive and

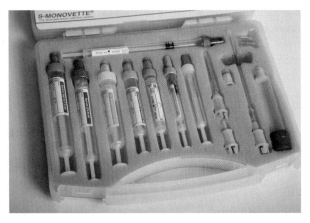

FIGURE 8-32 **S-Monovette Blood Collection System** *(Sarstedt, Inc., Newton, NC).*

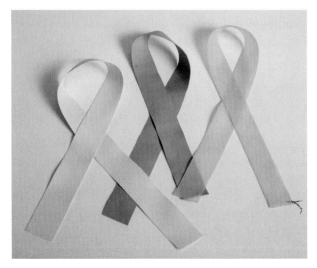

FIGURE 8-33 **Various types of tourniquets.**

may be disposed of between patients or reused if disinfected. Flat nonlatex strips are available for patients or phlebotomists allergic to latex.

 Technical Tip 8-20. Latex-free tourniquets are available on a roll that is perforated and should always be carried on the phlebotomist's tray. The stretch tourniquet is used and discarded.

Tourniquets with Velcro and buckle closures are easier to apply but are more difficult to decontaminate. The advantage of the buckle closure is that it stays on the patient's arm after release and can be retightened if necessary.

Blood pressure cuffs can be used as tourniquets. They are used primarily for veins that are difficult to locate. The cuff should be inflated to a pressure of 40 mm Hg. This allows blood to flow into but not out of the affected veins.

The application of tourniquets and their effects on blood tests are discussed in Chapters 9 and 10.

VEIN LOCATING DEVICES

A variety of portable devices are available to locate veins that are not easily visible, particularly in the infant, pediatric, and elderly patient where every attempt should be made to avoid multiple needlesticks. The Venoscope II (Fig. 8-34) and Neonatal

Transilluminator (Venoscope, L. L. C., Lafayette, LA) and the Transillumination Vein Locator (VL-U) (Promedic, McCordsville, IN) use high-intensity LED lights that shine through the patient's subcutaneous tissue to highlight the veins by absorbing the light rather than reflecting it. The vein stands out as a dark line enabling the phlebotomist to note the direction of the vein. The phlebotomist then marks the vein for needle insertion. The Wee Sight Transilluminator (Philips Children's Medical Ventures, Monroeville, PA) is designed for a baby's tiny veins. It does not emit heat, making it safe for an infant's delicate skin. The Vena-Vue (Biosynergy, Elk Grove Village, IL) uses liquid crystal thermography to locate veins. The device is placed on the skin like a bandage to cool the skin. Veins, because they emit heat, will become visible to the phlebotomist. The Vein Entry Indicator Device (VEID) (Vascular Technologies, Ness-Ziona, Israel) uses a sensor technology to indicate correct insertion of a catheter needle in a vein. The device emits a continuous beeping signal indicating a change of pressure when the needle penetrates a vein. The beeping signal stops when the needle exits the vein.

GLOVES

OSHA mandates that gloves must be worn when collecting blood and must be changed after each patient. Under routine circumstances, gloves do not need to be sterile. To provide maximal manual dexterity, they should fit securely.

Gloves are available in several varieties, including powdered and powder-free, and latex and nonlatex (vinyl, nitrile, neoprene, and polyethylene) (Fig. 8-35). Gloves with powder are not recommended because the powder can contaminate patient samples and cause falsely elevated calcium values. The glove powder can also cause a sensitization to latex. Allergenic latex proteins are absorbed on the glove powder, which become airborne and can be inhaled when the gloves are put on and taken off. As discussed in Chapter 4, allergy to latex is increasing among health-care workers.

3 important questions to ask patient

★ are you allergic to latex?

★ have you been fasting?

★ are you any blood thinners?

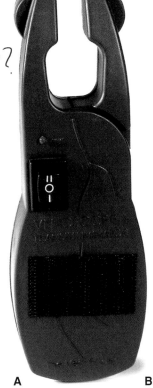
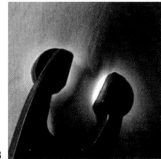

FIGURE 8-34   **A, Venoscope II transilluminator device.** *(With permission from Di Lorenzo, MS and Strasinger, SK: Blood Collection: A Short Course, ed. 2. FA Davis, 2010, Philadelphia.)* **B, A vein appears as a dark line between the light-emitting arms of the Venoscope.** *(Courtesy of Venoscope, LLC.)*

A   B

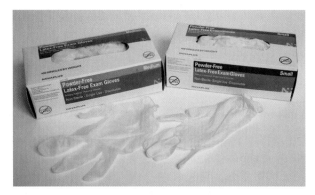

FIGURE 8-35 **Gloves.**

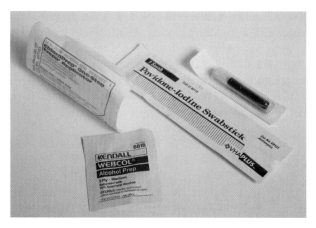

FIGURE 8-36 **Antiseptics.**

 Safety Tip 8-9. Persons who develop symptoms of allergy to latex should avoid latex gloves and other latex products, such as tourniquets, at all times.

Cotton glove liners can be worn under latex gloves for persons that develop an allergic dermatitis to gloves. Hands must be washed after removing gloves to prevent the transmission of bloodborne pathogens and to decrease the time of latex exposure and transmission of latex proteins to other parts of the body.

▶ *Technical Tip 8-21.* To avoid sample contamination and latex allergy, do not use powdered gloves. Wash hands immediately after removing gloves between each patient.

PUNCTURE SITE PROTECTION SUPPLIES

The primary antiseptic used for cleansing the skin in routine phlebotomy is 70 percent isopropyl alcohol. This is a bacteriostatic antiseptic used to prevent contamination by normal skin bacteria during the short period required to perform collection of the sample.

For collections that require additional sterility, such as blood cultures and arterial punctures, the stronger antiseptics such as iodine or chlorhexidine gluconate (for patients allergic to iodine) are used to cleanse the area (Fig. 8-36). To prevent skin discomfort, iodine should always be removed from the patient's skin with alcohol after a phlebotomy procedure.

2×2-inch gauze pads are used for applying pressure to the puncture site after the needle has been removed. Gauze pads can also serve as additional protection when folded in quarters and placed under a bandage. A bandage or adhesive tape is placed over the puncture site when the bleeding has stopped. Latex-free tape should be used for persons who are allergic to adhesive bandages. Self-adhering gauze bandages (Coban) are available for elderly patients, for use after arterial punctures or for patients with prolonged bleeding after venipuncture. It is not recommended to use cotton balls to apply pressure because the cotton ball fibers can stick to the venipuncture site and may cause bleeding to begin again when the cotton is removed. Patients should be instructed to remove the bandage in about an hour (Fig. 8-37).

ADDITIONAL SUPPLIES

Clean glass slides may be needed to prepare blood films for certain hematology tests. This procedure is discussed in Chapter 12. Biohazard bags should be available for transport of samples based on institutional protocol.

Alcohol-based hand sanitizers are an acceptable substitute for hand washing when the hands are not visibly soiled. Wall-mounted hand sanitizers are available in all health-care settings with either gels or foams. Carrying personal bottles of hand sanitizers provides a convenient method of decontamination that is readily available (Fig. 8-38).

The final piece of equipment needed by the phlebotomist is a pen for labeling tubes, initialing computer-generated labels, or noting unusual circumstances on the requisition form.

QUALITY CONTROL

Ensuring the sterility of needles and puncture devices and the stability of evacuated tubes, anticoagulants, and additives is essential to patient safety and sample quality. Disposable needles and puncture devices are individually packaged in tightly sealed sterile containers.

> **! Safety Tip 8-10.** Phlebotomists should not use puncture equipment if the seal has been broken.

Visual inspection for nonpointed or barbed needles may detect manufacturing defects. Manufacturers of evacuated tubes must ensure that tubes, anticoagulants, and additives meet the standards established by the CLSI. Evacuated tubes produced at the same time are referred to as a lot and have a distinguishing lot number printed on the packages. There is also an expiration date printed on each package. The expiration date represents the last day the manufacturer guarantees the stability of the specified amount of vacuum in the tube and the reactivity of the anticoagulants and additives. The expiration date should be checked each time a new package of tubes is opened, and outdated tubes should not be used.

> ▶ *Technical Tip 8-22.* Use of expired tubes may cause incompletely filled tubes (short draws), clotted anticoagulated samples, improperly preserved samples, and insecure gel barriers.

Failure to completely fill tubes (short draws) containing anticoagulants and additives affects sample quality because the amount of anticoagulant or additive present in the tube is based on the assumption that the tube will be completely filled. Possible errors include excessive dilution of the sample by liquid anticoagulants and distortion of cellular structure by increased chemical concentrations.

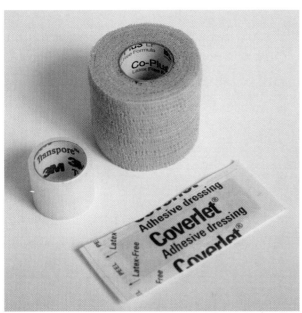

FIGURE 8-37 **Bandages.**

(handwritten notes)
- glass slides
- biohazard transport bags
- hand sanitizers
- pen - never pencil

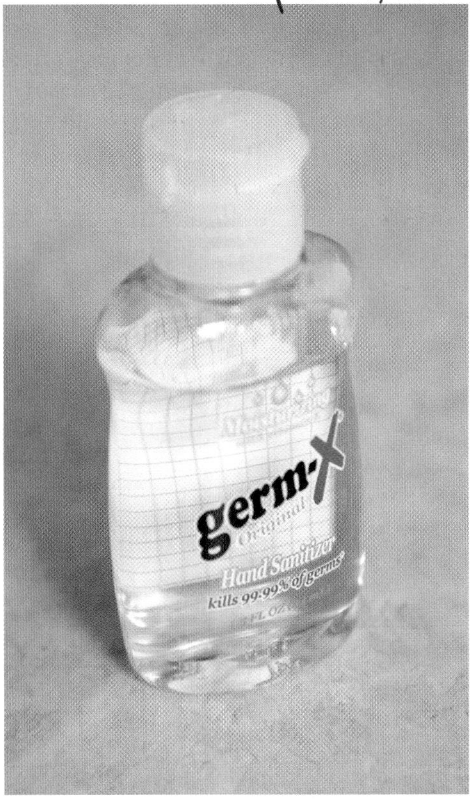

FIGURE 8-38 **Hand-held personal hand sanitizer.**

Preexamination Consideration 8-6.

Underfilled sodium citrate tubes (light blue stopper) will have an incorrect anticoagulant-to-blood ratio, which can cause a falsely lengthened aPTT result.

Technical Tip 8-23. Avoid manual filling of tubes with anticoagulant to maintain the correct blood-to-anticoagulant ratio.

Preexamination Consideration 8-7.

Underfilled EDTA tubes cause red blood cell shrinkage, which will affect hematology tests.

Key Points

✦ A well-stocked phlebotomy tray contains racks with evacuated blood collection tubes, tube holders and multisample needles, syringes with safety hypodermic needles, winged blood collection sets, blood transfer devices, tourniquets, alcohol pads, gauze, bandages, gloves, microcollection equipment, and a biohazard sharps container.

✦ Needle size varies by length and gauge. The needle gauge refers to the diameter of the needle lumen; the lower the number, the larger the needle. Needles used for blood collection range from 16 to 23 gauge. Standard needles used for venipuncture are 21 and 22 gauge with a 1-inch or 1.5-inch length. Needles of 23 gauge with a $^{3}/_{4}$-inch length may be used for children and patients with small, fragile veins.

✦ Needles for venipuncture have a bevel (angled point), hollow shaft, and a hub that attaches to a holder or syringe. Double-pointed needles are used with the ETS.

✦ OSHA requires the use of safety needles or holders with engineered safety devices that include self-sheathing needles, retractable needles, and blunting needles. Manufacturer's recommendations must be followed in the correct operation of the safety device. Needles should never be manually recapped or removed from the holder. Needles must be disposed of in an approved sharps container.

✦ The ETS consists of a double-pointed multisample needle, a holder, and color-coded evacuated blood collection tubes. Blood is collected directly into the tube, eliminating the need to transfer samples.

✦ Color-coded evacuated tubes are labeled with the type of anticoagulant or additive, the draw volume, and the expiration date. Each laboratory department has specific sample requirements for the analysis of particular blood constituents.

✦ EDTA, sodium citrate, and potassium oxalate prevent clotting by binding or chelating calcium. Heparin prevents clotting by inhibiting thrombin in the coagulation cascade. Tubes must be gently inverted three to eight times to ensure adequate mixing.

✦ Blood collection tubes should be collected in a specific order to prevent carryover of anticoagulants or additives that cause contamination of the sample. The correct order is (1) blood culture (SPS); (2) light blue (sodium citrate); (3) gold, red/gray (serum gel separator tube); red (glass or plastic); (4) green, light green, green/black (plasma gel separator tube with heparin); (5) lavender, pink, (EDTA), and white (plasma gel separator tube with EDTA; (6) gray (sodium fluoride); and (7) yellow/gray and orange (thrombin).

✦ Syringes attach to a hypodermic needle and are used for small and fragile veins. The phlebotomist is able to control the suction on the vein.

✦ Winged blood collection sets (butterflies) can be attached to a holder, a syringe, or an IV setup. They are used for performing venipuncture from very small fragile veins and are often used with children and the elderly. The wings can be used to guide the needle in the vein and to lower the needle insertion angle.

✦ Tourniquets are used to make the vein more visible by impeding venous blood but not arterial blood flow. Flat latex or nonlatex strips, tourniquets, with Velcro or buckle closures, and blood pressure cuffs may be used. Portable vein-locating devices are available.

✦ Substances used to cleanse the skin before venipuncture include 70 percent isopropyl alcohol for routine venipuncture and iodine or chlorhexidine gluconate for additional sterility in blood collections for blood cultures and arterial punctures.

✦ OSHA mandates that gloves must be worn when collecting blood and must be changed after each patient.

✦ Gauze pads are used to apply pressure to the puncture site after the needle has been removed.

✦ Additional blood collection supplies include a pen, slides, alcohol-based hand sanitizers, and biohazard bags.

✦ Quality control of venipuncture equipment is essential to patient safety and sample quality. Needles must be sterile and visibly inspected for nonpointed or barbs. The expiration date should be checked each time a new package of tubes is opened. Use of expired tubes may cause short draws, clotted anticoagulated samples, improperly preserved samples, and insecure gel barrier

BIBLIOGRAPHY

Becton, Dickinson Vacutainer Evacuated Blood Collection System. http://www.bd.com/vacutainer/productinserts.

CLSI. Procedures for the Collection of Diagnostic Blood Specimens by Venipuncture, ed. 6. Approved Guideline H3-A6. CLSI, 2007, Wayne, PA.

CLSI. Procedures for the Handling and Processing of Blood Specimens, ed. 3. Approved Guideline, H18-A4. CLSI, 2010, Wayne, PA.

CLSI. Tubes and Additives for Venous Blood Specimen Collection, ed. 5. Approved Guideline H01-A5. CLSI, 2003, Wayne, PA.

Greiner Bio-One. Venous Blood Collection. http://www.gbo.com/documents/1b_Vacuette_IFU_GB_rev08_hcys_internet.pdf

Greiner Bio-One. Widespread Errors Made During Blood Collection. http://www.gbo.com/documents/VACUETTE_Pre-analytics_Manual.pdf

International Sharps Injury Prevention Society. Safety Products. http://www.isips.org

Occupational Safety and Health Administration. Disposal of Contaminated Needles and Blood Tube Holders Used in Phlebotomy. Safety and Health Information Bulletin, http://www.osha.gov/dts/shib/shib101503.html.

http://www.gavenmedical.com

http://www.smiths-medical.com/brands/jelco

http://www.vanishpoint.com

http://www.vascular.co.il

http://www.venoscope.com

http://www.weesight.respironics.com

 ## Study Questions

1. Which of the following needles has the smallest diameter?
   a. 16-gauge needle
   b. 22-gauge needle
   c. 21-gauge needle
   d. 23-gauge needle

2. Which of the following tubes contains an anticoagulant that inhibits thrombin?
   a. lavender stopper
   b. white stopper
   c. light blue stopper
   d. green stopper

3. EDTA, sodium citrate, and potassium oxalate anticoagulants prevent blood clotting in blood collection tubes by:
   a. binding calcium
   b. binding fibrinogen
   c. acting as an antithrombin agent
   d. releasing heparin

4. All of the following can be used to collect a serum specimen **EXCEPT:**
   a. red stopper tube
   b. PST
   c. SST
   d. orange stopper tube

5. Which tube additive preserves glucose?
   a. sodium citrate
   b. sodium heparin
   c. sodium polyanethol sulfonate
   d. sodium fluoride

6. The stopper colored tube that must always be filled to the correct ratio is:
   a. light blue stopper tube
   b. light green PST
   c. gold SST
   d. tan stopper tube

7. Which of the following is the CLSI acceptable order of tube draw?
   a. light blue, light green, and lavender
   b. red, light blue, and lavender
   c. lavender, red, and yellow
   d. yellow, green, and light blue

8. The winged blood collection set is primarily used for:
   a. heel sticks
   b. large antecubital veins
   c. finger sticks
   d. difficult and hand veins

9. The primary antiseptic for routine venipuncture is:
   a. iodine
   b. chlorhexidine gluconate
   c. isopropyl alcohol
   d. Betadine

10. Using evacuated tubes past their expiration date may result in:
    a. clotted samples
    b. incompletely filled tubes
    c. insecure gel barriers
    d. all of the above

Clinical Scenarios

1 At Healthy Hospital laboratory, the information on a requisition form requesting a liver panel, an amylase, and a theophylline level tells the phlebotomist to collect a gold SST and a red stopper tube.

   a. Which test must be performed on the red stopper tube?

   b. Serum from which tube could be used by the serology department if an additional test was requested?

   c. Why is a gold SST preferred over a red stopper tube for most chemistry tests?

   d. State a reason why a different laboratory would require a green PST instead of a gold SST.

2 The phlebotomy supervisor is investigating the following complaints. State a technical phlebotomy error that could be the cause of each problem.

   a. The coagulation laboratory rejects a light blue stopper tube for a prothrombin time (PT). The phlebotomist used a winged blood collection set.

   b. The chemistry laboratory rejects an SST into which blood from a syringe has been transferred.

   c. A phlebotomist complains about getting short draws with lavender stopper tubes but not red stopper tubes during morning collections.

3 The phlebotomist was called to the Emergency Department (ED) to collect blood for a glucose and CBC from a patient. The phlebotomist collected a lavender stopper and gray stopper tube. The doctor then suspected the patient was having a MI and ordered a MI panel, PT, APTT, and type and crossmatch. Because the phlebotomist had a difficult time obtaining the first samples, the nurse asked if the tests could be performed on blood already collected.

   a. Can a lavender stopper tube be used to perform a PT and APTT? Why or why not?

   b. Can a glucose and an MI panel be performed on a gray stopper tube? Why or why not?

   c. What tube is used to perform a crossmatch?

Venipuncture Equipment Exercise

Instructions

State or assemble (if requested) the appropriate equipment for the situations described in this exercise. Include the number and stopper color of evacuated tubes, needle size, syringe size, or winged blood collection set, if appropriate. Instructors may specify the inclusion of other supplies.

1. Collection of a CBC from a 35-year-old woman.

2. Collection of a CBC from a 3-year-old boy.

3. Collection of a CBC and electrolytes from a 40-year-old man.

4. Collection of an amylase from the hand of a patient who is taking anticoagulants.

5. Collection of a PT from an elderly patient.

6. Collection of a chemistry profile from a patient with a latex allergy.

7. Assemble the equipment to collect a type and crossmatch on a 50-year-old man.

8. Assemble the equipment to collect a cardiac risk profile and ESR from a patient with fragile veins.

9. Assemble the equipment to collect a lead level from a 2-year-old patient.

10. Assemble the tubes in the order they would be drawn for a CBC, APTT, and a glucose using an evacuated tube system.

Evaluation of Equipment Selection and Assembly Competency

RATING SYSTEM

2 = Satisfactorily Performed,   **1** = Needs Improvement,   **0** = Incorrect/Did Not Perform

_____   **1.**   Collects all necessary equipment and supplies

_____   **2.**   Selects appropriate tubes for requested tests

_____   **3.**   Selects correct number of tubes or syringe size

_____   **4.**   Correctly attaches needle to holder or syringe

_____   **5.**   Does not uncap needle prematurely

_____   **6.**   Advances tube correctly into holder or checks plunger movement

_____   **7.**   Arranges supplies and extra tubes conveniently

TOTAL POINTS _____

MAXIMUM POINTS = 14

Comments:

CHAPTER 9

Routine Venipuncture

Learning Objectives

Upon completion of this chapter, the reader will be able to:

1. List the required information on a requisition form.
2. Discuss the appropriate procedure to follow when greeting and reassuring a patient.
3. Describe correct patient identification procedures for inpatients and outpatients.
4. Describe patient preparation and positioning.
5. Correctly assemble venipuncture equipment and supplies.
6. Name and locate the three most frequently used veins for venipuncture.
7. Correctly apply a tourniquet and state why the tourniquet can be applied for only 1 minute.
8. Describe vein palpation.
9. Discuss the venipuncture site cleansing procedure.
10. State the steps in a venipuncture procedure, and correctly perform a routine venipuncture using an evacuated tube system.
11. Demonstrate safe disposal of contaminated needles and supplies.
12. List the information required on a sample tube label.
13. Explain the importance of delivering samples to the laboratory in a timely manner.

Key Terms

Antecubital fossa
Bar codes
Basilic vein
Cephalic vein
Hematoma
Hemoconcentration
Hemolysis
Identification band
Median cubital vein
Palpation
Radio frequency identification
Requisition

The most frequently performed procedure in phlebotomy is the venipuncture. The ability to perform this technique in an organized, patient-considerate manner is the key to success as a phlebotomist. Each phlebotomist develops his or her own style for dealing with patients and performing the actual venipuncture. Administrative protocols vary among institutions and, of course, every patient is different; however, many basic rules are the same in all situations. These basic rules must be followed to ensure the safety of the patient and the phlebotomist, produce samples that are representative of the patient's condition, and create an efficient phlebotomy service for the institution.

In this chapter, the routine venipuncture technique is presented for the beginning phlebotomist in the recommended step-by-step procedure. The procedure is outlined again in Chapter 10 with a presentation of the complications that may occur at each step.

Preexamination Consideration 9-1.

According to the CLSI, a standardized venipuncture procedure can reduce or eliminate errors that can affect sample quality and patient test results.

REQUISITIONS

All phlebotomy procedures begin with the receipt of a test *requisition* form that is generated by or at the request of a health-care provider. The requisition becomes part of the patient's medical record and is essential to provide the phlebotomist with the information needed to correctly identify the patient, organize the necessary equipment, collect the appropriate samples, and provide legal protection. Phlebotomists should not collect a sample without a requisition form, and this form must accompany the sample to the laboratory.

The method by which a phlebotomist receives a requisition varies with the setting. Requisitions from outpatients may be hand carried by the patient, or requests may be telephoned or faxed to the central processing or accessioning area by the health-care provider's office staff, where the laboratory staff generates a requisition form. In some health-care providers' offices, the health-care provider will use a prescription pad to write the names of lab tests ordered. The patient then takes the prescription to a clinical lab where the requisition is then prepared following the health-care providers' orders. Inpatient requisitions may be delivered to the laboratory, sent by pneumatic tube system, or entered into the hospital computer at the nursing station and printed out by the laboratory computer.

Phlebotomists should carefully examine all requisitions for which they are responsible before leaving the laboratory. The requisition should be reviewed to verify the tests to be collected and the time and date of collection, and to determine whether any special conditions such as fasting or patient preparation requirements must be met before the venipuncture. They should check to be sure that all requisitions for a particular patient are together so that all tests are collected with one venipuncture. They must be sure they have all the necessary equipment.

The actual format of a requisition form may vary. Patient information may be handwritten or imprinted by an imprinter on color-coded forms with test check-off lists for different departments (Fig. 9-1). There may be multiple copies for purposes of record keeping and billing. Computer-generated forms can include not only the patient information and tests requested but also tube labels and **bar codes** for sample processing, the number and type of collection tubes needed, and special collection instructions (Fig. 9-2). Figure 9-3

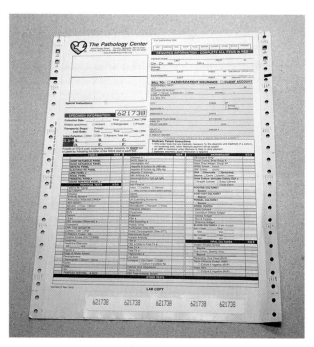

FIGURE 9-1 Manual requisition.

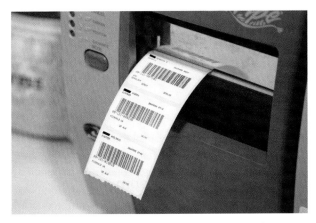

FIGURE 9-2 Computer requisitions printing in the laboratory.

FIGURE 9-3 Sample requisition form and labels.

shows a sample computer-generated requisition form with accompanying labels.

Requisitions must contain certain basic information to ensure that the sample drawn and the test results are correlated with the appropriate patient and that these can be correctly interpreted with regard to any special conditions, such as the time of collection. The required information on a requisition includes the following:

- Patient's first and last names
- Identification number (The identification number may be a hospital-generated number that is

also present on the patient's wrist *identification (ID) band* and in all hospital documents; in an outpatient setting it may be a laboratory-assigned number.)
- Patient's date of birth
- Patient's location
- Ordering health-care provider's name
- Tests requested
- Requested date and time of sample collection (When the sample is collected, the phlebotomist must write the actual date and time on the requisition and the sample label. Most hospitals have adopted the military time system because they operate continuously for 24 hours. Standard time and military time are similar between midnight and noon. Afternoon standard time repeats but military time is standard time plus 12. (See Table 9-1.)
- Status of sample (stat, timed, routine)
- Other information that may be present includes the following:
  - Number and type of collection tubes
  - Special collection information (such as fasting sample or latex sensitivity)
  - Special patient information (such as areas that should not be used for venipuncture)
- Billing information and ICD-9 codes

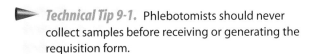

Technical Tip 9-1. Phlebotomists should never collect samples before receiving or generating the requisition form.

TABLE 9-1 ● **Standard and Military Time Comparison**	
STANDARD	**MILITARY**
12:00 midnight	0000
1:00 a.m.	0100
6:00 a.m.	0600
11:00 a.m.	1100
12:00 noon	1200
1:15 p.m.	1315
5:00 p.m.	1700
10:00 p.m.	2200
11:59 p.m.	2359

GREETING THE PATIENT

A phlebotomist's professional demeanor instills confidence and trust in the patient, which can effectively ease patient apprehension about the procedure. When approaching patients, phlebotomists should introduce themselves, say that they are from the laboratory, and explain that they will be collecting a blood sample. The procedure must be explained in nontechnical terms and in a manner the patient can understand. It is helpful to explain to the patient that his or her health-care provider has ordered the laboratory tests. The patient then can give the phlebotomist permission to collect the sample. Carefully listen to the patient and observe the patient's body language. Consent may be verbal or nonverbal indicated by the patient extending his or her arm or rolling up his or her sleeve. In the outpatient setting, the patient usually knows what is about to occur (Fig. 9-4).

 Technical Tip 9-2. The more relaxed and trusting your patient, the greater chance of a successful atraumatic venipuncture.

Room Signs

Observe any signs on the patient's door or in the patient's room relaying special instructions, such as allergic to latex, nothing by mouth (NPO), do not resuscitate (DNR), do not draw blood from (a particular) arm, infection control precautions, or patient expired (Fig. 9-5). A sign with a picture on it may be used in place of written warnings.

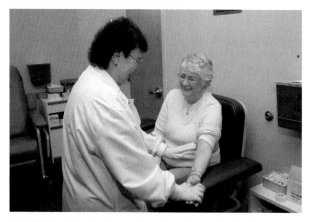

FIGURE 9-4 A phlebotomist greeting a patient in an outpatient setting.

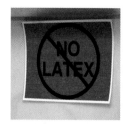

FIGURE 9-5 Warning sign in patient room to not use latex.

Entering a Patient's Room

When entering a patient's room, it is polite to knock lightly on the open or closed door to make your presence known. If the curtain is closed around the bed, speak to the patient first through the curtain. This will avoid any embarrassment or invasion of the patient's privacy if the patient happens to be bathing or using the bedpan. In the hospital setting, a variety of other circumstances may be present that require additional consideration when greeting the patient. These circumstances are discussed in Chapter 10.

PATIENT IDENTIFICATION

The most important procedure in phlebotomy is correct identification of the patient. Serious diagnostic or treatment errors and even death can occur when blood is drawn from the wrong patient. The Clinical and Laboratory Standards Institute (CLSI) recommends two identifiers for patient identification. The College of American Pathologists (CAP) and the Joint Commission (JC) patient safety goals require a minimum of two patient identifiers when collecting blood. To ensure that blood is drawn from the right patient, identification is made by comparing information obtained verbally and from the patient's wrist ID band with the information on the requisition form (Fig. 9-6).

Inpatient Identification

Verbal identification is made after the patient greeting by asking the patient to state his or her full name. Always have patients state their names. Do not ask, "Are you John Jones?" because many patients who are medicated, seriously ill, or hard of hearing have a tendency to say "yes" to anything. Examining the information on the patient's wrist ID band, which should always be present on hospitalized patients, follows verbal identification. Information on the wrist ID band should include patient's name, hospital identification

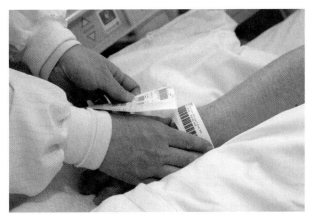

FIGURE 9-6 Phlebotomist checking an inpatient identification band.

number, date of birth, and physician. All information on the wrist ID band should match the information on the requisition form. Particular attention should be paid to the hospital identification number, because it is possible for two patients to have the same name, date of birth, and physician; however, they could not have the same identification number.

Preexamination Consideration 9-2.

Discrepancies between the patient's ID band the requisition must be verified before blood is drawn. It is estimated that 16 percent of ID bands contain erroneous information.

It is essential that identification of hospitalized patients be made from an ID band attached to the patient. Wristbands are sometimes removed when IV fluids are being administered in the wrist or when fluids have infiltrated the area. They should be reattached to the patient's ankle. Ankle bands are frequently used with pediatric patients and newborns. A wristband lying on the bedside table cannot be used for identification—it could belong to anyone. Likewise, a sign over the patient's bed or on the door cannot be relied on because the patient could be in the wrong bed.

Outpatient Identification

In an outpatient setting, ask the patient to state his or her full name, address, birth date, and/or unique identification number after calling him or her back to the drawing area. Compare the verbal information with the requisition form to verify the patient's identification. A person that is hard of hearing or nervous about the procedure may stand and follow you to the blood collection area from the waiting room just because you looked at him or her when calling the patient's name even when it was a different person's name called. Outpatients traditionally have not worn ID bands; however, facilities are beginning to assign an ID band for outpatient procedures to avoid patient identification errors. Photo identification may be a requirement for certain legal tests. Clinics may provide a patient ID card that can be imprinted or scanned for patient identification and to generate a requisition. Written policies must be available for outpatient centers.

Preexamination Consideration 9-3.

CLSI requires that a caregiver or family member must provide information on a cognitively impaired patient's behalf before collecting the sample. Document the name of the verifier.

Bar Code Technology

Positive patient identification can be made using barcode technology. Using a wireless hand-held computer, the phlebotomist positively identifies the patient by scanning the bar code on the patient's hospital ID band. The patient's identification is matched against a blood collection order on the mobile computer, which verifies that a blood sample is required and the correct patient has been identified. The system, which is interfaced with the laboratory information system (LIS), specifies the tests ordered, which kind of tube should be used, and special handling instructions. Following confirmation of the patient identification and test requests, the mobile computer directs a lightweight hand-held printer to create a bar code label that can be affixed to the tube before leaving the bedside. The system detects duplicate draw orders, new test requests, or cancellation of tests. Labels for a specific patient are printed only after the patient has been identified; therefore, eliminating the possibility of placing the wrong label to a sample.

The newest identification technology is *radio frequency identification* (RFID). It is an automated wireless technology that uses radio waves to transmit data for patient identification and sample tracking. The advantage of RFID is that patient data can be updated at any time versus with a bar code the data is set and nothing can be added until a new wristband is created.

Technical Tip 9-3. A hospitalized patient must always be correctly identified by an ID band that is attached to the patient.

 Safety Tip 9-1. Personnel already familiar with a patient must never become lax with regard to patient identification.

 Preexamination Consideration 9-4.
Failure to properly identify the patient may result in patient medication and treatment mismanagement.

PATIENT PREPARATION

Reassurance of the patient actually begins with the greeting and continues throughout the procedure. Phlebotomists should demonstrate both concern for the patient's comfort and confidence in their own ability to perform the procedure. Patients should be given a brief explanation of the procedure, including any nonroutine techniques that will be used, such as the additional site preparation performed when collecting blood cultures. They should not be told that the procedure will be painless.

Patients often question the phlebotomist about what tests are being performed or why their blood is being drawn so frequently. The best policy is to politely suggest that they ask their health-care provider these questions. Even listing the names of tests can cause problems, because many medical books and Internet sites are available to the general public. The patient may reach erroneous conclusions, because many tests have several diagnostic purposes; or the patient may misunderstand the test name and look up an inappropriate test associated with a very severe condition.

When patients are having repeated bedside tests performed such as glucose testing, the patient may ask for the result. It is often written on a paper in the room visible to the patient. Confirm the institutional procedure before telling the patient test results.

The phlebotomist's conversation with the patient should include verifying that the appropriate pretest preparation such as fasting or abstaining from medications has occurred. When these procedures have

not been followed, this problem should be reported to the nurse before drawing the blood. If the sample is still required, the irregular condition, such as "not fasting," should be written on the requisition form and the sample. Ask the patient if he or she has a latex sensitivity. Use nonlatex supplies where appropriate. Other preexamination variables will be discussed in Chapter 10.

 Technical Tip 9-4. When necessary, writing down information or using sign language or an interpreter will help the patient to understand the procedure and to give permission for the blood collection.

 Technical Tip 9-5. Good verbal, listening, and nonverbal skills are very important for patient reassurance.

Positioning the Patient

When patient identification is completed, the patient must be positioned conveniently and safely for the procedure. Always ask the patient if he or she is allergic to latex.

Blood should never be drawn from a patient who is in a standing position. Outpatients are seated or reclined at a drawing station as shown in Figure 9-7. In some drawing stations, the movable arm serves the dual purposes of providing a solid surface for the patient's arm and preventing a patient who faints from falling out of the chair. The patient's arm should be firmly supported and extended downward in a straight line, allowing the tubes to fill from the bottom up to prevent

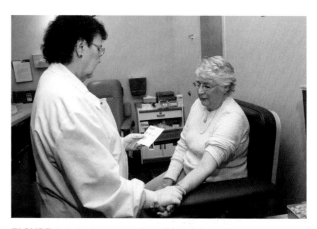

FIGURE 9-7 Patient seated in a blood drawing chair.

reflux and anticoagulant carryover between tubes. Asking the patient to make a fist with the hand of the arm not being used and placing it behind the elbow will provide support and make the vein easier to locate (Fig. 9-8). Phlebotomists should always be alert for any changes in the patient's condition while the procedure is being performed. Some patients know that they experience difficulties during venipuncture, and provisions should be made to allow them to lie down for the procedure.

When collecting a blood sample in a home setting, the patient must be seated in a chair with armrests and the patient's arm placed on a hard surface. A sofa or bed may be used if the patient is anxious or has had previous difficulties during venipuncture.

 Technical Tip 9-6. When supporting the patient's arm, do not hyperextend the elbow. This may make vein palpation difficult. Sometimes bending the elbow very slightly may aid in vein palpation.

It may be necessary to move a hospitalized patient slightly to make the arm more accessible, or to place a pillow or towel under the patient's arm for better support and to position the arm in a straight line downward. If bed rails are lowered, they must always be returned to the raised position before the phlebotomist leaves the room.

Patients should remove any objects such as food, drink, gum, or a thermometer from their mouths before performance of the venipuncture. Any foreign object in the mouth could cause choking.

EQUIPMENT SELECTION

Before approaching the patient for the actual venipuncture, the phlebotomist should collect all necessary supplies (including collection equipment, antiseptic pads, gauze, bandages, and needle disposal system) and place them close to the patient (Fig. 9-9). The blood collection tray should not be placed on the bed or on the patient's eating table. Place supplies on the same side as your free hand during blood collection to avoid reaching across the patient and causing unnecessary movement of the needle in the patient's vein. The requisition form is re-examined, and the appropriate blood collection system (evacuated tube system, syringe, or winged blood collection set) and the number and type of collection tubes are selected taking into consideration the age of the patient and the amount of blood to be collected. Check the expiration date on each tube and discard any tube that is expired.

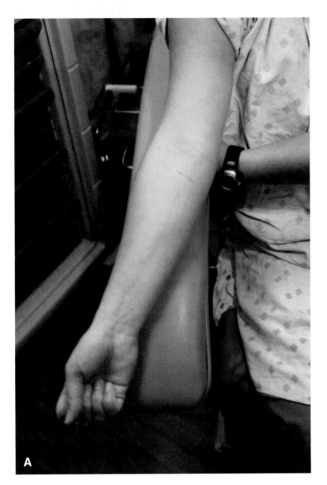

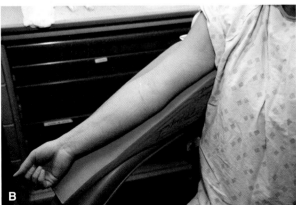

FIGURE 9-8 Positioning the patient's arm. A, Using the patient's fist. B, Using a phlebotomy wedge.

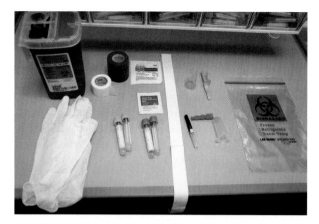

FIGURE 9-9 Venipuncture collection equipment.

Place the tubes in the correct order for sample collection, and have additional tubes readily available for possible use during the procedure. It is not uncommon to find an evacuated tube that does not contain the necessary amount of vacuum to collect a full tube of blood. Accidentally pushing a tube past the indicator mark on the holder before the vein is entered also results in loss of vacuum.

WASH HANDS AND APPLY GLOVES

In front of the patient, the phlebotomist should wash his or her hands using the procedure described in Chapter 4 and apply clean gloves. The gloves are pulled over the cuffs of protective clothing. Gloves are changed between each patient.

Safety Tip 9-2. Occupational Safety and Health Administration (OSHA) regulations mandate that gloves be worn when performing a venipuncture procedure.

Technical Tip 9-7. Patients are often reassured that proper safety measures are being followed when gloves are donned in their presence.

 TOURNIQUET APPLICATION

The tourniquet serves two functions in the venipuncture procedure. By impeding venous, but not arterial, blood flow, the tourniquet causes blood to accumulate in the veins making them more easily located and provides a larger amount of blood for collection. Use of a tourniquet can alter some test results by increasing the ratio of cellular elements to plasma (**hemoconcentration**) and by causing **hemolysis.** Therefore, the maximum amount of time the tourniquet should remain in place is 1 minute. This requires that the tourniquet be applied twice during the venipuncture procedure, first when vein selection is being made and then immediately before the puncture is performed. When the tourniquet is used during vein selection, the CLSI recommends that it should be released for 2 minutes before being reapplied.

The tourniquet should be placed on the arm 3 to 4 inches above the venipuncture site. Application of the commonly used flat vinyl or latex strip requires practice to develop a smooth technique and can be difficult if properly fitting gloves are not worn. Procedure 9-1 shows the technique used with vinyl and latex strip tourniquets. To achieve adequate pressure, both sides of the tourniquet must be grasped near the patient's arm, and while maintaining tension, the left side is tucked under the right side. The loop formed should face downward toward the patient's antecubital area, and the free end should be away from the venipuncture area but in a position that allows it to be easily pulled to release the pressure. Left-handed persons would reverse this procedure. The tourniquet should be flat around the arm and not rolled or twisted.

Tourniquets that are folded or applied too tightly are uncomfortable for the patient and may obstruct blood flow to the area. The appearance of small, reddish discolorations (**petechiae**) on the patient's arm, blanching of the skin around the tourniquet, and the inability to feel a radial pulse are indications of a tourniquet that is tied too tightly.

Technical Tip 9-8. A tourniquet applied too close to the venipuncture site may cause the vein to collapse.

 Safety Tip 9-3. The use of disposable one-time use tourniquets is advised, although not required, as part of good infection control practice to avoid health-care acquired infections (HAIs) for patients.

EQUIPMENT:

Vinyl or latex strip tourniquet

PROCEDURE:

Step 1. Position the vinyl or latex strip 3 to 4 inches above the venipuncture site. Avoid areas with a skin lesion or apply the tourniquet over the patient's gown.

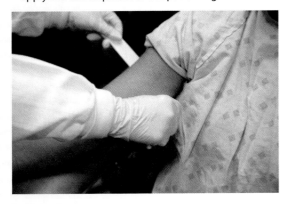

Step 2. Grasp both sides of the tourniquet and, while maintaining tension, cross the tourniquet over the patient's arm.

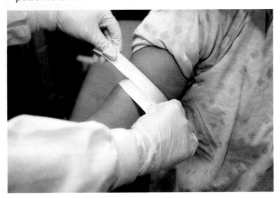

Step 3. Hold both ends between the thumb and forefinger of one hand close to the arm.

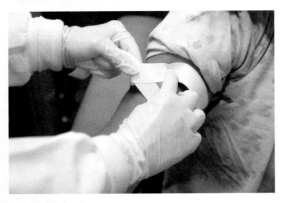

Step 4. Tuck a portion of the left side under the right side to make a partial loop facing the antecubital area.

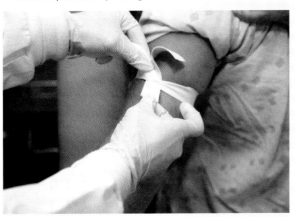

Step 5. A properly applied tourniquet will have the ends pointing up away from the venipuncture site.

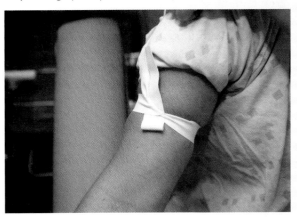

Step 6. Pull the end of the loop to release the tourniquet with one hand. The tourniquet should only be on for 1 minute.

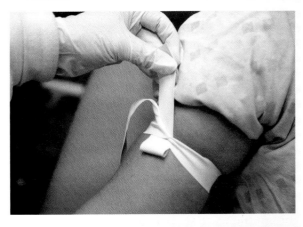

SITE SELECTION

The preferred site for venipuncture is the ***antecubital fossa*** located anterior and below the bend of the elbow. As shown in Figure 9-10, three major veins—the ***median cubital,*** the ***cephalic,*** and the ***basilic***—are located in this area and, in most patients, at least one of these veins can be easily located. Vein patterns vary among individuals. The most often seen arrangement of veins in the antecubital fossa are referred to as the "H-shaped" and "M-shaped" patterns. The H pattern includes the cephalic, median cubital, and basilic veins in a pattern that looks like a slanted H. The most prominent veins in the M pattern are the cephalic, median cephalic, median basilic, and basilic veins. The H-shaped pattern is seen in approximately 70 percent of the population (Fig. 9-11). Notice that the veins continue down the forearm to the wrist area; however, in these areas, they become smaller and less well anchored, and punctures are more painful to the patient. Small prominent veins are also located in the back of the hand (Fig. 9-12). When necessary, these veins can be used for venipuncture, but they may require a smaller needle or winged blood collection set (Fig. 9-13). The veins of the lower arm and hand are also the preferred site for administering IV fluids because they allow the patient more arm flexibility. Frequent venipuncture in these veins could make them unsuitable for IV use. Some institutions have special ID bands that indicate the restricted use of veins being used for other procedures. Veins on the underside of the wrist must not be used for venipuncture, because of the chance of accidentally puncturing arteries, nerves, or tendons.

 Safety Tip 9-4. Veins on the underside of the wrist must never be used according to the CLSI standard.

Median Cubital Vein

Of the three veins located in the antecubital area, the median cubital is the vein of choice because it is large and does not tend to move when the needle is inserted. It is often closer to the surface of the skin, more isolated from underlying structures, and the least painful to puncture as there are fewer nerve endings in this area.

Cephalic Vein

The cephalic vein located on the thumb side of the arm is usually more difficult to locate, except possibly in larger patients, and has more tendencies to move. The cephalic vein should be the second choice if the median cubital is inaccessible in both arms.

 Technical Tip 9-9. Because the cephalic vein is closer to the surface, there is the possibility of a blood spurt when the needle is inserted in to the vein. This often is controlled by decreasing the angle of needle insertion to 15 degrees.

Basilic Vein

The basilic vein is located on the inner edge of the antecubital fossa near the median nerve and brachial artery. The basilic vein is the least firmly anchored; therefore, it has a tendency to "roll" and hematoma formation is more likely. The basilic vein should be used as the last choice because the median nerve and brachial artery are in close proximity to it, increasing the risk of permanent injury. Care must be taken not to accidentally puncture the brachial artery.

 Technical Tip 9-10. Use of the basilic vein is discouraged; however, if necessary, the CLSI standard recommends locating the brachial pulse before accessing the basilic vein.

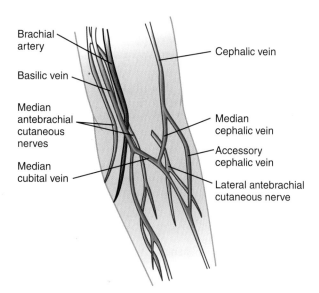

FIGURE 9-10 **The veins in the arm most often chosen for venipuncture.**

Brachial artery
Basilic vein
Median antebrachial cutaneous nerves
Median cubital vein
Cephalic vein
Median cephalic vein
Accessory cephalic vein
Lateral antebrachial cutaneous nerve

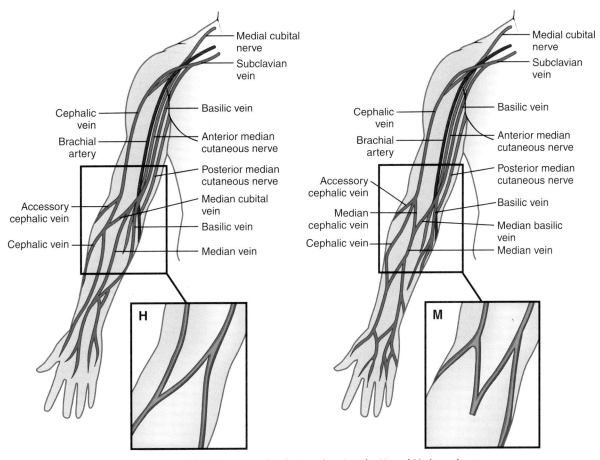

FIGURE 9-11 **Major antecubital veins showing the H- and M-shaped patterns.**

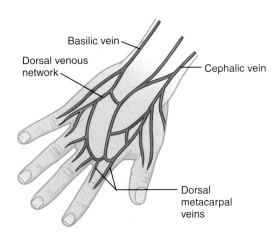

FIGURE 9-12 **Veins on the back of the hand and wrist.**

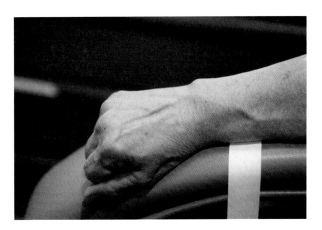

FIGURE 9-13 **Prominent hand and wrist veins.**

▶ *Technical Tip 9-11.* Using a syringe method for blood collection from the basilic vein offers more control over a "rolling" vein.

❗ **Safety Tip 9-5.** Collecting blood from the basilic vein has caused more complaints and legal actions against phlebotomists than any other vein.

Two routine steps in the venipuncture procedure aid the phlebotomist in locating a suitable vein. These steps are applying a tourniquet and asking the patient to clench his or her fist. Continuous clenching or pumping of the fist should not be encouraged because it will result in hemoconcentration and alter some test results. The difference in vein prominence before and after these procedures are used is usually remarkable, and phlebotomists examining an arm before they have been done should not become overly concerned about finding a vein. Most phlebotomists prefer to apply the tourniquet before examining the arm. As discussed earlier, the tourniquet can only be applied for 1 minute; therefore, after the vein is located, the tourniquet is removed while the site is being cleansed and is reapplied immediately before the venipuncture.

▶ *Technical Tip 9-12.* Patients often think they are helping by pumping their fists, because this is an acceptable practice when donating blood. In contrast to laboratory samples, a donated unit of blood is even better when it is hemoconcentrated.

📋 *Preexamination Consideration 9-5.* Asking the patient to pump his or her fist may cause elevated potassium levels in the sample. Based on those erroneous results, the patient's medication might be changed in a way that would adversely affect the patient.

Veins are located by sight and by touch (referred to as *palpation*). The ability to feel a vein is much more important than the ability to see a vein—a concept that is often difficult for beginning phlebotomists to accept. Palpation is usually performed using the tip of the index finger of the nondominant hand to probe the antecubital area with a pushing motion rather than a stroking motion. Feel for the vein in both a vertical and horizontal direction. The pressure applied by palpating locates deep veins; distinguishes veins, which feel like spongy, resilient, tube-like structures, from rigid tendon cords; and differentiates veins from arteries, which produce a pulse (Fig. 9-14). The thumb should not be used to palpate because it has a pulse beat.

Turning the arm slightly helps distinguish veins from other structures. Select a vein that is easily palpated and large enough to support good blood flow. Once an acceptable vein is located, palpation is used to determine the direction and depth of the vein to aid the phlebotomist during needle insertion. It is often helpful to find a visual reference for the selected vein, such as its location near a mole, freckle, or skin crease, to assist in relocating the vein after cleansing the site.

▶ *Technical Tip 9-13.* According to the CLSI standard, an attempt must have been made to locate the median cubital vein on both arms before considering other veins.

▶ *Technical Tip 9-14.* Using the nondominant hand routinely for palpation may be helpful when additional palpation is required immediately before performing the puncture.

▶ *Technical Tip 9-15.* Often, a patient has veins that are more prominent in the dominant arm.

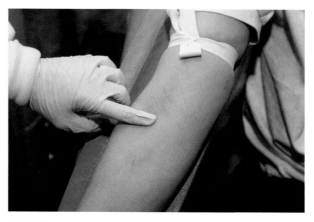

FIGURE 9-14 Palpating for a vein using the fingers, not the thumb.

CLEANSING THE SITE

When an appropriate vein has been located, the tourniquet is released and the area cleansed using a 70 percent isopropyl alcohol prep pad to prevent bacterial contamination of either the patient or the sample. Cleansing is performed with a circular motion, starting at the inside of the venipuncture site and working outward in widening concentric circles about 2 to 3 inches. Repeat this procedure using a new alcohol pad for particularly dirty skin. For maximum bacteriostatic action to occur, the alcohol should be allowed to dry for 30 to 60 seconds on the patient's arm rather than being wiped off with a gauze pad. The drying process helps kill the bacteria. Performing a venipuncture before the alcohol has dried will cause a stinging sensation for the patient and may hemolyze the sample. Do not reintroduce microbial contaminants by blowing on the site, fanning the area, or drying the area with nonsterile gauze.

 Preexamination Consideration 9-6.
Alcohol contamination may cause sample hemolysis affecting the integrity of the sample.

 Technical Tip 9-16. Patients are quick to complain about a painful venipuncture. The stinging sensation caused by undry alcohol is a frequent, yet easily avoided, cause of complaints.

ASSEMBLY OF PUNCTURE EQUIPMENT

While the alcohol is drying, the phlebotomist can make a final survey of the supplies at hand to be sure everything required for the procedure is present and can then assemble the equipment.

 Technical Tip 9-17. Place assembled venipuncture equipment within easy reach; however, do not place the collection tray on the patient's bed.

The stopper-puncturing end of the double-ended evacuated tube needle is screwed into the needle holder. The needle and holder may come preassembled by the manufacturer. The sterile cap is not removed from the other end of the needle. The first tube to be collected can be inserted into the needle holder up to the designated mark. After the tube is pushed up to the mark, it may retract slightly when pressure is released. This is acceptable.

Visual examination cannot detect defective evacuated tubes; therefore, extra tubes should be near at hand. It is not uncommon for the vacuum in a tube to be lost.

PERFORMING THE VENIPUNCTURE

Reapply the tourniquet, and confirm the puncture site. If necessary, cleanse the gloved palpating finger for additional vein palpation. Again, ask the patient to make a fist.

Examine the Needle

Immediately before entering the vein, the plastic cap of the needle is removed and the point of the needle is visually examined for any defects such as a non-pointed or rough (barbed) end. The needle is then positioned for entry into the vein with the bevel facing up.

Anchoring the Vein

Use the thumb of the nondominant hand to anchor the selected vein while inserting the needle (Fig. 9-15). Place the thumb 1 or 2 inches below and slightly to the left of the insertion site and the four fingers on the back of the arm and pull the skin taut. This will keep

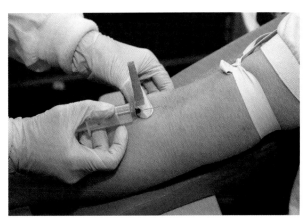

FIGURE 9-15 **Placement of the fingers when anchoring the vein.**

the skin tight, which will help prevent the vein from slipping to the side when the needle enters. A vein that moves to the side is said to have "rolled." Patients often state that they have "rolling veins"; however, all veins will roll if they are not properly anchored. These patients are really saying that they have had blood drawn by phlebotomists who were not anchoring the veins well enough. As mentioned previously, the median cubital vein is the easiest to anchor and the basilic vein the most difficult. In general, the closer a vein is to the surface, the more likely it is to roll. Anchor hand veins by having the patient make a fist or grasp the end of a table or drawing chair arm. Pull the skin tightly over the knuckles with the thumb of the nondominant hand (Fig. 9-16).

> **Safety Tip 9-6.** Anchoring the vein above and below the site using the thumb and index finger is not an acceptable technique, because sudden patient movement could cause the index finger to be punctured.

Inserting the Needle

The evacuated tube holder or syringe is held securely in the dominant hand with the thumb on top close to the needle hub and the remaining fingers below the holder. When the vein is securely anchored, align the needle with the vein and insert it, bevel up, at an angle of 15 to 30 degrees depending on the depth of the vein. This should be done in a smooth movement so the patient feels the stick only briefly. The phlebotomist will

notice a feeling of lessening of resistance to the needle movement when the vein has been entered. After insertion is made, the fingers are braced against the patient's arm to provide stability while tubes are being changed in the holder, or the plunger of the syringe is being pulled back.

 Technical Tip 9-18. Tell the patient that "there will be a little stick" before needle insertion to alert the patient to hold very still.

 Technical Tip 9-19. Entering the vein too slowly is more painful for the patient and may cause a spurt of blood to appear at the venipuncture site, which can be disconcerting for both phlebotomist and patient.

Filling the Tubes

Once the vein has been entered, the hand anchoring the vein can be moved and used to push the evacuated tube completely into the holder. Use the thumb to push the tube onto the back of the evacuated tube needle, while the index and middle fingers grasp the flared ends of the holder. Blood should begin to flow into the tube and the fist and tourniquet can be released, although if the procedure does not last more than 1 minute, the tourniquet can be left on until the last tube is filled. Some phlebotomists prefer to change hands at this point so that the dominant hand is free for performing the remaining tasks. This method of operating is usually better suited for use by experienced phlebotomists because holding the needle steady in the patient's vein is often difficult for beginners.

The hand used to hold the needle assembly should remain braced on the patient's arm. This is of particular importance when evacuated tubes are being inserted or removed from the holder, because a certain amount of resistance is encountered and can cause the needle to be pushed through or pulled out of the vein. Tubes should be gently twisted on and off the puncturing needle using the flared ends of the holder as an additional brace.

 Technical Tip 9-20. Pulling up or pressing down on the needle while it is in the vein can cause pain to the patient or a hematoma formation if blood leaks from the enlarged hole.

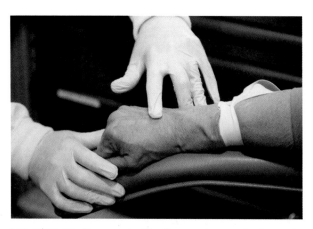

FIGURE 9-16 Placement of the fingers when anchoring and palpating a hand vein.

To prevent any chance of blood refluxing back into the needle, tubes should be held at a downward angle while they are being filled and have slight pressure applied to them. Be sure to follow the prescribed order of draw when multiple tubes are being collected, and allow the tubes to fill completely before removing them. Gentle inversion of the evacuated tubes for three to eight times, depending on the type of tube, should be done as soon as the tube is removed, before another tube is placed in the assembly. The few seconds that this procedure requires does not cause additional discomfort to the patient and ensures that the sample will be acceptable.

When the last tube has been filled, it is removed from the assembly and mixed before completing the procedure. Failure to remove the evacuated tube before removing the needle causes blood to drip from the end of the needle, resulting in unnecessary contamination and possible damage to the patient's clothes.

▶ *Technical Tip 9-21.* Vigorous mixing of the sample can cause hemolysis and make the sample unacceptable for testing.

▶ *Technical Tip 9-22.* Poor mixing may produce a sample with microclots that could yield erroneous test results.

▶ *Technical Tip 9-23.* Allow tubes to fill until the vacuum is exhausted to ensure the correct blood-to-anticoagulant ratio.

REMOVAL OF THE NEEDLE

Before removing the needle, remove the tourniquet by pulling on the free end and tell the patient to relax his or her hand. Failure to remove the tourniquet before removing the needle may produce a bruise (*hematoma*).

Activate the needle safety device if it is designed to function while the needle is the vein. Place folded gauze over the venipuncture site and withdraw the needle in a smooth swift motion and activate the safety device if it is designed to function after the needle is removed from the vein. Apply pressure to the site as soon as the needle is withdrawn. Do not apply pressure while the needle is still in the vein.

To prevent blood from leaking into the surrounding tissue and producing a hematoma, pressure must be applied until the bleeding has stopped, usually about 2 to 3 minutes. The arm should be held in a raised, outstretched position. Bending the elbow to apply pressure allows blood to leak more easily into the tissue, causing a hematoma. A capable patient can be asked to apply the pressure, thereby freeing the phlebotomist to dispose of the used needle and label the sample tubes. If this is not possible, the phlebotomist must apply the pressure and perform the other tasks after the bleeding has stopped.

DISPOSAL OF THE NEEDLE

On completion of the venipuncture, the first thing the phlebotomist must do is dispose of the contaminated needle and holder in an acceptable sharps container conveniently located near the patient. As discussed in Chapter 4, the method by which this is done will depend on the type of disposal equipment selected by the institution. Under no circumstance should the needle be bent, cut, placed on a counter or bed, or manually recapped.

▶ *Technical Tip 9-24.* Follow manufacturer's guidelines when activating needle safety devices. Some are activated when the needle is in the vein and some must be activated immediately upon removal of the needle from the vein.

LABELING THE TUBES

Tubes are labeled by writing with an indelible pen on the attached label or by applying a computer-generated label that may also contain a designated bar code. Tubes must be labeled at the time of collection, before leaving the patient's room or before accepting another outpatient requisition. Tubes must be labeled after the sample has been collected to prevent confusion of samples when additional tubes are needed because of lost vacuum or a re-stick is necessary or when more than one patient is having blood drawn. All preprinted labels must be carefully checked with the patient's identification before being attached to the sample. Mislabeled samples, just like misidentified patients, can result in serious patient harm.

Information on the sample label must include the following:

- Patient's name and identification number
- Date and time of collection
- Phlebotomist's initials

Additional information may be present on computer-generated labels. Samples for the blood bank may require an additional label obtained from the patient's blood bank ID band.

After labeling the tubes and before leaving the patient, the tubes must be compared with the patient's ID band. For an outpatient, verify correct labeling of the tube by showing the labeled tube to the patient and verbally asking the patient to confirm the name on the label.

Samples sent to the lab via a pneumatic tube system are placed in a biohazard bag. Samples requiring special handling, such as cooling or warming, are placed in the appropriate container when labeling is complete.

BANDAGING THE PATIENT'S ARM

Bleeding at the venipuncture site should stop within 5 minutes. Before applying the adhesive bandage, the phlebotomist should examine the patient's arm to be sure the bleeding has stopped. Paper tape should be used for patients allergic to adhesive bandages. For additional pressure, an adhesive bandage or tape is applied over a folded gauze square. A self-adhering gauze-like material (Coban) may be placed over the folded gauze square and wrapped around the arm for patients with fragile skin or when additional pressure is needed. The patient should be instructed to remove the bandage within an hour and to avoid using the arm to carry heavy objects during that period.

 Technical Tip 9-25. The practice of quickly applying tape over the gauze without checking the puncture site frequently produces a hematoma.

 Safety Tip 9-7. The CLSI standard H3-A6 recommends that the phlebotomist observe for hematoma formation by releasing pressure to the puncture and visually observing for subcutaneous bleeding BEFORE applying a bandage. Hematoma formation can place pressure on the nerves and cause a disabling compression nerve injury.

DISPOSING OF USED SUPPLIES

Before leaving the patient's room, the phlebotomist disposes of all contaminated supplies such as alcohol pads and gauze in a biohazard container and needle caps and paper in the regular waste container, removes gloves and disposes of them in the biohazard container, and washes his or her hands.

LEAVING THE PATIENT

Return the bed and bed rails to the original position if they have been moved. Failure to replace bed rails that results in patient injury can result in legal action.

In the outpatient setting, patients can be excused when the arm is bandaged and the tubes are labeled. If patients have been fasting and no more procedures are scheduled, they should be instructed to eat. Before calling the next patient, the phlebotomist cleans up the area as described earlier. In both the inpatient and outpatient settings, patients should be thanked for their cooperation.

COMPLETING THE VENIPUNCTURE PROCEDURE

The venipuncture procedure is complete when the sample is delivered to the laboratory in satisfactory condition and all appropriate paperwork has been completed. These procedures vary depending on institutional protocol and the types of samples collected. The phlebotomist needs to be familiar with procedures such as verifying collection in the computer system, making entries in the logbook, stamping the time of sample arrival in the laboratory on the requisition form, and informing the nursing station that the procedure has been completed.

Transporting Samples to the Laboratory

Deliver each sample to the laboratory as soon as possible. Follow procedures for samples requiring special handling, which is covered in the following chapters, and in stat situations. When possible, the phlebotomist should try to schedule patients so that a sample requiring special handling is collected last.

Use designated biohazard containers for transport, and securely attach the requisitions with the sample when using the pneumatic tube system. Verify that the pneumatic tube has been sent before leaving.

Blood samples should be transported to the laboratory for processing in a timely manner. The stability of analytes varies greatly, as do the accepted methods of preservation. This is why delivery to the laboratory or following laboratory prescribed sample-handling protocols is essential.

 Technical Tip 9-26. Gel separation tubes must always be stored and transported in an upright position to facilitate clotting and prevent hemolysis.

CLSI recommends centrifugation of clotted tubes and anticoagulated tubes and separation of the serum or plasma from the cells within 2 hours. Ideally, the sample should reach the laboratory within 45 minutes and be centrifuged on arrival. Tests most frequently affected by improper processing include glucose, potassium, and coagulation tests. Glycolysis caused by the use of glucose in cellular metabolism causes falsely lower glucose values. Hemolysis and leakage of intracellular potassium into the serum or plasma falsely elevates potassium results. Coagulation factors are destroyed in samples remaining at room temperature for extended periods of time. Appendix A summarizes the requirements of some routinely encountered analytes. The routine venipuncture procedure is illustrated in Procedure 9-2.

 Technical Tip 9-27. Verification of the sample collection recorded either into the computer or in a log book completes the collection process.

PROCEDURE 9-2 ✦ **Venipuncture Using an Evacuated Tube System**

EQUIPMENT:

Requisition form

Gloves

Tourniquet

70 percent isopropyl alcohol pad

Evacuated tube needle with safety device

Evacuated tube holder with safety device if the needle
does not have one

Evacuated tubes

2 × 2 gauze

Sharps container

Indelible pen

Bandage

Biohazard bag

PROCEDURE:

Step 1. Obtain and examine the requisition form.

Step 2. Greet and reassure the patient and explain the
procedure to be performed.

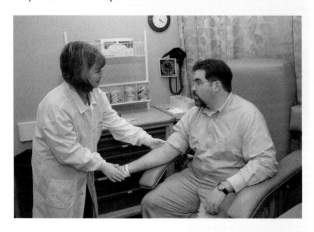

Step 3. Identify the patient verbally by having him or her
state both the first name and last name and compare
the information on the patient's ID band with the
requisition form.

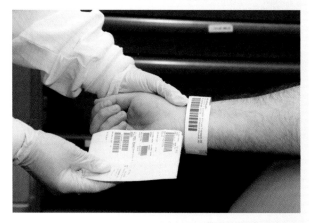

PROCEDURE 9-2 ✦ **Venipuncture Using an Evacuated Tube System** (Continued)

Step 4. Verify if the patient has fasted, has allergies to latex, or has had previous problems with venipuncture.

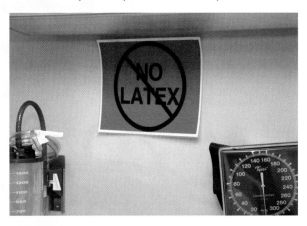

Step 5. Select correct tubes and equipment for the procedure. Have extra tubes available.

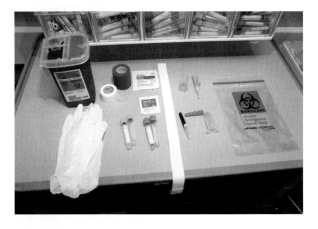

Step 6. Wash hands and apply gloves.

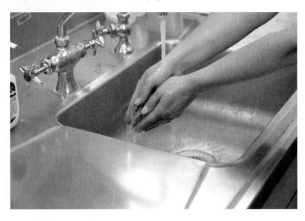

Step 7. Position the patient's arm slightly bent in a downward position so that the tubes fill from the bottom up. Do not allow blood to touch the stopper-puncturing needle. Do not let the patient hyperextend the arm. Ask the patient to make a fist.

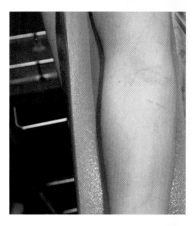

Step 8. Apply the tourniquet 3 to 4 inches above the antecubital fossa. Palpate the area in a vertical and horizontal direction to locate a large vein and to determine the depth, direction, and size. The median cubital is the vein of choice followed by the cephalic vein. The basilic vein should be avoided if possible. Remove the tourniquet and have the patient open his or her fist.

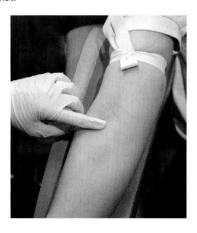

Continued

PROCEDURE 9-2 ✦ **Venipuncture Using an Evacuated Tube System** (Continued)

Step 9. Clean the site with 70 percent isopropyl alcohol in concentric circles moving outward and allow it to air dry.

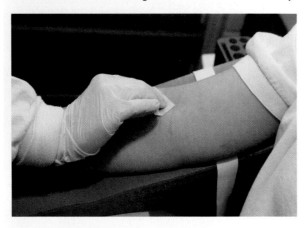

Step 10. Assemble the equipment while the alcohol is drying. Attach the multisample needle to the holder.

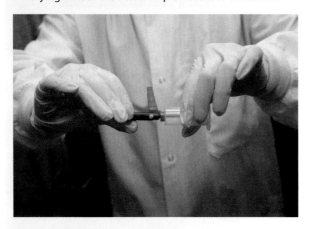

Step 11. Insert the tube into the holder up to the tube advancement mark.

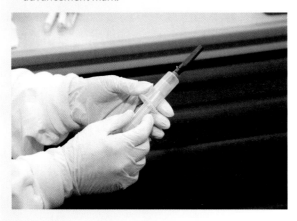

Step 12. Reapply the tourniquet. Do not touch the puncture site with an unclean finger. Ask the patient to remake a fist. Patient should be instructed not to "pump" or "continuously clench" the fist to prevent hemoconcentration.

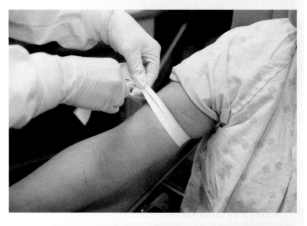

Step 13. Remove the plastic needle cap and examine the needle for defects such as nonpointed or barbed ends.

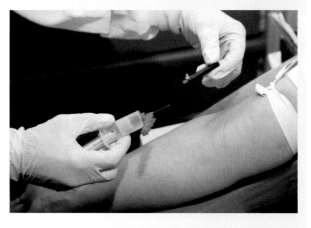

PROCEDURE 9-2 ✦ **Venipuncture Using an Evacuated Tube System** (Continued)

Step 14. Anchor the vein by placing the thumb of the nondominant hand 1 to 2 inches below the site and pulling the skin taut.

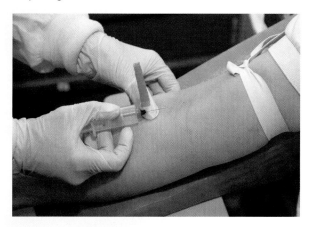

Step 15. Grasp the assembled needle and tube holder using your dominant hand with the thumb on the top near the hub and your other fingers beneath. Smoothly insert the needle into the vein at a 15- to 30-degree angle with the bevel up until you feel a lessening of resistance. Brace the fingers against the arm to prevent movement of the needle when changing tubes.

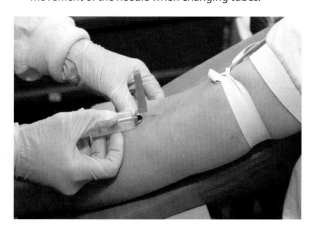

Step 16. Using the thumb, advance the tube onto the evacuated tube needle, while the index and middle fingers grasp the flared ends of the holder.

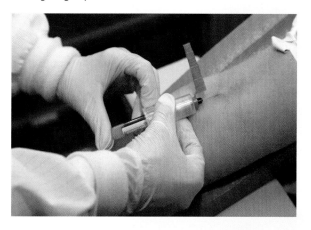

Step 17. When blood flows into the tube, release the tourniquet, and ask the patient to open the fist.

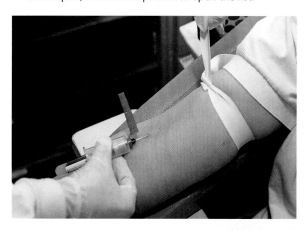

Continued

[handwritten note:] ※ once the last tube is although filled up, take off tourneaguet, tube, needle

PROCEDURE 9-2 ✦ **Venipuncture Using an Evacuated Tube System** (Continued)

Step 18. Gently remove the tube when the blood stops flowing into it. Gently invert anticoagulated tubes promptly. Insert the next tube using the correct order of draw. Fill tubes completely.

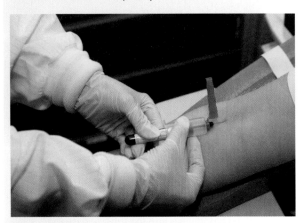

Step 19. Remove the last tube collected from the holder and gently invert.

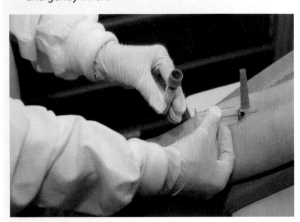

Step 20. Cover the puncture site with clean gauze. Remove the needle smoothly and apply pressure or ask the patient to apply pressure.

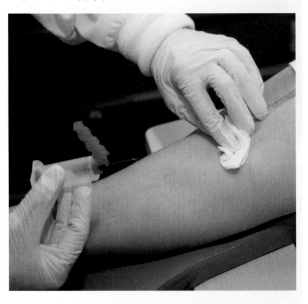

Step 21. Activate the safety device.

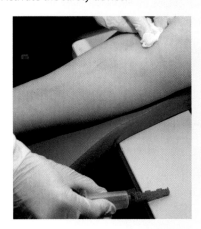

PROCEDURE 9-2 ✦ **Venipuncture Using an Evacuated Tube System** (Continued)

Step 22. Dispose the needle/holder assembly with the safety device activated into the sharps container.

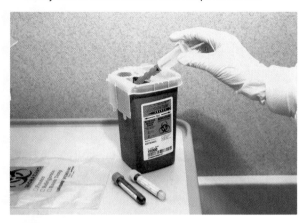

Step 23. Label the tubes before leaving the patient and verify identification with the patient ID band or verbally with an outpatient. Observe any special handling procedures. Complete paperwork.

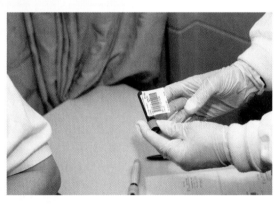

Step 24. Examine the puncture site and apply bandage. Place bandage over folded gauze for additional pressure.

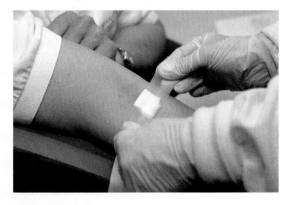

Step 25. Prepare sample and requisition for transportation to the laboratory. Dispose of used supplies.

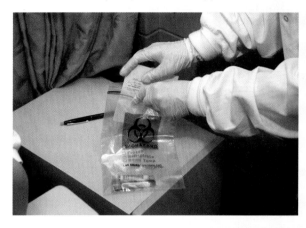

Step 26. Thank the patient, remove gloves, and wash hands.

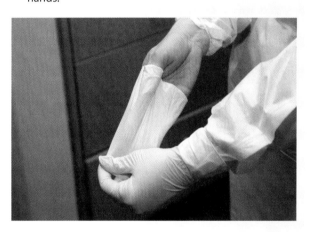

Key Points

- The required information on a requisition form includes the patient's name and identification number, patient's date of birth, patient's location, ordering health-care provider's name, tests requested, requested date and time of sample collection, number and type of collection tubes, status of sample, special collection information, special patient information, and billing information.

- The phlebotomist should introduce himself or herself to the patient, say that he or she is from the laboratory, and explain that he or she will be collecting a blood sample for a test that the patient's health-care provider has requested. The phlebotomist must obtain permission from the patient before collecting the sample.

- Patient identification is the most important step in the venipuncture procedure. The JC, CAP, and CLSI require a minimum of two identifiers. Identifiers may include comparing the patient's name and ID number on the requisition form with the patient's ID band and having the patient verbally state his or her first and last name and date of birth.

- The patient must be seated or reclining with the arm in a downward position for blood collection. Verify that the pretest preparation such as fasting and abstaining from medications has occurred. Ask the patient if he or she has a latex sensitivity. Use nonlatex supplies when appropriate.

- Choose the appropriate blood collection system (evacuated tube systems [ETS], syringe, or winged blood collection set) and the number and type of collection tubes and other supplies, taking into consideration the age of the patient and the amount of blood to be collected.

- The three major veins for venipuncture are the median cubital, the cephalic, and the basilic. The median cubital is the vein of choice for venipuncture, followed by the cephalic vein located on the thumb side, and, lastly, the basilic vein located on the inner edge of the antecubital fossa near the median nerve and brachial artery. The dorsal veins of the hand may be used.

- Tourniquets are placed snugly on the arm 3 to 4 inches above the venipuncture site with the loop facing toward the patient's antecubital area and the free end facing up away from the venipuncture area in a position that allows it to be easily pulled to release the pressure. Leaving the tourniquet on for longer than 1 minute results in hemoconcentration that can adversely affect test results.

- Palpation is performed using the tip of the index finger of the nondominant hand to probe the antecubital area with a pushing motion rather than a stroking motion to determine the size, depth, and direction of the vein. The area is felt in both a vertical and horizontal direction to differentiate veins, which feel bouncy and resilient, from rigid tendon cords and from arteries that produce a pulse. The thumb should not be used to palpate because it has a pulse beat.

- The area is cleansed with 70 percent isopropyl alcohol in a circular motion, starting at the inside of the venipuncture site and working outward in widening concentric circles about 2 to 3 inches and allowed to dry for 30 to 60 seconds. Confirm the alcohol has dried before venipuncture to avoid sample hemolysis and a stinging sensation for the patient.

- The phlebotomist examines the needle, anchors the vein 2 to 3 inches below the site with the thumb of the nondominant hand, inserts the needle at a 15- to 30-degree angle, collects the blood tubes in the correct order, removes the tourniquet, removes the last tube in the holder, covers the needle with gauze, removes needle and activates the safety feature, applies pressure to the site, and applies a bandage when bleeding has stopped.

- Contaminated needles and holders with safety feature activated are disposed in an acceptable sharps container conveniently located near the patient.

- Tubes are labeled at the time of collection—before leaving the patient's room or before accepting another outpatient requisition—with the patient's name, ID number, date, time, and initials of the phlebotomist.

- Samples must be delivered to the laboratory in a timely manner because some analytes are affected by glycolysis (glucose) or hemolysis (potassium). CLSI recommends centrifugation of clotted tubes and anticoagulated tubes and separation of the serum or plasma from the cells within 2 hours.

BIBLIOGRAPHY

CLSI. Procedures for Collection of Diagnostic Blood Specimens by Venipuncture; Approved Standard, ed. 6. CLSI document H3-A6. Clinical and Laboratory Standards Institute, 2007, Wayne, PA.

CLSI. Procedures for the Handling and Processing of Blood Specimens for Common Laboratory Tests; Approved Guideline, ed 4. CLSI document H18-A4. Clinical and Laboratory Standards Institute, 2010, Wayne, PA.

Study Questions

1. What information is required on a requisition form?
   a. patient's first and last name
   b. patient's identification number
   c. the test requested
   d. all of the above

2. Before you draw a blood sample from a patient you must always:
   a. check the patient's ID number and name on the wristband
   b. ask the patient his or her first and last name
   c. tell the patient what type of blood test that you are going to collect
   d. a and b
   e. all of the above

3. The maximum length of time the tourniquet should be applied is:
   a. 1 minute
   b. 3 minutes
   c. 5 minutes
   d. 10 minutes

4. The vein of choice for venipuncture is the:
   a. basilic
   b. cephalic
   c. median cubital
   d. radial

5. A properly tied tourniquet:
   a. permits arterial flow and blocks venous flow
   b. blocks arterial and venous flow
   c. prevents backflow
   d. permits venous flow and blocks arterial flow

6. Correct palpation of a vein includes all of the following **EXCEPT:**
   a. determining the depth of the vein
   b. detecting a pulse using the thumb
   c. determining the direction of the vein
   d. probing with the index finger

7. Failure to allow the alcohol to dry on the patient's arm after site cleansing can cause all of the following **EXCEPT:**
   a. increased bacteriostatic action
   b. a stinging sensation for the patient
   c. a possible unsterile site
   d. sample hemolysis

8. The venipuncture step of primary importance to prevent rolling veins is:
   a. tightly applying the tourniquet
   b. selecting the median cubital vein
   c. using a 23-gauge needle
   d. anchoring the vein while inserting the needle

9. The needle is inserted into the vein:
   a. bevel up at a 45- to 50-degree angle
   b. bevel up at a 15- to 30-degree angle
   c. bevel down at a 15- to 30-degree angle
   d. bevel down at a 45- to 50-degree angle

10. Prior to bandaging the puncture site, the phlebotomist should:
    a. thank the patient
    b. instruct a fasting patient to eat
    c. examine the site for bleeding
    d. apply pressure for at least 5 minutes

Clinical Situations

1 A phlebotomist enters a patient's room. The phlebotomist asks, "Are you Sandra Jones?" The patient answers, "Yes." The phlebotomist applies the tourniquet, selects a vein, assembles the equipment, labels the tubes, cleanses the site, blows on the site to dry the alcohol, and performs the venipuncture.

   a. What is wrong with this situation?
   b. State three ways the patient or sample in this scenario could be affected.

2 An outpatient arrived at the Cancer Center with her requisition from the doctor's office. She handed the requisition to the secretary and waited for her turn to be called to have her blood drawn. The phlebotomist prepared to draw her blood using the computer labels handed to her by the secretary. The label indicated that a CBC was ordered and the phlebotomist prepared her equipment. The phlebotomist collected a lavender stopper tube and labeled the tube with the computer label. The outpatient was released. When the sample was received in the laboratory for testing, it was rejected because it was a lavender stopper tube instead of a green stopper tube. When the phlebotomist compared the information from the manual requisition form from the doctor's office with the computer labels, she noticed that on the manual requisition form a TSH test was ordered. The phlebotomist investigated the discrepancy with the secretary. The secretary said that she was used to ordering and printing CBC tests on cancer patients that she hadn't actually looked at the requisition. The patient had to be called to return to the lab for another sample collection.

   a. How could have this mistake been avoided?
   b. What assumptions were made by the secretary and phlebotomist?
   c. How will this affect patient treatment?
   d. What might the patient's reaction be to find out that she had to have another blood collection?

3 A phlebotomist is assigned to the pre-op, post-op, and ED. She collected a light blue stopper tube and a plasma separator tube (PST) on the patient in post-op and then gets called to the ED for a stat collection and then for several more pre-op patients. The phlebotomist forgot about the sample she drew at 7 a.m. in post-op and it is now 10 a.m.

   a. Name two tests that will have falsely decreased values.
   b. Name a test that will have a falsely increased value.
   c. What is the recommended time frame for delivering samples to the laboratory?

Evaluation of Tourniquet Application and Vein Selection Competency

RATING SYSTEM
2 = Satisfactorily Performed,   **1** = Needs Improvement,   **0** = Incorrect/Did Not Perform

_____   1.   Positions arm correctly for vein selection

_____   2.   Selects appropriate tourniquet application site

_____   3.   Places tourniquet in flat position behind arm

_____   4.   Smoothly positions hands when crossing and tucking tourniquet

_____   5.   Fastens tourniquet at appropriate tightness

_____   6.   Tourniquet is not folded into arm

_____   7.   Loop and loose end do not interfere with puncture site

_____   8.   Asks patient to clench fist

_____   9.   Selects antecubital area to palpate

_____ 10.   Performs palpation using correct fingers

_____ 11.   Palpates entire area or both arms if necessary

_____ 12.   Checks size, depth, and direction of veins

_____ 13.   Removes tourniquet smoothly

_____ 14.   Removes tourniquet in a timely manner

TOTAL POINTS _____

MAXIMUM POINTS = 28

Comments:

Evaluation of Venipuncture Competency Using an Evacuated Tube Competency

RATING SYSTEM
2 = Satisfactorily Performed,   **1** = Needs Improvement,   **0** = Incorrect/Did Not Perform

_____ 1. Examines requisition form

_____ 2. Greets patient and states procedure to be done

_____ 3. Identifies patient verbally

_____ 4. Examines patient's ID band

_____ 5. Compares requisition information with ID band

_____ 6. Selects correct tubes and equipment for procedure

_____ 7. Washes hands

_____ 8. Puts on gloves

_____ 9. Positions patient's arm

_____ 10. Applies tourniquet

_____ 11. Identifies vein by palpation

_____ 12. Releases tourniquet

_____ 13. Cleanses site and allows it to air dry

_____ 14. Assembles equipment

_____ 15. Reapplies tourniquet

_____ 16. Does not touch puncture site with unclean finger

_____ 17. Removes needle cap and examines the needle

_____ 18. Anchors vein below puncture site

_____ 19. Smoothly enters vein at appropriate angle with bevel up

_____ 20. Does not move needle when changing tubes

_____ 21. Collects tubes in correct order

_____ 22. Mixes tubes promptly

_____ 23. Fills tubes completely

_____ 24. Releases tourniquet within 1 minute

_____ 25. Removes last tube collected from holder

_____ 26. Covers puncture site with gauze

_____ 27. Removes the needle smoothly and applies pressure

_____ 28. Activates any safety feature

_____ 29. Disposes of the needle in sharps container with the safety device activated and attached to the holder

Evaluation of Venipuncture Competency Using an Evacuated Tube Competency (Continued)

_____ **30.** Labels tubes

_____ **31.** Confirms labeled tube to the patient ID band or has patient verify that the information is correct

_____ **32.** Examines puncture site

_____ **33.** Applies bandage

_____ **34.** Disposes of used supplies

_____ **35.** Removes gloves and washes hands

_____ **36.** Thanks patient

_____ **37.** Converses appropriately with patient during procedure

TOTAL POINTS _____

MAXIMUM POINTS = 74

Comments:

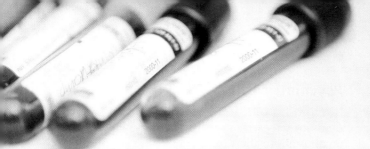

CHAPTER 10

Venipuncture Complications and Preexamination Variables

Learning Objectives

Upon completion of this chapter, the reader will be able to:

1. State the procedure for coordinating requisition forms, patient identification, and labeling of tubes for unidentified patients.
2. Discuss the procedures to follow when patients are asleep, not in their rooms, or being visited by a physician, member of the clergy, or friend.
3. Describe the identification procedure for patients that are too young, are cognitively impaired, or do not speak the language.
4. Describe the preexamination variables that affect laboratory tests.
5. Identify patient complications and describe methods to handle each situation.
6. Discuss the procedure to follow when a patient develops syncope during the venipuncture procedure.
7. State the policy regarding patients who refuse to have their blood drawn.
8. State the reasons why a tourniquet can only be applied for 1 minute.
9. Describe methods used to locate veins that are not prominent.
10. Describe conditions when it is not advisable to draw from veins in the legs or feet.
11. State reasons why blood should not be drawn from a hematoma, burned or scarred area, or an arm adjacent to a mastectomy.
12. State the procedure to follow when drawing blood from a patient with a fistula.
13. Describe the venipuncture procedure using a syringe, including equipment examination, technique for exchanging syringes, transfer of blood to evacuated tubes, and disposal of the equipment.
14. Describe the venipuncture procedure using a winged blood collection set, the technique involved, and disposal of equipment.
15. Identify technical complications and describes remedies for each situation.
16. State reasons why blood may not be immediately obtained from a venipuncture and describe the procedures to follow to obtain blood.
17. List 15 venipuncture errors that may produce hemolysis and the tests affected.
18. List nine causes of hematomas.
19. List nine reasons for rejecting a sample.

Key Terms

Basal state
Cannula
Fistula
Heparin lock
Iatrogenic
Lipemia
Lymphostasis
Mastectomy
Occluded
Preexamination variable
Syncope

The venipuncture procedure discussed in Chapter 9 describes the procedure under normal circumstances; however, complications to the routine procedure can occur at any step. The phlebotomist must be aware of surroundings and patient conditions that warrant a change in the routine procedure. In this chapter, the procedure is reviewed in the same order with emphasis on the complications that may be encountered.

REQUISITIONS

In the emergency department or other emergency situations, the request for phlebotomy may be telephoned to the laboratory and the labels automatically printed for the phlebotomist to take to the patient's location. A requisition picked up in an emergency situation must still contain all pertinent information for patient identification. The patient ID number from the patient's wristband may have to be written on the requisition form when a temporary identification system has been used.

GREETING THE PATIENT

Sleeping Patients

Patients are frequently asleep and should be gently awakened and given time to become oriented and have their identity verified before the venipuncture is performed. Blood collection from a sleeping patient may result in identification errors or physical injury to the patient. A sleeping patient would not be able to give informed consent to the procedure, which could result in a charge of assault and battery.

Unconscious Patients

Unconscious patients should be greeted in the same manner as conscious patients, because they may be capable of hearing and understanding even though they cannot respond. In this circumstance, nursing personnel are often present and can assist with the patient, if necessary.

Safety Tip 10-1. A sleeping or unconscious patient may move or jerk unexpectedly when the needle is inserted into the vein or while the needle is in the vein during the venipuncture procedure and cause injury to the patient and the phlebotomist.

Psychiatric Units

It is usually preferable to have a nurse assist with patients on the psychiatric unit. These patients are often anxious about the venipuncture procedure and feel more comfortable when a caregiver with whom they are familiar is present. Be sure to place blood collection equipment away from the patient.

Physicians, Clergy, Visitors

Physicians, members of the clergy, and visitors may be present when the phlebotomist enters the room. When the physician or clergy member is with the patient, it is preferable to return at another time, unless the request is for a stat or timed sample. When this occurs, the phlebotomist should explain the situation and request permission to perform the procedure at that time.

Visitors and family members should be greeted in the same manner as the patient and given the option to step outside. If they choose to stay, the phlebotomist should assess their possible reactions and may elect to pull the curtain around the bed. Visitors and family members can sometimes be helpful in the case of pediatric or very apprehensive patients.

Unavailable Patient

Patients are not always in the room when the phlebotomist arrives. The phlebotomist should attempt to locate the patient by checking with the nursing station. The patient may be in the lounge or walking in the hall, or may have been taken to another department. If the sample must be collected at a particular time, it may be possible to draw blood from the patient in the area to which he or she has been taken. If this is not possible, the nursing station must be notified and the appropriate forms completed so that the test can be rescheduled. The requisition form is usually left at the nursing station. Message boards in the patient's room can be used to alert the nurse to call the lab for blood collection when the patient returns to the room.

PATIENT IDENTIFICATION

Missing ID Band

The phlebotomist will occasionally encounter a patient who has no ID band on either the wrist or the ankle. In this circumstance, the phlebotomist must contact the nurse and request that the patient be banded before the drawing of blood. The nurse's signature on the requisition form verifying identification should be accepted in only emergency situations or according to hospital policy. Patients in psychiatric units often do not wear an identification band. Positive identification by the nursing staff is required with these patients. Follow strict institutional protocol in all special situations.

Unidentified Emergency Department Patients

Unidentified patients are sometimes brought into the emergency department, and a system must be in place to ensure that they are correctly matched with their laboratory work. The American Association of Blood Banks (AABB) requires that the patient be positively identified with a temporary but clear designation attached to the body. Some hospitals generate identification bands with an identification number and a tentative name, such as John Doe or Patient X. When the patient identity is known, a permanent identification number is assigned to the patient. The temporary identification number is cross-referenced to the permanent number for patient identification and correlation of patient and test result information.

▶ *Technical Tip 10-1.* Both the temporary and permanent identification band must be attached to the patient and confirmed before blood may be collected.

Commercial identification systems are particularly useful when blood transfusions are required. In these systems, the identification band that is attached to the patient comes with matching identification stickers. The stickers are placed on the sample tubes, requisition form, and any units of blood designated for the patient. Many hospitals use this type of system, in addition to the routine identification system, for all patients receiving transfusions. In some institutions, patients are required to wear the blood bank identification band for 48 hours during their inpatient stay to indicate how long the sample that has been drawn can be used. Follow institutional protocol.

Identification of Young, Cognitively Impaired, or Patients Who Do Not Speak the Language

If a patient is too young, cognitively impaired, or does not speak the language of the phlebotomist, ask the patient's nurse, relative, or a friend to identify the patient

by name, address, and identification number or date of birth. Document the name of the verifier. This information must be compared with the information on the requisition and the patient's identification band. Any discrepancies must be resolved before collecting the sample.

PATIENT PREPARATION

The preexamination stage of laboratory testing involves processes that occur before testing of the specimen. Errors that occur during this stage often happen during blood collection and are primarily controlled by the phlebotomist. Numerous variables in patient preparation can affect sample quality, and the phlebotomist cannot be expected to control and monitor all variables. However, phlebotomists should be aware of the critical variables that can affect sample quality and consequently laboratory results and report them to the nursing staff or phlebotomy supervisor. The phlebotomist should also be able to recognize various patient conditions and complications that may occur during or after blood collection.

Numerous *preexamination variables* associated with the patient's activities before sample collection can affect the quality of the sample. These variables can include diet, posture, exercise, stress, alcohol, smoking, time of day, and medications. Physiological variables, such as age, altitude, and gender affect normal values for test results. Other patient conditions that may influence laboratory test results are dehydration, fever, and pregnancy.

Basal State

The ideal time to collect blood from a patient is when the patient is in a *basal state* (has refrained from strenuous exercise and has not ingested food or beverages except water for 12 hours [fasting]). Normal values (reference ranges) for laboratory tests are determined from a normal, representative sample of volunteers who are in a basal state. Not all tests are affected by fasting and exercise, as evidenced by the collection and testing of samples throughout the day, and many diagnostic results can be obtained at any time. However, the best comparison of a patient's results with the normal values can be made while the patient is in the basal state. This explains why phlebotomists begin blood collection in the hospital very early in the morning while the patient is in a basal state and why the majority of outpatients arrive in the laboratory as soon as the drawing station opens. Table 10-1 summarizes the major tests affected

TABLE 10-1 • Major Tests Affected by Patient Preexamination Variables

VARIABLE	INCREASED RESULTS	DECREASED RESULTS
Nonfasting	Glucose, triglycerides, aspartate aminotransferase (AST), bilirubin, blood urea nitrogen (BUN), phosphorus, uric acid, growth hormone, cholesterol, lipoproteins (high-density lipoprotein [HDL], low-density lipoprotein [LDL]	
Prolonged fasting	Bilirubin, ketones, lactate, fatty acids, glucagon, and triglycerides	Glucose, insulin, cholesterol, and thyroid hormones
Posture	Albumin, aldosterone, bilirubin, calcium, cortisol, enzymes, cholesterol, total protein, triglycerides, red blood cells (RBCs), white blood cells (WBCs), thyroid (T_4), plasma renin, serum aldosterone, and catecholamines	
Short-term exercise	Creatinine, fatty acids, lactate, AST, creatine kinase (CK), lactate dehydrogenase (LD), uric acid, bilirubin, HDL, hormones, aldosterone, renin, angiotensin, and WBCs	Arterial pH and P_{CO_2}
Long-term exercise	Aldolase, creatinine, sex hormones, AST, CK, and LD	
Stress	Adrenal hormones, aldosterone, renin, thyroid-stimulating hormone (TSH), growth hormone (GH), prolactin, P_{O_2}, and WBCs	Serum iron and P_{CO_2}
Alcohol	Glucose, aldosterone, prolactin, cortisol, cholesterol, triglycerides, luteinizing hormone (LH), catecholamine, AST, alanine transaminase (ALT), estradiol, mean corpuscular volume (MCV), HDL, and iron	Testosterone
Caffeine	Fatty acids, hormone levels, glycerol, lipoproteins, and serum gastrin	
Smoking	Glucose, BUN, triglycerides, cholesterol, alkaline phosphatase (ALP), catecholamines, cortisol, IgE, hemoglobin, hematocrit, RBCs, and WBCs	Immunoglobulins IgA, IgG, and IgM
Altitude	RBCs, hemoglobin, and hematocrit	
Age	Cholesterol and triglycerides	Hormones
Pregnancy	Protein, ALP, estradiol, free fatty acids, iron, and RBCs	Erythrocyte sedimentation rate (ESR), and factors II, V, VII, IX, X
Dehydration	Calcium, coagulation factors, enzymes, iron, RBCs, and sodium (NA)	
Diurnal variation (a.m.)	Cortisol, testosterone, bilirubin, hemoglobin, insulin, potassium, renin, RBCs, TSH, LH, follicle-stimulating hormone (FSH), estradiol, aldosterone, and serum iron	Eosinophils, creatinine, glucose, phosphate, and triglyceride

by variables that change the basal state. Phlebotomists should be aware of the effects these conditions have on test results and document them to help avoid a misdiagnosis.

PREEXAMINATION VARIABLES

Diet

The ingestion of food and beverages alters the level of certain blood components. The tests most affected are glucose and triglycerides. Serum or plasma collected from patients shortly after a meal may appear cloudy or turbid (lipemic) due to the presence of fatty compounds such as meat, cheese, butter, and cream. *Lipemia* will interfere with many test procedures (see Fig. 2-7).

Certain beverages can also affect laboratory tests. Alcohol consumption can cause a transient elevation in glucose levels, and chronic alcohol consumption affects tests associated with the liver and increases triglycerides. Caffeine has been found to affect hormone levels, whereas hemoglobin levels and electrolyte balance can be altered by drinking too much liquid.

Because of these dietary interferences in laboratory testing, fasting samples are often requested. When a fasting sample is requested, it is the responsibility of the phlebotomist to determine whether the patient has been fasting for the required length of time. If the patient has not, this must be reported to a supervisor or the nurse and noted on the requisition form. For most tests, the patient is required to fast for 8 to 12 hours. As shown in Table 10-1, prolonged fasting, however, can also alter certain blood tests.

Posture

Changes in patient posture from a supine to an erect position cause variations in some blood constituents, such as cellular elements, plasma proteins, compounds bound to plasma proteins, and high molecular weight substances. The large size of these substances prevents their movement between the plasma and tissue fluid when body position changes. Therefore, when a person moves from a supine to an erect position and water leaves the plasma, the concentration of these substances increases in the plasma. Tests most noticeably elevated by the decreased plasma volume are cell counts, protein, albumin, bilirubin, cholesterol, triglycerides, calcium, and enzymes. The concentration of these analytes can increase 4 percent to 15 percent within 10 minutes after changing from a supine position to standing. After returning to the supine position from the standing, it takes about 30 minutes for the analytes to decrease back to the original level. Plasma renin, serum aldosterone, and catecholamines can double in 1 hour; therefore, patients are required to be lying down for 30 minutes before blood collection. The National Institutes of Health recommends that patients be lying or sitting for 5 minutes prior to blood collection for lipid profiles to minimize the effects caused by posture. The increase is most noticeable in patients with disorders such as congestive heart failure and liver diseases that cause increased fluid to remain in the tissue. When inpatient and outpatient results are being compared, the physician may request that an outpatient lie down before sample collection.

Preexamination Consideration 10-1.

Lab results in elderly patients may be more affected by changes in posture.

Exercise

Moderate or strenuous exercise affects laboratory test results by increasing the blood levels of creatinine, fatty acids, lactic acid, aspartate aminotransferase (AST), creatine kinase (CK), lactic dehydrogenase (LD), aldolase, hormones (antidiuretic hormone, catecholamines, growth hormone, cortisol, aldosterone, renin, angiotensin), bilirubin, uric acid, high-density lipoprotein (HDL), and white blood cell (WBC) count and decreasing arterial pH and P_{CO_2}. The effects of exercise depend on the physical fitness and muscle mass of the patient, the strenuousness and intensity of the exercise, and the time between the exercise and blood collection. Vigorous exercise has been associated with a temporary activation of coagulation factors and platelet function. Transient short-term exercise and prolonged exercise or weight training affect test results differently. In short-term exercise, muscle contents are released into the blood. Anaerobic glycolysis and metabolic changes interfere with laboratory results. Short-term exercise elevates the enzymes associated with muscles (AST, CK, LD) and the WBC count because WBCs attached to the venous walls are released into the circulation. The values usually return to normal within several hours of relaxation in a healthy person; however, skeletal muscle enzymes, aldosterone, renin, and angiotensin may be elevated for 24 hours. Prolonged exercise also increases the muscle-related waste products (AST, CK, and LD) and hormones, and they will remain more consistently elevated.

Preexamination Consideration 10-2.

Well-trained athletes are more resistant to exercise-related changes because of their consistently elevated level of skeletal muscle enzymes.

Stress

Failure to calm a frightened, nervous patient before sample collection may increase levels of adrenal hormones (cortisol and catecholamines), increase WBC counts, decrease serum iron, and markedly affect arterial blood gas (ABG) results. It has been shown that WBC counts collected from a violently crying newborn may be markedly elevated. This is caused by the release of WBCs attached to the blood vessel walls into the circulation. In contrast, WBC counts on early morning samples collected from patients in a basal state will be decreased until normal activity is resumed. Elevated WBC counts return to normal within 1 hour.

Preexamination Consideration 10-3.

For an accurate WBC count, discontinue blood collection from a crying child until after the child has been calm for at least 1 hour.

Severe anxiety that results in hyperventilation may cause acid-base imbalances and increased lactate and fatty acid levels.

Smoking

The immediate effects of nicotine include increases in plasma catecholamines, cortisol, glucose, blood urea nitrogen (BUN), cholesterol, and triglycerides. The extent of the effect depends on the type and the number of cigarettes smoked and the amount of smoke inhaled. Glucose and BUN can increase by 10 percent and triglycerides by 20 percent. Chronic smoking increases hemoglobin, red blood cell (RBC) counts, the mean corpuscular volume (MCV),

and immunoglobulin (Ig) E. Immunoglobulins IgA, IgG, and IgM are decreased, lowering the effectiveness of the immune system.

Altitude

RBC counts and hemoglobin (Hgb) and hematocrit (Hct) levels are increased in high-altitude areas such as the mountains where there are reduced oxygen levels. The body produces increased numbers of RBCs to transport oxygen throughout the body. Normal ranges for RBC parameters must be established for populations living at 5,000 to 10,000 feet above sea level. It is important to note this information if when speaking with the patient you realize that he or she has just traveled from another geographical area.

Age and Gender

Laboratory results vary between infancy, childhood, adulthood, and the elderly because of the gradual change in the composition of body fluids. Hormone levels vary with age and gender. RBC, Hgb, and Hct values are higher for males than for females. Normal reference ranges are established for the different patient age and gender groups; therefore, the age and gender of the patient should be present on the requisition.

Pregnancy

Pregnancy-related differences in laboratory test results are caused by the physiological changes in the body including increases in plasma volume. The increased plasma volume may cause a dilutional effect and cause lower RBC counts, protein, alkaline phosphatase, estradiol, free fatty acids, and iron values. The erythrocyte sedimentation rate and coagulation factors II, V, VII, VIII, IX, and X may be increased.

Other Factors Influencing Patient Test Results

Other factors caused by certain medical conditions such as shock, malnutrition, fever, burns, and trauma may influence blood and body fluid composition and can affect laboratory test results. Malnutrition may cause increased ketones, bilirubin, lactate, and triglycerides and decreased glucose, cholesterol, thyroid hormones, total protein, and albumin. Fever may cause increases in insulin, glucagon, and cortisol levels.

Environmental factors associated with geographical location, such as temperature and humidity, can change body fluid composition and laboratory test results. Acute exposure to heat that causes sweating may cause dehydration and hemoconcentration.

Diurnal Variation

The concentration of some blood constituents is affected by the time of day. Diurnal rhythm is the normal fluctuation in blood levels at different times of the day based on a 24-hour cycle of eating and sleeping. Blood analytes are released into the bloodstream intermittently. Cortisol, aldosterone, renin, luteinizing hormone, follicle-stimulating hormone, estradiol, thyroid-stimulating hormone (TSH), testosterone, bilirubin, hemoglobin, insulin, potassium, RBC count, and serum iron levels are highest in the morning, whereas eosinophil counts, creatinine, glucose, triglyceride, and phosphate levels are lower.

Preexamination Consideration 10-4.

Cortisol and iron levels can differ by 50 percent between 8 a.m. and 4 p.m.; therefore, it is important to collect samples for analytes that exhibit diurnal variation at the correct scheduled time.

Medications

Administration of medication prior to sample collection may affect tests results, either by changing a metabolic process within the patient or by producing interference with the testing procedure. IV administration of dyes used in diagnostic procedures, including radiographic contrast media for kidney disorders and fluorescein used to evaluate cardiac blood vessels, can interfere with testing procedures. In general, understanding the effect of medications and diagnostic procedures on laboratory test results is the responsibility of the health-care provider, pathologist, or clinical laboratory testing personnel. Phlebotomists, however, should be aware of any procedures being performed at the time they are collecting a sample and note this on the requisition form. For example, samples collected while a patient is receiving a blood transfusion may not represent the patient's true condition.

A variety of medications, both prescription and over-the-counter, can influence laboratory test results. Physicians frequently order tests to evaluate the effect of certain prescribed medications on body systems. In other cases, test results may be affected by over-the-counter medications not reported to the physician by the patient. Medications that are toxic

to the liver can cause an increase in blood liver enzymes and abnormal coagulation tests. Elevated BUN levels or imbalanced electrolytes may be noted in patients taking medications that impair renal function. Patients taking corticosteroids, estrogens, or diuretics can develop pancreatitis and would have elevated serum amylase and lipase levels. Chemotherapy drugs cause a decrease in WBC counts and platelets. Patients taking diuretics may have elevated calcium, glucose, and uric acid levels, and decreased potassium levels. Oral contraceptives can cause a decrease in apoprotein, cholesterol, HDL, triglycerides, and iron levels (Table 10-2). Aspirin, medications that contain salicylate, and certain herb use can interfere

TABLE 10-2 ● **Common Medications Affecting Laboratory Tests**	
MEDICATION	**AFFECTED TESTS/SYSTEMS**
Acetaminophen and certain antibiotics	Elevated liver enzymes and bilirubin
Cholesterol-lowering drugs	Prolonged PT and APTT
Certain antibiotics	Elevated BUN, creatinine, and electrolyte imbalance
Corticosteroids and estrogen diuretics	Elevated amylase and lipase
Diuretics	Increased calcium, glucose, and uric acid and decreased sodium and potassium
Chemotherapy	Decreased RBCs, WBCs, and platelets
Aspirin, salicylates, and herbal supplements	Prolonged PT and bleeding time
Radiographic contrast media	Routine urinalysis
Fluorescein dye	Increased creatinine, cortisol, and digoxin
Oral contraceptives	Decreased apoproteins, transcortin, cholesterol, HDL, triglycerides, LH, FSH, ferritin, and iron

APTT = activated partial thromboplastin time; BUN = blood urea nitrogen; FSH = follicle-stimulating hormone; HDL = high-density lipoprotein; LH = luteinizing hormone; PT = prothrombin time; RBCs = red blood cells; WBCs = white blood cells.

with platelet function or Coumadin anticoagulant therapy and may cause increased risk of bleeding. Herbs, vitamins, and dietary supplements that have been reported to have effects on coagulation by the National Institutes of Health are listed in Box 10-1.

The College of American Pathologists recommends that drugs known to interfere with blood tests should be discontinued 4 to 24 hours before blood tests and 48 to 72 hours before urine tests.

 Technical Tip 10-2. Patients taking herbs often do not realize the side effect of bleeding that can occur. When excessive post venipuncture bleeding occurs, question the patient about herbal medications and document this on the requisition.

BOX 10-1 Herbs, Vitamins, and Dietary Supplements Having Effects on Coagulation and Blood Clotting

Garlic
Ginkgo biloba
Ginseng
Anise
Dong Quai
Omega-3 fatty acids in fish oil
Ginger
Vitamin E
Fucus
Danshen
St. John's wort
Alfalfa
Coenzyme Q10
Bilberry
Bladder wach
Bromelain
Cat's claw
Celery
Coleus
Cordyceps
Evening primrose
Fenugreek
Feverfew
Grape seed
Green tea
Guarana
Guggu
Horse chestnut seed
Horseradish
Horsetail rush
Licorice
Prickly ash
Red clover
Reishi
Sweet clover
Turmeric
White willow

PATIENT COMPLICATIONS

Apprehensive Patients

It is common to encounter extremely apprehensive patients. Enlisting the help of the nurse who has been caring for the patient may help to calm the person's fears. It may also be necessary to ask for assistance from the nurse to hold the patient's arm steady during the procedure. Assistance from a nurse or parent is frequently required when working with children. Phlebotomists also may require nursing assistance when encountering patients in fixed positions, such as those in traction or body casts.

Fainting (Syncope)

Fainting (*syncope*) is the spontaneous loss of consciousness caused by insufficient blood flow to the brain. A part of the involuntary nervous system that regulates heart rate and blood pressure malfunctions in response to a trigger that causes a vasovagal reaction. In response, the heart rate suddenly drops; blood vessels in the legs dilate causing blood to pool in the legs and lower blood pressure. Triggers such as the sight of blood, having blood drawn, fear of bodily injury, standing for long periods of time, heat exposure, and exertion can cause vasovagal syncope. Other conditions that can cause a person to faint include postural hypotension, dehydration, low blood pressure, heart disease, anemia, hypoglycemia, and neurological disorders. Symptoms before fainting or a syncope episode include paleness of the skin, hyperventilation, lightheadedness, dizziness, nausea, a feeling of warmth, or cold, clammy skin. The phlebotomist must be aware of these symptoms and monitor the patient throughout the entire venipuncture procedure.

Apprehensive patients and fasting patients may be prone to fainting, and the phlebotomist should be alert to this possibility. It is sometimes possible to detect such patients during vein palpation because their skin feels cold and damp. The phlebotomist should ask the patient if he or she has had problems with blood collection or a tendency to faint. Keeping their minds off the procedure through conversation can be helpful. If a patient begins to faint during the procedure, immediately remove the tourniquet and needle, and apply pressure to the venipuncture site. In the inpatient setting, notify the nursing station as soon as possible. In the outpatient area, make sure the patient is supported and that the patient lowers his or her head. The phlebotomist must watch the patient carefully as patients have a tendency to fall forward while fainting and can easily slip out of the phlebotomy chair. Ask the patient to take deep breaths. If possible, lay the patient flat and loosen tight clothing. Cold compresses applied to the forehead and back of the neck will help to revive the patient. Outpatients who have been fasting for prolonged periods should be given something sweet to drink (if the blood has been collected) and required to remain in the area for 15 to 30 minutes. All incidents of syncope should be documented following institutional policy.

 Technical Tip 10-3. Patients frequently mention previous adverse reactions. If these patients are sitting up, it may be wise to have them lie down before collection. It is not uncommon for patients with a history of fainting to faint again.

 Technical Tip 10-4. According to the CLSI standards, the use of ammonia inhalants may be associated with adverse effects and is not recommended.

Seizures

It is rare for patients to develop seizures during venipuncture. If this situation occurs, the tourniquet and needle should be removed, pressure applied to the site, and help summoned. Restrain the patient only to the extent that injury is prevented. Do not attempt to place anything in the patient's mouth. Any very deep puncture caused by sudden movement by the patient should be reported to the physician. Document the time the seizure started and stopped according to institutional policy.

 Technical Tip 10-5. In both a syncope or seizure situation, notify the designated first-aid–trained personnel immediately.

Petechiae

Patients who present with small, nonraised red hemorrhagic spots (petechiae) may have prolonged bleeding following venipuncture. Petechiae can be an indication of a coagulation disorder, such as a low platelet count or abnormal platelet function. Additional pressure should be applied to the puncture site following needle removal.

Allergies

Patients are occasionally allergic to alcohol, iodine, latex, or the glue used in adhesive bandages. Necessary precautions must be observed by using alternate antiseptics, paper tape or self-adhering wrap (Coban), and nonlatex products.

Vomiting

A patient may experience nausea or vomiting before, during, or after blood collection. If the patient is nauseated, instruct the patient to breathe deeply and slowly and apply cold compresses to the patient's forehead. If the patient vomits, stop the blood collection and provide the patient with an emesis basin or wastebasket and tissues. Give an outpatient water to rinse out his or her mouth and a damp washcloth to wipe the face. Notify the patient's nurse or designated first-aid personnel.

Additional Patient Observations

Phlebotomists must be alert for changes in a patient's condition and notify the nursing station. Such changes could include the presence of vomitus, urine, or feces; infiltrated or removed IV fluid lines; extreme breathing difficulty; and possibly a patient who has expired.

Patient Refusal

Some patients may refuse to have their blood drawn, and they have the right to do this. The phlebotomist can stress to the patient that the results are needed by the health-care provider for treatment and discuss the problem with the nurse, who may be able to convince the patient to agree to have the test performed.

If the patient continues to refuse, this decision should be written on the requisition form and the form should be left at the nursing station or the area stated in the institution policy.

 Safety Tip 10-2. Carefully listen to the patient and observe the patient's body language. The patient has the right to refuse to have his or her blood drawn. The phlebotomist may be guilty of assault if the patient perceives that his or her refusal is being ignored.

EQUIPMENT ASSEMBLY

When positioning the needed equipment and supplies within easy reach, the phlebotomist should include extra evacuated collection tubes. Occasionally, an evacuated tube does not contain the proper amount of vacuum necessary to collect a full tube of blood. Accidentally pushing a tube past the indicator mark on the needle holder before the vein is entered will also result in loss of vacuum.

Rarely, the phlebotomist may encounter an evacuated tube that pops off the back of the holder needle while blood is being collected. Readvancing the tube onto the needle in the holder and holding it in this position until the tube is filled will remedy this situation. When using the evacuated tube system, always screw the needle onto the holder tightly. Needles have become unscrewed from the holder during venipuncture. If this happens, release the tourniquet immediately, and carefully remove the needle and activate the safety device.

As discussed in Chapter 4, remember that only the necessary amount of equipment is brought into isolation rooms. For patients on the psychiatric unit, leave the phlebotomy tray at the nursing station and take only the necessary equipment into the room. Do not leave any type of equipment in the patients' room.

TOURNIQUET APPLICATION

As discussed in Chapter 8, a blood pressure cuff is sometimes used to locate veins that are difficult to find. The cuff should be inflated to a pressure of 40 mm Hg. Too much pressure affects the flow of arterial blood.

When dealing with patients with skin conditions or sensitivity and open sores, it may be necessary to place the tourniquet over the patient's gown or to cover the area with gauze or a dry cloth before application. If possible, another area should be selected for the venipuncture.

▶ *Technical Tip 10-6.* Consider routinely using latex-free, single-use tourniquets.

Hemoconcentration

Application of the tourniquet for more than 1 minute will interfere with some test results, which is why the Clinical and Laboratory Standards Institute (CLSI) set the limit on tourniquet application time to be 1 minute and states that the tourniquet should be released as soon as the vein is accessed. Prolonged tourniquet time causes hemoconcentration because the plasma portion of the blood passes into the tissue, which results in an increased concentration of protein-based analytes in the blood. Tests most likely to be affected are those measuring large molecules, such as plasma proteins and lipids, RBCs, and substances bound to protein such as iron, calcium, magnesium, or analytes affected by hemolysis, including potassium, lactic acid, and enzymes. Tourniquet application and fist clenching are not recommended when drawing samples for lactic acid determinations.

Releasing the tourniquet as soon as blood begins to flow into the first tube can sometimes result in the inability to fill multiple collection tubes. Phlebotomists may have to make a decision regarding immediately removing the tourniquet based on the size of the patients' veins or the difficulty of the puncture. Regardless of the situation, the tourniquet should not remain in place for longer than 1 minute.

Other causes of hemoconcentration are excessive squeezing or probing a site, long-term IV therapy, sclerosed or *occluded* veins, and vigorous fist pumping (Box 10-2).

 Preexamination Consideration 10-5.
Repeated fist pumping can increase the blood potassium level 1 to 2 mmol/L.

 Preexamination Consideration 10-6.
Prolonged tourniquet application can increase hemoglobin levels 3 percent after 1 minute and 7 percent after 3 minutes, which can mislead health-care providers in diagnosing anemia.

BOX 10-2 Cellular Elements Increased by Hemoconcentration

Ammonia
Bilirubin
Calcium
Enzymes
Iron
Lactic acid
Lipids
Potassium
Proteins
Red blood cells

Preexamination Consideration 10-7.

Cholesterol levels can increase 2 percent to 5 percent after the tourniquet is applied for 2 minutes and up to 10 percent to 15 percent after 5 minutes.

Technical Tip 10-7. According to the CLSI standard H3-A6, tourniquet use is recommended unless it interferes with test results, such as lactate.

SITE SELECTION

Not all patients have a median cubital, cephalic, or basilic vein that becomes immediately prominent when the tourniquet is applied. In fact, a high percentage of patients have veins that are not easily located, and the phlebotomist may have to use a variety of techniques to locate a suitable puncture site. Many patients have prominent veins in one arm and not in the other; therefore, checking the patient's other arm should be the first thing done when a site is not easily located. Patients with veins that are difficult to locate often point out areas where they remember previous successful phlebotomies. Palpation of these areas may prove beneficial and is also good for patient relations.

Technical Tip 10-8. Never be reluctant to check both arms and to listen to the patient's suggestions.

Other techniques used by phlebotomists to enhance the prominence of veins include massaging the arm upward from the wrist to the elbow, briefly hanging the arm down, and applying heat to the site for 3 to 5 minutes. Remember that when performing these techniques, the tourniquet should not remain tied for more than 1 minute at a time.

If no palpable veins are found in the antecubital area, the wrist and hand should be examined (Fig. 10-1A). The tourniquet is retied on the forearm. Because the veins in these areas are smaller, it may be necessary to change equipment and use a smaller needle with a syringe or winged blood collection set or a smaller evacuated tube. Wrist veins must be tightly anchored as they tend to roll to the side easily. Veins on the underside of the wrist should never be used because nerves, tendons, and the ulnar and radial arteries lie close to the veins and can be injured if accidentally punctured (Fig. 10-1B).

Safety Tip 10-3. Nerve damage caused by drawing on the underside of the wrist may cause a patient to lose his or her ability to open or close the hand.

Veins in the legs and feet are sometimes used as venipuncture sites when veins in the arms or hands are unsuitable (Fig. 10-2). They should be used only with physician approval. Leg or foot veins are more susceptible to infection and the formation of thrombi (clots), particularly in patients with diabetes, cardiac problems, and coagulation disorders.

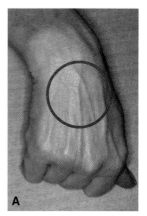
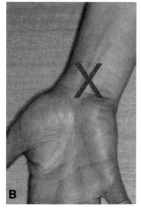

FIGURE 10-1 Alternate site for venipuncture. A, The back (posterior side) of the hand. B, Do not use the underside of the wrist.

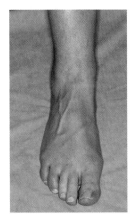

FIGURE 10-2 **Veins in the foot.**

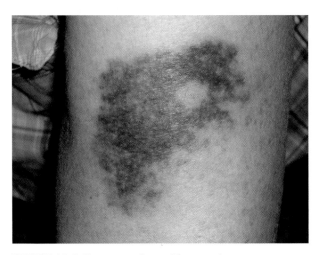

FIGURE 10-3 Hematoma formed from venipuncture.

Areas to Be Avoided

Certain areas must be avoided for venipuncture because of the possibility of decreased blood flow, infection, hemolysis, or sample contamination. Sample contamination affects the integrity of the specimen causing invalid test results. The laboratory personnel may not know that contamination has occurred and consequently can report erroneous test results that adversely affect overall patient care. Incorrect blood collection techniques that cause contamination include blood collected from edematous areas, blood collected from veins with hematomas, blood collected from arms containing an IV, sites contaminated with alcohol or iodine, or anticoagulant carryover between tubes.

Damaged Veins

Veins that contain thrombi or have been subjected to numerous venipunctures often feel hard (sclerosed) and should be avoided as they may be blocked (occluded) and have impaired circulation. Chemotherapy patients, chronically ill patients, and illegal IV drug users may have hardened veins. Probing or using a lateral needle direction when redirecting the needle also can cause vein damage. Areas that appear blue or are cold may also have impaired circulation.

Hematoma

The presence of a hematoma indicates that blood has accumulated in the tissue surrounding a vein during or following venipuncture (Fig. 10-3). Puncturing into a hematoma is not only painful for the patient but will result in the collection of old, hemolyzed blood from the hematoma rather than circulating venous blood that is representative of the patient's current condition.

If a vein containing a hematoma must be used, blood should be collected below the hematoma to ensure sampling of free-flowing blood.

Edema

Drawing from areas containing excess tissue fluid (**edema**) also is not recommended because the sample will be contaminated with tissue fluid and yield inaccurate test results. Edema may be caused by heart failure, renal failure, inflammation, or infection. Edema also may be caused by IV fluid infiltrating into the surrounding tissue. Phlebotomists should notify nursing personnel if they encounter this situation.

Burns, Scars, and Tattoos

Extensively burned and scarred areas, including tattoos, are more susceptible to infection. They also have decreased circulation and can yield inaccurate test results. Veins in these areas are difficult to palpate and penetrate. Tattooed areas contain dyes that can interfere in testing.

Mastectomy

Applying a tourniquet to or drawing blood from an arm located on the same side of the body as a recent *mastectomy* can be harmful to the patient and produce erroneous test results. Removal of lymph nodes in the mastectomy procedure interferes with the flow of lymph fluid (*lymphostasis*) and increases the blood level of lymphocytes and waste products normally contained in the lymph fluid. Patients are in danger of developing lymphedema in the affected area, and this could be increased by application of a tourniquet. The protective functions of the lymphatic system are also lost, so that the area becomes more prone to infection. For these reasons, blood should be drawn from the other arm. In the case of a double mastectomy, the physician should be consulted as to an appropriate site, such as the hand. It may be possible to perform the tests from a fingerstick with a physician's permission.

 Technical Tip 10-9. Most mastectomy patients have been told never to have blood drawn from the affected side. Make sure they receive appropriate reassurance in cases of a double mastectomy.

Obesity

Veins on obese patients are often deep and difficult to palpate. Often, the cephalic vein is more prominent and easier to palpate. A blood pressure cuff may work better as a tourniquet when a vinyl or latex tourniquet is too short. It is important to not probe to find the vein as that can be painful to the patient and cause hemolysis by destroying red blood cells that can alter test results. Using a syringe with a 1½-inch needle may offer more control.

IV Therapy

Frequently, the phlebotomist encounters patients receiving IV fluids in an arm vein. Whenever possible, blood should then be drawn from the other arm because the sample maybe contaminated with IV fluid. If an arm containing an IV must be used for sample collection, the site selected must be below the IV insertion point and preferably in a different vein. CLSI recommends having the nurse turn off the IV infusion for 2 minutes, the phlebotomist then may apply the tourniquet between the IV and the venipuncture site and perform the venipuncture. Document the location of the venipuncture (right or left arm) and that it was drawn below an infusion site. Certain "add on tests" may not be acceptable from this sample. It is preferred, however, that a dermal puncture be performed to collect the sample if possible.

A nurse may choose to collect blood from an IV line that is inserted into the vein. If blood is collected from the IV line, the nurse should turn off the IV drip for at least 2 minutes. The first 5 mL of blood drawn must be discarded, because it may be contaminated

with IV fluid. A new syringe is then used for the sample collection. If a coagulation test is ordered, an additional 5 mL (total of 10 mL) of blood should be drawn before collecting the coagulation test sample because IV lines are frequently flushed with heparin. This additional blood can be used for other tests if they have been requested. Collections from an IV site are usually performed by the nursing staff to ensure proper care of the site. Whenever blood is collected from an arm containing an IV line, the type of fluid and location of IV must be noted on the requisition form. Avoid collecting blood at the same time dye for a radiological procedure or a unit of blood is being infused.

 Technical Tip 10-10. Avoid drawing blood from the site of a previous IV for 24 hours after the IV was disconnected.

 Preexamination Consideration 10-8.
Inappropriate collection of blood from an arm containing an IV is a major cause of erroneous test results. Unless the sample is highly contaminated, the error may not be detected.

Heparin and Saline Locks

Heparin or saline *locks* are winged infusion sets connected to a stopcock or cap with a diaphragm that can be left in a vein for up to 48 hours to provide a means for administering frequently required medications and for obtaining blood samples. The devices must be flushed with heparin or saline periodically and after use to prevent blood clots from developing in the line. The first 5 mL of blood drawn must be discarded from either device. It is not recommended to collect blood through these devices for coagulation testing because residual heparin can affect test results. Only specifically trained personnel are authorized to draw blood from heparin and saline locks.

Cannulas and Fistulas

Patients receiving renal dialysis have a permanent surgical fusion of an artery and a vein called a *fistula* in one arm, and this arm should be avoided for venipuncture because of the possibility of infection. Accidental puncture of the area around the fistula can cause prolonged bleeding.

The dialysis patient also may have a temporary external connection between the artery and a vein formed by a *cannula* that contains a special T-tube connector with a diaphragm for drawing blood. Only specifically trained personnel are authorized to draw blood from a cannula or fistula.

 Technical Tip 10-11. Be sure to check for the presence of a fistula or cannula before applying a tourniquet to the arm, because this can compromise the patient.

CLEANSING THE SITE

Certain procedures, primarily blood cultures and ABGs, require that the site be cleansed with a stronger antiseptic than isopropyl alcohol (see Chapter 11). The most frequently used solutions are povidone-iodine and tincture of iodine or chlorhexidine gluconate for persons who are allergic to iodine.

Alcohol should not be used to cleanse the site before drawing a sample for blood alcohol level test. Thoroughly cleansing the site with soap and water will ensure the least amount of interference. Some institutions use benzalkonium chloride (Zephiran Chloride) to cleanse the site or find povidone-iodine to be acceptable.

EXAMINATION OF PUNCTURE EQUIPMENT

When using a syringe, the plunger is pulled back and pushed forward while the protective cap is still on the needle to ensure that it will move freely when the vein has been entered. The protective cap on the needle is then removed, and the needle point is examined for imperfections just before insertion. Syringe and winged blood collection needles should be examined for flaws in the same manner as evacuated tube needles.

PERFORMING THE VENIPUNCTURE

Although venipuncture is most frequently performed using an evacuated tube system, it may be necessary to use a syringe or winged blood collection set to better control the pressure applied to the delicate veins found in pediatric and elderly patients, or when drawing from hand veins.

Using a Syringe

Except for a few minor differences, the procedure for drawing blood using a syringe is the same as when using an evacuated tube system. Blood is withdrawn from the vein by slowly pulling on the plunger of the syringe, using the hand that is free after the anchored vein is entered. The advantage of using a syringe is that when the vein is entered, blood will appear in the hub of the needle and the plunger can then be pulled back at a speed that corresponds to the rate of blood flow into the syringe. Pulling the plunger back faster than the rate of blood flow may cause the walls of the vein to collapse and can cause hemolysis. It is important to anchor the hand holding the syringe firmly on the patient's arm so that the needle will not move when the plunger is pulled.

 Technical Tip 10-12. Pulling the plunger of the syringe back too slowly can cause the blood to begin to clot before the collection is completed.

Ideally, the size of the syringe used should correspond with the amount of blood needed. However, with small veins that easily collapse, it may be necessary to fill two or more smaller syringes. This procedure will require assistance, because blood from the filled syringe must be transferred to the appropriate tubes while the second syringe is being filled. Before exchanging syringes, gauze must be placed on the patient's arm under the needle because blood will leak from the hub of the needle during the exchange.

 Technical Tip 10-13. In many circumstances, the use of small evacuated tubes with a winged blood collection set instead of a syringe can prevent the need to change syringes.

As discussed in Chapter 8, blood is transferred from the syringe to evacuated tubes, following the correct order of draw, using a blood transfer device. After removing the needle from the vein, activate the needle safety device and remove the needle and discard it in the sharps container. The blood transfer device is attached to the syringe and the evacuated tubes are pushed onto the internal rubber sheathed needle. Allow the tubes to fill according to the vacuum in the tube. Pushing on the plunger can hemolyze the red blood cells or cause the tube stopper to pop off, risking an aerosol spray. After the tubes are filled, the syringe and blood transfer device are discarded into a sharps container. For hypodermic needles without a safety shield, insert the needle into a Portex Point-Lok device and remove the needle. Then, using the blood transfer device, the sample is placed into tubes. After transferring the sample, the needle, Point-Lok device, syringe, and transfer device are discarded into a sharps con-

tainer. The venipuncture procedure using a syringe is shown in Procedure 10-1.

 Technical Tip 10-14. Transfer the blood quickly from the syringe to the evacuated tube to avoid the possibility of the blood clotting. Do not lay the syringe aside to complete the venipuncture procedure before transferring the blood.

PROCEDURE 10-1 ✦ **Venipuncture Using a Syringe**

EQUIPMENT:

Requisition form
Gloves
Tourniquet
70 percent isopropyl alcohol pad
Syringe needle with safety device
Blood transfer device
Evacuated tubes
2 × 2 gauze
Sharps container
Indelible pen
Bandage
Biohazard bag

PROCEDURE:

Step 1. Perform steps 1 to 9 of Procedure 9-2, "Venipuncture Using an Evacuated Tube System."

Step 2. Assemble the equipment as the alcohol is drying. Attach the hypodermic needle to the syringe. Pull the plunger back to ensure that it moves freely and then push it forward to remove any air in the syringe.

Step 3. Reapply the tourniquet, remove the needle cap, and inspect the needle.

Step 4. Ask the patient to remake a fist, and anchor the vein by placing the thumb of the nondominant hand 1 to 2 inches below the site and pulling the skin taut.

Step 5. Hold the syringe in the dominant hand with the thumb on top near the hub and the other fingers underneath. Smoothly insert the needle into the vein at a 15- to 30-degree angle with the bevel up until you feel a lessening of resistance. A flash of blood will appear in

the syringe hub when the vein has been entered. Brace the fingers against the arm to prevent movement of the needle when pulling back on the plunger.

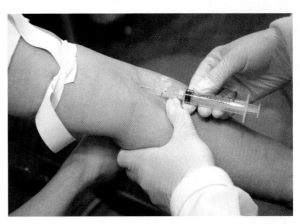

Step 6. Pull back the syringe plunger slowly using the non-dominant hand to collect the appropriate amount of blood.

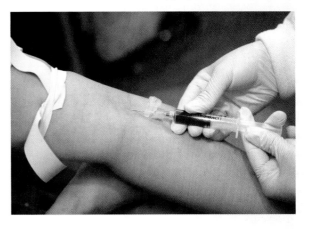

PROCEDURE 10-1 ✦ **Venipuncture Using a Syringe** (Continued)

Step 7. Release the tourniquet and have the patient open the fist.

Step 8. Cover the puncture site with gauze, remove the needle smoothly, activate the safety shield, and apply pressure.

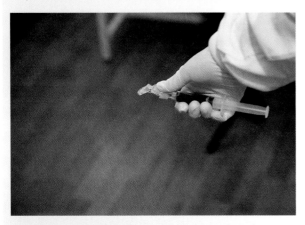

Step 9. Remove the needle from the syringe and discard it in the sharps container.

Step 10. Attach a blood transfer device to the syringe.

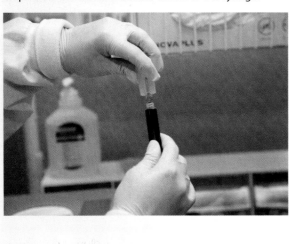

Step 11. Holding the syringe vertically with the blood transfer device at the bottom, advance the evacuated tube onto the internal needle in the blood transfer device. Tubes will fill by the vacuum in the tube. Keep the tube in a vertical position to ensure that the tubes fill from the bottom up to avoid cross-contamination. Do not push on the plunger.

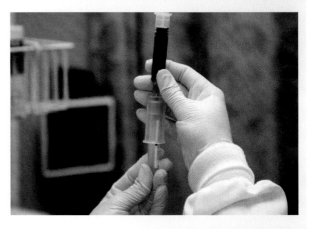

Step 12. Fill tubes in the correct order. Mix anticoagulated tubes as soon as they are removed from the transfer device.

Step 13. After tubes are filled, the entire syringe and blood transfer device are discarded into a sharps container.

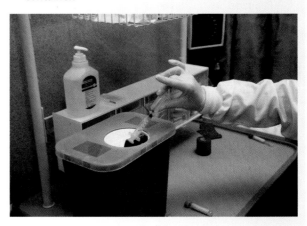

Continued

PROCEDURE 10-1 ✦ Venipuncture Using a Syringe (Continued)

Step 14. Label the tubes and confirm identification with the patient.

Step 15. Examine the puncture site and apply a bandage.

Step 16. Remove gloves and wash hands.

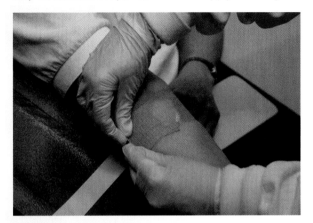

USING A WINGED BLOOD COLLECTION SET

All routine venipuncture procedures used with evacuated tubes and syringes also apply to blood collection using a winged blood collection set (butterfly). This method is used for difficult venipuncture and is often less painful to patients. By folding the plastic needle attachments ("wings") upward while inserting the needle, the angle of insertion can be lowered to 10 to 15 degrees, thereby facilitating entry into small veins. Blood will appear in the tubing when the vein is entered. The needle can then be threaded securely into the vein and kept in place by holding the plastic wings against the patient's arm.

Depending on the type of winged blood collection set used, blood can be collected into evacuated tubes or into a syringe. The tubing contains a small amount of air that will cause underfilling of the first tube; therefore, a discard tube should be collected before an anticoagulated tube to maintain the correct blood-to-anticoagulant ratio. To prevent hemolysis when using a small (23-gauge) needle, small-volume evacuated tubes should be used. Tubes are positioned downward to fill from the bottom up and in the same order of draw as in routine venipuncture. If blood has been collected into a syringe, the winged blood collection needle safety device is activated and removed from the syringe. A blood transfer device is attached to the syringe and the evacuated tubes are filled in the correct order.

 Safety Tip 10-4. When using a winged blood collection set, be sure to attach the holder and do not just push the tubes onto the back of the rubber-sheathed needle. This will avoid an accidental needlestick exposure from the stopper-puncturing needle.

When disposing of the winged blood collection set, use extreme care, because many accidental sticks result from unexpected movement of the tubing. Immediately activating the needle safety device and placing the needle into a sharps container before removing the syringe, and then allowing the tubing to fall into the container when the syringe is removed can prevent accidents. Always hold a winged blood collection set by the wings, not by the tubing. Using an apparatus with automatic resheathing capability or activating a device on the needle set that advances a safety blunt before removing the needle from the vein is recommended to prevent accidental needle punctures. Do not push the apparatus manually into a full sharps container.

> ▎**Safety Tip 10-5.** When removing the winged
> ◆ blood collection needle from the vein, always hold
> the base of the needle or the wings until it has been
> placed in the biohazard sharp container. The needle
> safety mechanism should be activated immediately.

The venipuncture procedure using a winged blood collection set is shown in Procedure 10-2.

PROCEDURE 10-2 ✦ **Venipuncture Using a Winged Blood Collection Set**

EQUIPMENT:

    Requisition form
    Gloves
    Tourniquet
    70 percent isopropyl alcohol pad
    Winged blood collection set
    Blood transfer device
    Evacuated tubes
    2 × 2 gauze
    Sharps container
    Indelible pen
    Bandage
    Biohazard bag

PROCEDURE:

Step 1. Perform steps 1 to 6 of Procedure 9-2, "Venipuncture Using an Evacuated Tube System."

Step 2. Support the hand on the bed or drawing chair armrest and have the patient make a fist.

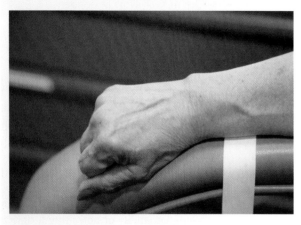

Step 3. Apply the tourniquet 3 to 4 inches above the wrist bone.

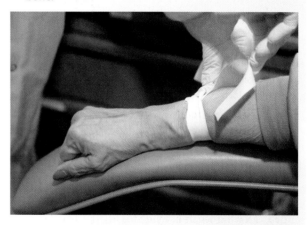

Step 4. Palpate the top of the hand or wrist. Select a vein that is large and straight and that can be easily anchored.

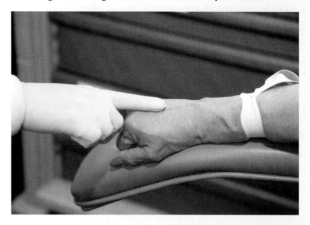

Step 5. Release the tourniquet, have the patient relax the fist, and clean the site with 70 percent isopropyl alcohol in concentric circles and allow to air dry.

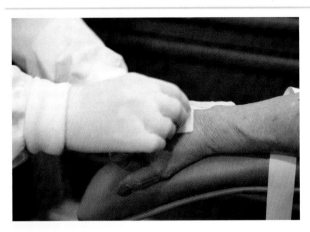

Step 6. Assemble the equipment as the alcohol is drying. Attach the winged blood collection set to the evacuated tube holder or the syringe. Stretch out the coiled tubing. Pull the plunger back to ensure that it moves freely and then push it forward to remove any air in the syringe. If using an evacuated tube holder, insert the first tube to the tube advancement mark.

Step 7. Reapply the tourniquet, remove the needle cap, and inspect the needle. Lay the syringe and tubing next to the patient's hand.

Step 8. Anchor the vein by placing the thumb of the nondominant hand below the knuckles and pulling the skin taut. Having the patient make a fist may be helpful.

Step 9. Grasp the needle between the thumb and index finger by holding the back of the needle or by folding the wings together. Smoothly insert the needle into the vein at a shallow 10- to 15-degree angle with the bevel up. Thread the needle into the lumen of the vein until the bevel is firmly "seated" in the vein. A flash of blood will appear in the tubing when the needle has entered the vein.

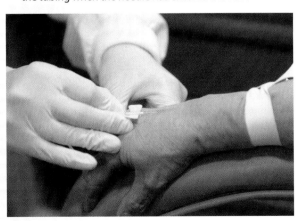

Step 10. Pull back on the plunger of the syringe slowly and smoothly with the nondominant hand to collect blood. Do not pull back on the syringe plunger if a blood flash does not appear. When using an evacuated tube holder, insert the tubes in the correct order of draw. Use a discard tube when collecting anticoagulated tubes to prime the tubing and maintain the correct blood-to-anticoagulant ratio. Invert anticoagulated tubes immediately.

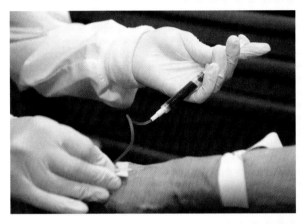

Step 11. Release the tourniquet.

Step 12. Cover the puncture site with gauze, remove the needle smoothly or activate the safety device on needles designed to be retracted while the needle is in the vein.

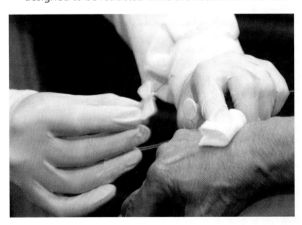

Continued

PROCEDURE 10-2 ✦ **Venipuncture Using a Winged Blood Collection Set** (Continued)

Step 13. Activate the safety shield for needles designed to be shielded when the needle is out of the vein, and apply pressure.

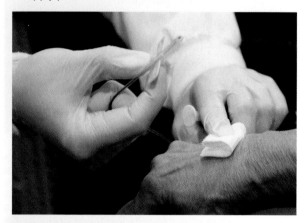

Step 14. Remove the winged blood collection set from the syringe and discard it in the sharps container.

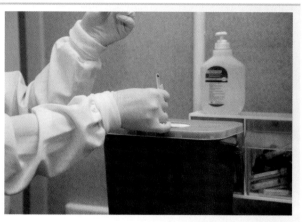

Step 15. Attach a blood transfer device to the syringe and fill the evacuated tubes in the correct order.

Step 16. After tubes are filled, the syringe and blood transfer device are discarded into a sharps container.

Step 17. Label the tubes and confirm identification with the patient.

Step 18. Examine the puncture site and apply a bandage.

Step 19. Remove gloves and wash hands.

TECHNICAL COMPLICATIONS

Technical complications with the venipuncture procedure result in the inability to obtain blood, a rejected sample, or discomfort to the patient. By identifying the types of complications encountered, the phlebotomist usually can remedy the situation without having to repuncture the patient.

Failure to Obtain Blood

Needle Position

Not all venipunctures result in the immediate appearance of blood; however, in many instances, this is only a temporary setback that can be corrected by slight movement of the needle. It is important for beginning phlebotomists to know these techniques, because they have a tendency to immediately remove the needle when blood does not appear. The patient must then be repunctured when it may not have been necessary.

Figure 10-4 illustrates possible causes of failure to obtain blood.

Bevel Against the Wall of the Vein

As shown in Figure 10-4B and C, the bevel of the needle may be resting against the upper or lower wall of the vein, obstructing blood flow. Often this occurs because the angle of the needle is incorrect; a too shallow angle of needle insertion can cause the needle to lay against the upper wall of the vein and a too steep angle can cause the needle to lay against the lower wall of the vein. Failure to insert the needle with the bevel up also can obstruct blood flow into the needle. Removing the evacuated tube and rotating the needle a quarter of a turn will allow blood to flow freely into a new evacuated tube (Figure 10-4D).

Needle Too Deep

When the angle of needle insertion is too steep (greater than 30 degrees) or while advancing the evacuated tube onto the tube stoppering needle when the holder is not firmly braced against the skin, the needle may penetrate through the vein into the tissue. Blood can leak into the tissues, forming a hematoma. Gently pulling the needle back may produce blood flow (Fig. 10-4E).

 Technical Tip 10-15. Failure to keep the holder steady by bracing the hand against the patient's arm may cause the needle to be pushed through the vein or pulled out of the vein when tubes are being changed.

Needle Too Shallow

If the needle angle is too shallow (less than 15 degrees), the needle may only partially enter the lumen of the vein, causing blood to leak into the tissues, forming a hematoma. Slowly advancing the needle into the vein may correct the problem. If a hematoma appears under the skin, remove the tourniquet and needle immediately and apply pressure to the site. Continuing to draw the sample may result in injury to the patient and a sample contaminated with tissue fluid and hemolysis (Figure 10-4F).

Collapsed Vein

Using too large an evacuated tube or pulling back on the plunger of a syringe too quickly creates suction pressure that can cause a vein to collapse and stop blood flow (Fig. 10-4G). Using a smaller evacuated tube may remedy the situation. If it does not, another puncture must be performed, possibly using a syringe or winged blood collection set.

Needle Beside the Vein

A frequent reason for the failure to obtain blood occurs when a vein is not well anchored before the puncture. The needle may slip to the side of the vein without actual penetration ("rolling vein") (Fig. 10-4H). Gentle touching of the area around the needle with the cleansed gloved finger may determine the positions of the vein and the needle, and allow the needle to be slightly redirected. To avoid having to repuncture the patient, withdraw the needle until the bevel is just under the skin, reanchor the vein, and redirect the needle into the vein.

Movement of the needle should not include vigorous probing because this is not only painful to the patient but also enlarges the puncture site so that blood can leak into the tissues and form a hematoma or cause an accidental nicking of an artery. CLSI recommends to never move the needle in a lateral direction to access the basilic vein because of the close proximity of the brachial artery and antebrachial cutaneous nerve.

Faulty Evacuated Tube

If the needle appears to be in the vein, a faulty evacuated tube (either by manufacturer error, age of the tube, dropping and cracking the tube, or accidental puncture when assembling the equipment) may be the problem, and a new tube should be used. Occasionally an evacuated tube will lose its vacuum if the needle bevel moves out of the skin during venipuncture. This will be detected by a splash of blood into the tube and sometimes a hissing sound before the blood flow stops. Remember always to have extra tubes within reach.

Collection Attempts

When blood is not obtained from the initial venipuncture, the phlebotomist should select another site, either in the other arm or below the previous site, and *repeat the procedure using a new needle.* If the second puncture is not successful, the same phlebotomist should not make another attempt. Following hospital policy, the phlebotomist should notify the nursing station and request that another phlebotomist perform the venipuncture.

 Technical Tip 10-16. Never attempt to stick a patient unless a vein can be seen and/or felt.

Nerve Injury

Temporary or permanent nerve damage can be caused by incorrect vein selection or improper venipuncture technique and may result in loss of movement to the arm or hand and the possibility of a lawsuit. The most critical permanent injury in the venipuncture procedure is damage to the median antebrachial cutaneous nerve.

Damage to the nerve can occur when a nerve is nicked during venipuncture. The patient may experience a shooting pain, electric-like tingling or numbness running up or down the arm or in the fingers of the arm used for venipuncture. Errors in technique that can cause injury include blind probing, selecting high-risk venipuncture sites (underside of the wrist, basilic vein), employing an excessive angle of needle insertion (greater than 30 degrees), lateral redirection of the needle, excessive manipulation (jerky

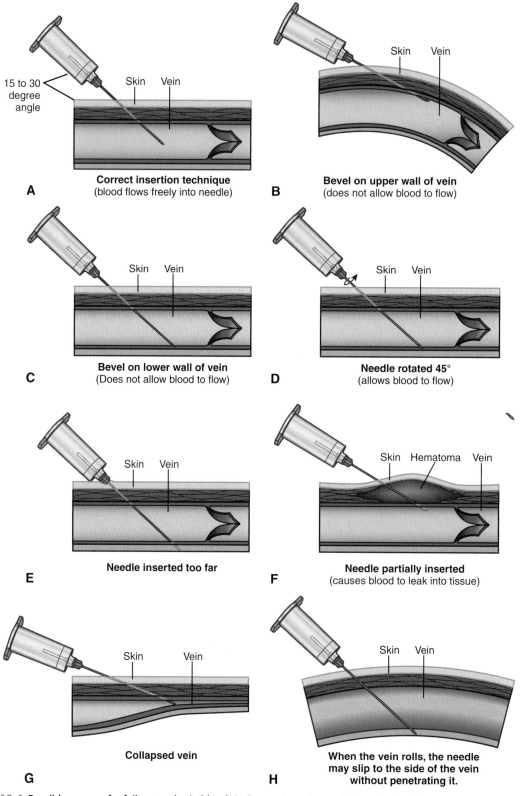

FIGURE 10-4 Possible reasons for failure to obtain blood. A, Correct insertion technique. B, Bevel on upper wall of vein (does not allow blood to flow). C, Bevel on lower wall of vein (does not allow blood to flow). D, Needle rotated 45 degrees (allows blood to flow). E, Needle inserted too far. F, Needle partially inserted (causes blood to leak into tissue). G, Collapsed vein. H, When the vein rolls, the needle may slip to the side of the vein without penetrating it.

movements) of the needle, and movement by the patient while the needle is in the vein.

The pressure from a hematoma, infiltrations of IV fluid, or a tourniquet that is on for too long or too tight can cause a nerve compression injury. Swelling and numbness may occur 24 to 96 hours later.

The symptoms of nerve injury are treated with a cold ice pack initially and then warm compresses to the area. Document the incident and direct the patient to medical evaluation if indicated, according to facility policy.

Iatrogenic Anemia

Iatrogenic anemia pertains to a condition of blood loss caused by treatment. An anemia can occur when large amounts of blood are removed for testing at one time or over a period of time. This is especially dangerous for infants and the elderly. Removal of over 10 percent of a patient's blood can be life-threatening in these patients. Collecting the minimum amount of blood, monitoring collection orders for duplicate requests, and the avoidance of redraws can reduce excessive blood collections. Some facilities have instituted a blood conservation program to minimize blood loss that can cause iatrogenic anemia.

Hemolyzed Samples

Hemolysis may be detected by the presence of pink or red plasma or serum (Fig. 10-5). Rupture of the red blood cell membrane releases cellular contents into the serum or plasma and produces interference with many test results so that the sample may need to be redrawn. Hemolysis that is not visibly noticeable may be present and will affect test results of analytes such as potassium and lactic acid that are particularly sensitive to hemolysis. Table 10-3 summarizes the major tests affected by hemolysis.

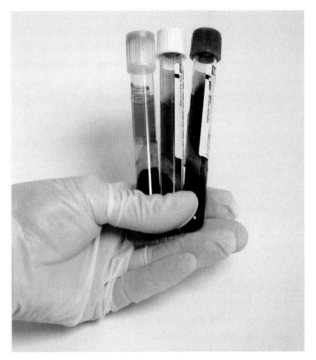

FIGURE 10-5 **Slight, moderate, and gross serum hemolysis.**

▶ *Technical Tip 10-17.* Samples collected following vigorous probing are frequently hemolyzed and must be recollected.

▶ *Technical Tip 10-18.* Hemolysis that is not evident to the naked eye can elevate critical potassium values.

▶ *Technical Tip 10-19.* Potassium values are higher in serum than in plasma due to the release of potassium from platelets during clotting.

TABLE 10-3 • Laboratory Tests Affected by Hemolysis		
SERIOUSLY AFFECTED	**NOTICEABLY AFFECTED**	**SLIGHTLY AFFECTED**
Potassium (K)	Serum iron (Fe)	Phosphorus (P)
Lactic dehydrogenase (LD)	Alanine aminotransferase (ALT)	Total protein (TP)
Aspartate aminotransferase (AST)	Thyroxine (T$_4$)	Albumin
Complete blood count (CBC)		Magnesium (Mg)
		Calcium (Ca)
		Acid phosphatase

Errors in performance of the venipuncture account for the majority of hemolyzed samples and include the following:

1. Using a needle with too small a diameter (above 23 gauge)
2. Using a small needle with a large evacuated tube
3. Using an improperly attached needle on a syringe so that frothing occurs as the blood enters the syringe
4. Pulling the plunger of a syringe back too fast
5. Drawing blood from a site containing a hematoma
6. Vigorously mixing tubes
7. Forcing blood from a syringe into an evacuated tube
8. Collecting samples from IV lines when not recommended by the manufacturer
9. Applying the tourniquet too close to the puncture site or for too long
10. Using fragile hand veins
11. Performing venipuncture before the alcohol is allowed to dry
12. Collecting blood through different internal diameters of catheter and connectors
13. Partially filling sodium fluoride tubes
14. Readjusting the needle in the vein (probing) or using occluded veins

Factors in processing, handling, or transporting the sample also can result in hemolyzed samples and include:

1. Rimming clots
2. Prolonged contact of serum/plasma with cells
3. Centrifuging at a higher than recommended speed and with increased heat exposure in the centrifuge
4. Elevated or decreased temperatures of blood
5. Using pneumatic tube systems with unpadded canisters, speed acceleration and/or deceleration, excessive agitation

Various patient physiological factors can cause hemolysis and include:

1. Metabolic disorders (liver disease, sickle cell anemia, autoimmune hemolytic anemia, blood transfusion reactions)
2. Chemical agents (lead, sulfonamides, antimalarial drugs, analgesics)
3. Physical agents (mechanical heart valve, third-degree burns)
4. Infectious agents (parasites, bacteria)

Reflux of Anticoagulant

Reflux of a tube anticoagulant can occur when there is blood backflow into a patient's vein from the collection tube. This can cause adverse reactions in patients. Keeping the patient's arm and the tube in a downward position, allowing the collection tubes to fill from the bottom up, eliminates this problem.

 Technical Tip 10-20. To ensure prevention of reflux, blood in the tubes should not come in contact with the stopper during collection.

REMOVAL OF THE NEEDLE

Hematoma Formation

Improper technique when removing the needle is a frequent (although not the only) cause of a hematoma appearing on the patient's arm. The skin discoloration and swelling that accompanies a hematoma is often a cause of anxiety and discomfort to the patient and in severe cases can cause disabling compression injury to nerves.

Errors in technique that cause blood to leak or be forced into the surrounding tissue and produce hematomas include:

1. Failure to remove the tourniquet before removing the needle
2. Applying inadequate pressure to the site after removal of the needle
3. Bending the arm while applying pressure
4. Excessive probing to obtain blood
5. Failure to insert the needle far enough into the vein
6. Inserting the needle through the vein
7. Selecting a needle too large for the vein
8. Using veins that are small and fragile
9. Accidentally puncturing the brachial artery

Under normal conditions, the elasticity of the vein walls prevents the leakage of blood around the needle during venipuncture. A decrease in the elasticity of the vein walls in older patients causes them to be more prone to developing hematomas. Using small-bore needles and firmly anchoring the veins before needle insertion may prevent a hematoma in older patients. If a hematoma begins to form while blood is being collected, immediately remove the tourniquet and needle and apply pressure to the site for 2 minutes. A cold compress may be offered to the patient to minimize hematoma swelling and pain. Follow institutional policy. An alternate site should be chosen for the repeat venipuncture, or if none is available, the venipuncture must be performed below the hematoma. The goal of successful blood collection is not only to obtain the sample but also to preserve the site for future venipunctures. It is critical to prevent hematoma formation.

DISPOSAL OF THE NEEDLE

There should be no deviations from the methods for needle disposal discussed in Chapter 9.

LABELING THE TUBES

Information contained on the labels of tubes from unidentified patients must follow the protocol used by the institution to provide a temporary but clear designation of the patient. When available, stickers from the patient's ID band should be attached to all samples for the blood bank.

If preprinted labels are being used, it is important to double check the name on the label while attaching it to the tube.

BANDAGING THE PATIENT'S ARM

Patients receiving anticoagulant medications or large amounts of aspirin or herbs, or patients with coagulation disorders, may continue to bleed after pressure has been applied for 5 minutes. The phlebotomist should continue to apply pressure until the bleeding has stopped. The nurse should be notified in cases of excessive bleeding. For patients who have bleeding problems, a self-adhering gauze (Coban) can be placed over a folded gauze to form a pressure dressing. Never leave the patient until the bleeding has stopped.

Compartment Syndrome

Some patients receiving anticoagulants or who have a coagulation disorder (hemophilia) may continue to bleed large amounts of blood into the subcutaneous tissue surrounding the puncture site. The blood can accumulate within the tissues of the muscles that surround the arm or hand and cause an increased pressure to build in the area, which can interfere with blood flow and cause muscle injury. This condition called "compartment syndrome" can cause pain, swelling, numbness, and permanent injury to the nerves. This is a serious condition and would require a surgical procedure to open the compartment to relieve the pressure and stop the bleeding. This syndrome can be prevented by checking the venipuncture site for bleeding and hematoma formation before applying the bandage.

 Technical Tip 10-21. Phlebotomists should routinely ask patients if they are taking blood thinners (anticoagulant therapy) and take extra care to maintain pressure on the site until bleeding has stopped.

Accidental Arterial Puncture

In the case of an accidental arterial puncture, which can usually be detected by the appearance of unusually red blood that spurts into the tube, the phlebotomist, not the patient, should apply pressure to the site for 5 minutes (10 minutes may be required if the patient is on anticoagulant therapy). A nick to the artery also can cause compartment syndrome and compression nerve injury due to the accumulation of blood in the tissue. The fact that the sample is arterial blood should be recorded on the requisition form because some test values are different for arterial blood versus venous blood.

 Technical Tip 10-22. Probing and lateral movement of the needle particularly near the basilic vein are the main causes of accidental arterial punctures.

Allergy to Adhesives

Some patients are allergic to adhesive bandages, and it may be necessary to wrap gauze around the arm before applying the adhesive tape or use paper tape. Omitting the bandage in these patients and those with hairy arms is another option, particularly if the patient requests it. Self-adhering bandages, such as Coban, may be used. Bandages are not recommended for children younger than 2 years because children may put bandages in their mouths.

Infection

Instruct the patient to keep the bandage on for at least 15 minutes post venipuncture to avoid the possibility of infection. Bandages should not be opened ahead of time and placed on the table or lab coat.

 Technical Tip 10-23. Practicing aseptic technique throughout the venipuncture procedure will minimize the risk of infection.

LEAVING THE PATIENT

Patients often request that the phlebotomist change the position of their bed or provide them with a drink of water. Because this may not be in the best interest of the patient, the phlebotomist should tell the patient that she or he will inform the nurse of the request. Leave the room in the condition in which you found it (bed and bed rails in the same position).

COMPLETING THE VENIPUNCTURE PROCEDURE

Samples brought to the laboratory may be rejected if conditions are present that would compromise the validity of the test results. Major reasons for sample rejection are the following:

1. Unlabeled or mislabeled samples
2. Inadequate volume
3. Collection in the wrong tube
4. Hemolysis
5. Lipemia
6. Clotted blood in an anticoagulant tube
7. Improper handling during transport, such as not chilling the sample
8. Samples without a requisition form
9. Contaminated sample containers
10. Delays in processing the sample
11. Use of outdated blood collection tubes

Phlebotomists should make sure that none of these conditions exist in the samples they deliver to the laboratory.

Key Points

✦ Unidentified patients must be identified with a temporary identification band that includes an identification number and tentative name. The requisition may be obtained at the emergency situation. The tubes are labeled with the temporary information. Patients that are not wearing an identification band must be positively identified by the nursing staff and their signature documented. Follow institutional policy.

✦ The patient's nurse, relative, or friend must identify anyone who is too young, cognitively impaired, or does not speak the language. Document the verifier.

✦ Patients sleeping should be gently awakened before venipuncture to ensure proper identification and informed consent. Do not interrupt a physician or clergy member visit with a patient to collect blood unless it is a stat or timed test. Visitors should be given the option of stepping outside the room during the venipuncture. The phlebotomist should attempt to locate a patient not in the room, particularly if it is a timed or stat request; otherwise notify the nursing staff.

✦ Preexamination variables that can affect laboratory tests include diet, posture, exercise, stress, alcohol, smoking, time of day, medications, gender, age, altitude, dehydration, fever, and pregnancy.

✦ Basal state describes a patient who has refrained from strenuous exercise and has not ingested food or beverages except water for 12 hours.

✦ If a patient faints during the venipuncture procedure, immediately remove the tourniquet and needle, apply pressure to the site, lower the patient's head, and keep the patient in the area for 15 to 30 minutes. Document the incident.

✦ Document refusal by a patient to have blood drawn on the requisition form and notify the nursing staff. Follow institutional policy.

✦ Tourniquet application of longer than 1 minute can alter test results by causing hemocentration and hemolysis. Tests primarily affected are plasma proteins, cholesterol, hemoglobin, iron, calcium, magnesium, potassium, lactic acid, and enzymes.

✦ Techniques used to locate veins that are not prominent include massaging the arm upward from the wrist to the elbow, hanging the arm down, and applying heat to the site for 3 to 5 minutes.

✦ It is not advisable to draw from leg or foot veins because they are more susceptible to infection and the formation of thrombi (clots), particularly in patients with diabetes, cardiac problems, and coagulation disorders. Requires physician approval.

✦ Unacceptable sites for venipuncture include damaged veins (sclerosed), hematomas, edematous areas, burns, scars, tattoos, above an IV, arms with a fistula or cannula, and arms adjacent to a mastectomy because of sample contamination, decreased blood flow, and risk of patient infection.

✦ A syringe or winged blood collection set can be used for difficult venipuncture to better control the pressure applied to the delicate veins found in pediatric and elderly patients, or when drawing from hand veins.

✦ Failure to obtain blood can be caused by incorrect needle position in the vein (bevel on lower wall of vein, bevel on upper wall of vein, needle inserted through the vein, needle partially inserted into the vein), collapsed vein, "rolling" vein, or a faulty evacuated tube.

✦ Venipuncture technique errors account for the majority of hemolyzed samples and include using a needle with too small a diameter, using a small needle with a large evacuated tube, using an improperly attached needle on a syringe so that frothing occurs as the blood enters the syringe, pulling the plunger of a syringe back too fast, drawing blood from a site containing a hematoma, vigorously mixing tubes, forcing blood from a syringe into an evacuated tube, collecting samples from IV lines when not recommended by the manufacturer, applying the tourniquet too close to the puncture site or for too long, using fragile hand veins, performing venipuncture before the alcohol is allowed to dry, collecting blood through different internal diameters of catheter and connectors, partially filling sodium fluoride tubes, and readjusting the needle in the vein or using occluded veins.

✦ The laboratory tests most seriously affected by hemolysis are potassium, lactic dehydrogenase, aspartate aminotransferase, and the complete blood count.

✦ A hematoma is caused by the leakage of blood into the tissues and is characterized by a black

Continued

Key Points—cont'd

and blue discoloration and swelling at the site. Errors in technique that are associated with needle insertion and removal are the primary causes of hematomas and include failure to remove the tourniquet before removing the needle, applying inadequate pressure to the site after removal of the needle, bending the arm while applying pressure, excessive probing to obtain blood, failure to insert the needle far enough into the vein, inserting the needle through the vein, selecting a needle too large for the vein, using veins that are small and fragile without additional precautions, and accidentally puncturing the brachial artery.

✦ Reasons to reject compromised samples by the laboratory include unlabeled or mislabeled samples, inadequate volume, collection in the wrong tube, hemolysis, lipemia, clotted blood in an anticoagulant tube, improper handling during transport, samples without a requisition form, and contaminated sample containers.

BIBLIOGRAPHY

Anderson, SC, and Cockayne, S: Method Evaluation and Pre-Analytical Variables. In Clinical Chemistry, Concepts and Applications. McGraw-Hill Professional, 2003, New York, NY.

American Dental Hygienists' Association. Blood Clotting: An Examination of the Bleeding Complications Associated with Herbal Supplements, Antiplatelet and Anticoagulant Mechanism. http://www.adha.org/CE_courses/course15/blood_clotting.htm.

CLSI. Collection, Transport, and Processing for Testing Plasma-Based Coagulation Assays and Molecular Hemostasis Assays; Approved Guideline-Fifth Edition. CLSI document H21-A5. Clinical and Laboratory Standards Institute, 2008, Wayne, PA.

CLSI. Procedures for Collection of Diagnostic Blood Specimens by Venipuncture; Approved Standard-Sixth Edition. CLSI document H3-A6. Clinical and Laboratory Standards Institute, 2007, Wayne, PA.

CLSI. Procedures for the Handling and Processing of Blood Specimens; Approved Guideline-Third Edition. CLSI document H18-A3. CLSI, 2004, Wayne, PA.

Holmes, WE: The Interpretation of Laboratory Tests. In McClatchey, KD: Clinical Laboratory Medicine, ed 2. Lippincott Williams & Wilkins, 2001, Philadelphia, PA.

Lusky, K: Safety Net: Juggling the Gains, Losses of Phlebotomy Routines. *CAP Today* June, 2004. http://www.cap.org/.

National Institutes of Health. 2005 Jan 13 [Cited 2006 Jun 5]. An NIH Conference on Dietary Supplements, Coagulation and Antithrombotic Therapies. http://www.nhlbi.nih.gov/meetings/coagulation/summary.htm.

Ogden-Grable, H, and Gill, GW: Phlebotomy Puncture Juncture, Preventing Phlebotomy Errors–Potential For Harming Your Patients. *Lab Medicine* 2005;36(7):430-433.

Patton, MT: Addressing Nerve Damage. *Advance for Medical Laboratory Professionals* April 21, 2003, p. 25-26.

Proytcheva, MA: Issues in Neonatal Cellular Analysis. *American Journal of Clinical Pathology* 2009;131:560–573.

Wyan, RL, Meiller, TF, and Crossley, HL: Drug Information Handbook for Dentistry, ed 10. Lexi-Comp, Inc., 2005, Hudson, NY.

Study Questions

1. A phlebotomist who encounters a comatose patient with no ID band should:
   a. notify the phlebotomy supervisor
   b. check the patient's identify with the patient's roommate
   c. leave the requisition at the nurse's station
   d. ask the nurse to band the patient

2. What should a phlebotomist do when the patient is sleeping?
   a. postpone the collection
   b. gently wake the patient
   c. allow the patient to become oriented
   d. both B and C

Study Questions—cont'd

3. Why do phlebotomists perform their routine blood collections early in the morning?
   a. the physician needs the results early
   b. patients are in a basal state
   c. patients will have had breakfast
   d. patients have a lower chance of fainting

4. Match the following patient variables with the possible effect on test results.

   Effect
   _____ a. Increased Hgb
   _____ b. Decreased glucose
   _____ c. Increased WBCs
   _____ d. Increased skeletal enzymes
   _____ e. Increased cholesterol

   Variable
   1. prolonged fasting
   2. stress
   3. erect posture
   4. long-term exercise
   5. tobacco

5. A patient who appears pale and has cold, damp skin may develop:
   a. coagulation problems
   b. septicemia
   c. sclerosis
   d. syncope

6. Hemoconcentration can be caused by:
   a. tourniquet applied for longer than 1 minute
   b. failure to clench the fist
   c. excessive probing
   d. vigorously mixing the tubes

7. Methods to locate veins that are not prominent include all of the following **EXCEPT:**
   a. massaging the arm upward
   b. hanging the arm down
   c. applying heat for 3 minutes
   d. applying a cold compress

8. Physician approval is required when collecting blood from:
   a. patients with diabetes
   b. lower arm veins
   c. foot and leg veins
   d. pediatric patients

9. Areas that should be avoided for venipuncture include all of the following **EXCEPT:**
   a. hematomas
   b. deep cephalic veins
   c. edematous tissue
   d. tattoos

10. When encountering a patient with a fistula, the phlebotomist should:
    a. apply the tourniquet below the fistula
    b. use the other arm
    c. collect the blood from the fistula
    d. attach a syringe to the T-tube connector

11. If the plunger of a syringe is pulled back too fast:
    a. the patient feels a stinging sensation
    b. the sample may be hemolyzed
    c. the patient will develop a hematoma
    d. both A and B

12. When collecting blood using a winged blood collection set, all of the following are acceptable **EXCEPT:**
    a. lowering the angle of insertion
    b. drawing blood into a syringe
    c. using a 15-mL evacuated tube
    d. threading the needle into the vein

13. All of the following may cause hematoma formation **EXCEPT:**
    a. removing the tourniquet after removing the needle
    b. bandaging the patient's arm immediately after needle removal
    c. firmly anchoring the vein in needle insertion
    d. having the patient bend the elbow and apply pressure

14. The puncture site may require additional pressure to stop bleeding when the patient:
    a. has low blood pressure
    b. is taking anticoagulants
    c. frequently takes aspirin
    d. both B and C

15. Samples are rejected by the laboratory for all of the following reasons **EXCEPT:**
    a. clots in a lavender stopper tube
    b. collection in the wrong tube
    c. incompletely filled light blue stopper tubes
    d. clots in a red stopper tube

Clinical Situations

1 A patient enters the outpatient drawing station, properly identifies herself, and states that she had a mastectomy 3 months ago. She holds her left arm out for the phlebotomist.

   a. What should the phlebotomist ask the patient?
   b. If blood is drawn from the wrong arm, state two possible dangers to the patient.
   c. If blood is drawn from the wrong arm, state two possible effects on laboratory tests.

2 While a CBC is being collected, the patient develops syncope and the phlebotomist immediately removes the needle and lowers the patient's head. When the patient has recovered, the phlebotomist labels the lavender stopper tube, which fortunately contains enough blood, and delivers it to the hematology section. Many results on this specimen are markedly lower than those on the patient's previous CBC.

   a. How could the quality of the sample have caused this discrepancy?
   b. How could the venipuncture complication have contributed to this error?
   c. Could the phlebotomist have done anything differently? Explain your answer.

3 The phlebotomist has a requisition to collect two serology tests and a prothrombin time. No blood is obtained from the left antecubital area. The phlebotomist then moves to the right antecubital area and obtains a full red stopper tube, but cannot fill the light blue stopper tube.

   a. What should the phlebotomist do next?
   b. State two things the phlebotomist should do before deciding that the needle must be removed without filling the second tube.

Evaluation of Venipuncture Using a Syringe Competency

RATING SYSTEM
2 = Satisfactorily Performed,　　**1** = Needs Improvement,　　**0** = Incorrect/Did Not Perform

_____　**1.** Examines requisition form

_____　**2.** Greets patient, states procedure to be done

_____　**3.** Identifies patient verbally

_____　**4.** Examines patient's ID band

_____　**5.** Compares requisition form with ID band

_____　**6.** Washes hands and puts on gloves

_____　**7.** Selects tubes and equipment for procedure

_____　**8.** Positions patient's arm

_____　**9.** Applies tourniquet

_____　**10.** Identifies vein by palpation

_____　**11.** Releases tourniquet

_____　**12.** Cleanses site and allows it to air dry

_____　**13.** Assembles and conveniently places equipment

_____　**14.** Reapplies tourniquet

_____　**15.** Does not touch puncture site with unclean finger

_____　**16.** Checks plunger movement

_____　**17.** Anchors vein below puncture site

_____　**18.** Smoothly enters vein at appropriate angle with bevel up

_____　**19.** Does not move needle when plunger is retracted

_____　**20.** Collects appropriate amount of blood

_____　**21.** Releases tourniquet

_____　**22.** Covers puncture site with gauze

_____　**23.** Removes needle smoothly, activates the safety device and applies pressure

_____　**24.** Uses a blood transfer device to fill tubes

_____　**25.** Fills tubes in correct order

_____　**26.** Mixes anticoagulated tubes promptly

_____　**27.** Disposes of needle, transfer device, and syringe in sharps container

_____　**28.** Labels tubes and confirms with patient

_____　**29.** Examines puncture site

_____　**30.** Applies bandage

Continued

Evaluation of Venipuncture Using a Syringe Competency (Continued)

_____ **31.** Disposes of used supplies

_____ **32.** Removes gloves and washes hands

_____ **33.** Thanks patient

_____ **34.** Converses appropriately with patient during procedure

TOTAL POINTS _____

MAXIMUM POINTS = 68

Comments:

Evaluation of Venipuncture Using a Winged Blood Collection Set Competency

RATING SYSTEM
2 = Satisfactorily Performed,   **1** = Needs Improvement,   **0** = Incorrect/Did Not Perform

_____ **1.** Examines requisition form

_____ **2.** Greets patient, states procedure to be done

_____ **3.** Identifies patient verbally

_____ **4.** Examines patient's ID band

_____ **5.** Compares requisition form with ID band

_____ **6.** Washes hands and puts on gloves

_____ **7.** Selects tubes and equipment for procedure

_____ **8.** Positions patient's hand

_____ **9.** Applies tourniquet

_____ **10.** Identifies vein by palpation

_____ **11.** Releases tourniquet

_____ **12.** Cleanses site and allows it to air dry

_____ **13.** Assembles and conveniently places equipment

_____ **14.** Reapplies tourniquet

_____ **15.** Does not touch puncture site with unclean finger

_____ **16.** Anchors vein below puncture site

_____ **17.** Holds needle appropriately

_____ **18.** Enters vein smoothly at appropriate angle with bevel up

_____ **19.** Maintains needle securely in vein

_____ **20.** Smoothly operates syringe or evacuated tube holder

_____ **21.** Fills tubes in the correct order

_____ **22.** Mixes anticoagulated tubes promptly

_____ **23.** Collects appropriate amount of blood

_____ **24.** Releases tourniquet

_____ **25.** Covers puncture site with gauze

_____ **26.** Removes needle smoothly, activates safety device and applies pressure

_____ **27.** Disposes of apparatus in sharps container

_____ **28.** Uses a blood transfer device to fill tubes in the correct order when syringe is attached

_____ **29.** Labels tubes and confirms with patient

_____ **30.** Examines puncture site

Continued

Evaluation of Venipuncture Using a Winged Blood Collection Set Competency (Continued)

_____ **31.** Applies bandage

_____ **32.** Disposes of used supplies

_____ **33.** Removes gloves and washes hands

_____ **34.** Thanks patient

_____ **35.** Converses appropriately with patient during procedure

TOTAL POINTS _____

MAXIMUM POINTS = 70

Comments:

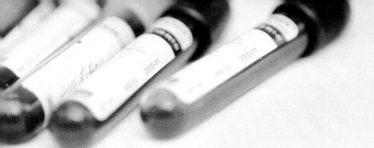

CHAPTER 11

Special Blood Collection

Learning Objectives

Upon completion of this chapter, the reader will be able to:

1. Define the various test collection priorities.
2. Define a fasting sample, and name three tests affected by not fasting.
3. List four reasons for requesting timed samples.
4. Describe the phlebotomist's duties when administering an oral glucose tolerance test for diabetes mellitus and gestational diabetes.
5. Discuss diurnal variation of blood constituents and list substances that would be affected.
6. Differentiate between a trough and a peak level in therapeutic drug monitoring and state the importance of collecting the sample at the prescribed time.
7. Discuss the timing sequences for the collection of blood cultures, the reasons for selecting a particular timing sequence, and the number of samples collected.
8. Describe the aseptic techniques required when collecting blood cultures.
9. Discuss blood collection from central venous access devices.
10. Describe the procedure for collecting samples for cold agglutinins and cryoglobulins.
11. List tests that must be chilled immediately after collection.
12. List tests that are affected by exposure to light.
13. Define chain of custody.
14. List three tests frequently requested for forensic studies.
15. Describe the physical and emotional changes in special patient populations and their effects on blood collection.

Key Terms

Aerobic
Anaerobic
Aseptic
Central venous access device
Chain of custody
Diurnal variation
Fasting
Forensic
Geriatric
Peak level
Postprandial
Septicemia
Trough level

Certain laboratory tests require the phlebotomist to use techniques that are not part of the routine venipuncture procedure. These special techniques may involve patient preparation, timing of sample collection, other blood collection techniques, and sample handling. Phlebotomists must know when these techniques are required, how to perform them, and how sample integrity is affected when they are not properly performed.

COLLECTION PRIORITIES

Each test order is designated as routine, ASAP, stat, or timed. Collections lists and turnaround times (TATs) for test results are based on these designations and will vary for different institutions. The phlebotomist must prioritize his or her workload accordingly to accommodate the various test priorities.

Routine Samples

Routine samples are tests that are ordered by the health-care provider to diagnose and monitor a patient's condition. Routine samples are usually collected early in the morning but can be collected throughout the day during scheduled "sweeps" (collection times) on the floors or from outpatients.

ASAP Samples

ASAP means "as soon as possible." The response time for the collection of this test sample is determined by each hospital or clinic and may vary by laboratory tests.

Stat Samples

Stat means the sample is to be collected, analyzed, and results reported immediately. Stat tests have the highest priority and are usually ordered from the emergency department or for a critically ill patient whose treatment will be determined by the laboratory result. The sample must be delivered to the laboratory promptly and the laboratory personnel notified.

FASTING SAMPLES

Certain laboratory tests must be collected from a patient who has been *fasting.* Fasting differs from a basal state condition in that the patient must only have refrained from eating and drinking (except water) for 12 hours, whereas in the basal state, the patient also must have refrained from exercise. Drinking water is encouraged to avoid dehydration in the patient, which can affect laboratory results. A patient who is NPO is not allowed to have food or water because of possible complications with anesthesia during surgery or certain medical conditions.

Test results most critically affected in a nonfasting patient are those for glucose, cholesterol, triglycerides, or lipid profiles. Prolonged fasting increases bilirubin and triglyceride values and markedly decreases glucose levels. When a fasting sample is requested, it is the responsibility of the phlebotomist to determine whether the patient has been fasting for the required length of time. If the patient has not, this must be reported to a supervisor or the nurse and noted on the requisition form if the decision is made to collect the sample nonfasting.

 Technical Tip 11-1. A sample that appears lipemic is an indication that the patient was not fasting and the lipemia may interfere with laboratory testing.

TIMED SAMPLES

Requisitions are frequently received requesting that blood be drawn at a specific time. Reasons for timed samples are shown in Box 11-1.

Phlebotomists should arrange their schedules to be available at the specified time and should record the actual time of collection on the requisition and sample tube. Results from samples collected too early

---

BOX 11-1 Reasons for Timed Samples

Measurement of the body's ability to metabolize a particular substance

Monitoring changes in a patient's condition (such as a steady decrease in hemoglobin)

Determining blood levels of medications

Measuring substances that exhibit diurnal variation (normal changes in blood levels at different times of the day)

Measurement of cardiac markers following acute myocardial infarction

Monitoring anticoagulant therapy

or too late may be falsely elevated or decreased. Misinterpretation of test results can cause improper treatment for the patient.

The most frequently encountered timed samples are discussed in this chapter. Other diagnostic procedures may also require timed samples, and any request for a timed sample should be strictly followed.

Glucose Tolerance Tests

A variety of methods have been available for the diagnosis of diabetes mellitus and gestational diabetes. Originally these included the 2-hour *postprandial* (pp) glucose test and the classic glucose tolerance test (GTT). The 2-hour pp glucose compared a patient's fasting glucose level with the glucose level 2 hours after eating a meal with a high carbohydrate content. The classic GTT required patients to drink a standard glucose load and return for testing on an hourly basis up to 6 hours in length.

Currently statistics and methods developed by the American Diabetes Association (ADA) and the World Health Organization (WHO) have standardized and shortened the methods used for the diagnosis of hyperglycemia. These methods include the 2-hour oral glucose tolerance test (OGTT) for diabetes mellitus and the 1-step and 2-step methods for diagnosing gestational diabetes.

Phlebotomists need to be aware of the variation in these procedures and follow their institutional protocol for instructing patients, administering the glucose loads, and setting up sample collection schedules. The basic instructions for these procedures are similar and are shown in Procedure 11-1.

GTT Preparation

Before the test, patients should be instructed to eat a balanced diet that includes 150 g per day of carbohydrates for 3 days and to fast for 12 hours but not more than 16 hours. Certain medications can interfere with the test results (Box 11-2), and the phlebotomist should ask the patient about medications before beginning the test. For glucose tolerance tests, the fasting patient should be instructed to abstain from food and drinks including coffee and unsweetened tea, except water, for 12 hours but not more than 16 hours before and during the test. Smoking, chewing tobacco, alcohol, sugarless gum, and vigorous exercise should be avoided before and during the test because they stimulate digestion and may cause inaccurate test results. Note on the requisition form if the patient is chewing gum.

BOX 11-2 Medications That May Interfere With Glucose Tolerance Test

Alcohol

Anticonvulsants

Aspirin

Birth control pills

Blood pressure medications

Corticosteroids

Diuretics

Estrogen-replacement pills

PROCEDURE 11-1 ✦ **GTT Procedure**

EQUIPMENT:

Requisition form
Flavored glucose solution
Gloves
Tourniquet
Alcohol pads
Evacuated tube holder and needles
Evacuated tubes
2 × 2 gauze
Sharps container
Indelible pen
Bandage
Biohazard bag

PROCEDURE:

Step 1. Identify the patient and explain the procedure.

Step 2. Confirm that the patient has fasted for 12 hours and not more than 16 hours.

Step 3. Draw a fasting glucose sample. The fasting blood sample is tested before continuing the procedure to determine whether the patient can safely be given a large amount of glucose.

Step 4. Ask the patient to drink the appropriate flavored glucose solution within 5 minutes. Small adults and children may have adjusted amounts based on 1 g of glucose per kilogram of weight. Oral glucose loads may vary when testing for gestational diabetes.

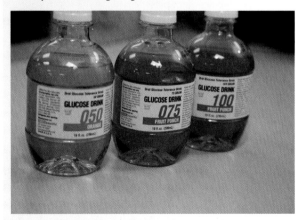

Step 5. Timing for the remaining collection times begins when the patient finishes drinking the glucose solution (Table 11-1). Outpatients are given a copy of the schedule and instructed to continue fasting, to drink water, and to remain in the drawing station area.

TABLE 11-1 • Sample Glucose Tolerance Test Schedule for 3-Hour Test	
TEST PROCEDURE	**3-HOUR TEST**
Fasting blood	0700
Patient finishes glucose	0800
1-Hour sample	0900
2-Hour sample	1000
3-Hour sample	1100

Step 6. Collect remaining samples at the scheduled times. Timing of sample collection is critical, because test results are related to the scheduled times; any discrepancies should be noted on the requisition.

Step 7. The type of evacuated tubes used for blood collection must be consistent. Blood samples that will not be tested until the end of the sequence should be collected in gray stopper tubes. Consistency of venipuncture or dermal puncture must also be maintained, because glucose values differ between the two types of blood. Venous blood samples are preferred.

Step 8. Corresponding labels containing routinely required information and sample order in the test sequence, such as 1-hour, 2-hour, and 3-hour are placed on the blood samples. Some health-care providers still request a ¹/₂-hour blood sample and urine samples to be collected and tested with each sample.

Step 9. During scheduled sample collections, phlebotomists should also observe patients for any changes in their condition, such as dizziness, which might indicate a reaction to the glucose, and should report any changes to a supervisor.

Step 10. Some patients may not be able to tolerate the glucose solution, and if vomiting occurs, the time of the vomiting must be reported to a supervisor and the health-care provider contacted for a decision concerning whether to continue the test. Vomiting early in the procedure is considered the most critical, and in most situations, the tolerance test is discontinued.

Step 11. Transport samples to the laboratory immediately. Samples not collected in gray stopper tubes must be centrifuged or tested within 2 hours of collection for reliable results.

▶ *Technical Tip 11-2.* Timing of inpatient glucose tolerance test collections is the responsibility of the phlebotomist.

▶ *Technical Tip 11-3.* Outpatients must understand the importance of adhering to the scheduled blood collection times for accurate results.

▶ *Technical Tip 11-4.* When collecting glucose tolerance test samples, closely observe the patient for symptoms of hyperglycemia or hypoglycemia.

2-Hour Oral Glucose Tolerance Test

The OGTT is now the recommended method for the diagnosis of diabetes mellitus. The procedure requires the collection of a fasting glucose sample, having the patient drink a 75-g glucose solution within 5 minutes and return for an additional glucose test in 2 hours. A result equal to or greater than 200 mg/dL is considered indicative of diabetes mellitus.

One- and Two-Step Method for Gestational Diabetes

Timing for these tests may vary with institutions and health-care providers. It is important for the phlebotomist to check with a supervisor for any requests that he or she is not familiar with.

The one-step method utilizes the same procedure as the diagnostic OGTT used to diagnose diabetes mellitus. A value equal to or less than 140mg/dL is considered normal. The two-step method requires the patient to receive two tests. First a 50-g glucose challenge load is administered to the fasting patient and blood collected and tested at 1-hour postingestion. The second test is administered on a different day and consists of either a 75-g OGTT or a 100-g 3-hour OGTT based on institutional protocol and health-care provider preferences. A value of 155 mg/dL in the 2-hour 75-g test is considered normal and a value of 140 mg/dL is considered normal in the 3-hour 100-g test.

❗ **Phlebotomist Alert 11-1.** It is essential that a phlebotomist take extra precautions to ensure that the requested methodology is being followed when administering the oral glucose tolerance tests (OGT Ts). Never hesitate to discuss the request with a supervisor or the chemistry department.

Lactose Tolerance Test

A lactose tolerance test evaluates a patient's ability to digest lactose, a milk sugar. The enzyme mucosal lactase converts lactose into glucose and galactose. Patients without this enzyme are unable to break down lactose from milk and milk products, which may result in gastrointestinal discomfort and diarrhea. Avoiding milk can reduce the symptoms.

Lactose intolerance can be diagnosed by a lactose tolerance test. The patient is asked to drink a standardized amount of lactose solution based on body weight in place of the glucose. A blood collection schedule is similar to a 2-hour GTT. Glucose levels will raise no more than 20 mg/dL from the fasting sample result if the patient is lactose intolerant.

Diurnal Variation

Substances and cell counts primarily affected by *diurnal variation* are corticosteroids, hormones, serum iron, glucose, and white blood cell counts, particularly eosinophils. Phlebotomists are often requested to draw samples for these tests at specific times, usually corresponding to the peak diurnal level. Certain variations can be substantial. Plasma cortisol levels drawn between 0800 and 1000 will be twice as high as levels drawn at 1600. Consequently, requests for plasma cortisol levels frequently specify that the test be drawn between 0800 and 1000, or at 1600. If the sample cannot be collected at the specified time, the health-care provider should be notified and the test rescheduled for the next day.

▶ *Technical Tip 11-5.* Patients must understand the importance of adhering to the scheduled blood collection times for accurate results.

Therapeutic Drug Monitoring

The fact that medications affect all patients differently frequently results in the need to change dosages or medications. Some medications can reach toxic levels in patients who do not metabolize or excrete them within an expected time frame. Likewise, there are patients who metabolize and excrete medications at an increased rate. The use of multiple medications also may interfere with the action of the medication being tested. To ensure patient safety and medication effectiveness, the blood levels of many therapeutic drugs are monitored.

Examples of frequently monitored therapeutic drugs are shown in Box 11-3. Random samples are

BOX 11-3 Frequently Monitored Therapeutic Drugs
Digoxin
Phenobarbital
Lithium
Gentamicin
Tobramycin
Vancomycin
Dilantin
Amikacin
Valproic acid
Theophylline
Methotrexate
Various antibiotics

occasionally requested; however, the most beneficial levels are those drawn before the next dosage is given (*trough level*) and shortly after the medication is given (*peak level*). Trough levels are collected immediately before the drug is to be given and represent the lowest level in the blood and ensure the drug is in the therapeutic (effective) range. Ideally, trough levels should be tested before administering the next dose to ensure that the level is low enough for the patient to receive more medication safely. The time for collecting peak levels varies with the medication and the method of administration (30 minutes after IV, 1 hour after intramuscular, or 1 to 2 hours after oral dosage) and ensures that the drug is not at a toxic level. Information from drug manufacturers provides the half-life, the toxicity level, and the recommended times for collection of peak levels.

To ensure correct documentation of the peak and trough levels, requisitions and sample tube labels should include the time and method of administration of the last dosage given, as well as the time that the sample is drawn. Therapeutic drug monitoring collections are often coordinated with the pharmacy, laboratory, and nursing staff.

Preexamination Consideration 11-1.

Collection of blood in gel serum separator tubes has caused falsely low levels for certain medications. Red stopper tubes are recommended for therapeutic drug monitoring and samples should be transported in an upright position.

 Technical Tip 11-6. Depending on the half-life of the medication, the timing of peak levels in therapeutic drug monitoring can be critical.

BLOOD CULTURES

One of the most difficult phlebotomy procedures is collection of blood cultures. This is because of the strict *aseptic* technique required and the need to collect multiple samples in special containers. The skin is covered with bacteria. If the venipuncture needle is contaminated with skin bacteria, the microorganisms can be inoculated into the collection bottles. A positive blood culture could be from skin contamination and not from an actual patient infection in the blood. Blood cultures are requested on patients when symptoms of fever and chills indicate a possible infection of the blood by pathogenic microorganisms (*septicemia*). The patient's initial diagnosis is often fever of unknown origin (FUO). A blood culture test can determine the microorganism causing the infection and the most effective antibiotic to treat the infection.

Timing of Sample Collection

Blood cultures are usually ordered stat or as timed collections. Isolation of microorganisms from the blood is often difficult due to the small number of organisms needed to cause symptoms. Samples are usually collected in sets of two drawn 30 or 60 minutes apart; however, timing of sample draws varies from institution to institution, or just before the patient's temperature reaches its highest point (spike). The concentration of microorganisms fluctuates and is often highest just before the patient's temperature spikes. This explains why collections may be ordered at specific intervals or ordered stat if a pattern has been observed in the patient's temperature chart. If antibiotics are to be started immediately, the sets are drawn at the same time from different sites. Samples collected from different sites at the same time serve as a control for possible contamination and must be labeled as to the collection site, such as right arm antecubital vein, and their number in the series (#1 or #2).

Collection Equipment

Blood can be drawn directly into bottles containing culture media or drawn into sterile, yellow stopper evacuated tubes containing the anticoagulant and sodium polyanethol sulfonate, and transferred to culture media in the laboratory. Each set should be collected in the same manner as the first set.

A winged blood collection set with a Luer adapter and a specially designed holder can be used to transfer blood directly from the patient to bottles containing culture media. The Luer adapter on the winged blood collection apparatus attaches to the transfer device that contains a stopper-puncturing needle. Blood flows from the vein through the winged blood collection set tubing, Luer adapter, and stopper-puncturing needle into the culture bottle.

Blood can be collected in a syringe and aseptically transferred to blood culture bottles at the bedside using a safety transfer device. Occupational Safety and Health Administration (OSHA) regulations do not allow direct inoculation from the syringe to the bottle.

A health-care provider may order blood cultures on a patient who is on antibiotic therapy, which would require the blood to be collected using special blood collection systems. Some blood culture collection systems have antimicrobial removal devices (ARDs) containing resin that inactivates antibiotics. The fastidious antimicrobial neutralization (FAN) blood collection system uses bottles that contain an activated charcoal that neutralizes the antibiotic.

Blood cultures may be collected from IV lines by specially trained personnel. The recommended procedure is to collect one blood culture from the IV line and a second culture by venipuncture. Both sources must be documented according to the facility's policy.

Blood Culture Anticoagulation

An anticoagulant must be present in the tube or blood culture bottle to prevent microorganisms from being trapped within a clot, where they might be undetected; therefore, blood culture bottles must be mixed after the blood is added. The anticoagulant sodium polyanethol sulfonate is used for blood cultures because it does not inhibit bacterial growth and may, in fact, enhance it by inhibiting the action of phagocytes, complement, and some antibiotics. Other anticoagulants should not be used because bacterial growth may be inhibited.

▶ *Technical Tip 11-7.* Blood collection bottles should be transported to the laboratory for testing as soon as possible, particularly the antimicrobial removal devices and fastidious antimicrobial neutralizations.

Cleansing the Site

The venipuncture technique for collecting blood cultures follows the routine procedures, except for the increased aseptic preparation of the puncture site. Contamination of the blood culture bottles with skin bacteria could interfere with the interpretation of the test results. Antiseptics for disinfecting the blood collection site include 2% iodine tincture, povidone-iodine, multiple isopropyl alcohol preps, and chlorhexidine gluconate, and all are equally effective in killing bacteria on the skin. Following institutional policy and strict adherence to aseptic technique during sample collection is essential to ensure that a positive blood culture is not caused by external contamination.

Cleansing of the site typically begins with vigorous scrubbing of the site for 1 minute using isopropyl alcohol. The alcohol is followed by scrubbing the site with 2% iodine tincture or povidone-iodine for another minute starting in the center of the venipuncture site and progressing outward 3 to 4 inches in concentric circles. Allow the iodine to dry on the site for at least 30 seconds. To prevent irritation of the patient's arm and iodine's possible adverse effect on the thyroid and liver, the iodine is removed with alcohol when the procedure is complete.

Chlorhexidine gluconate/isopropyl alcohol (ChloraPrep, Medi-Flex, Cardinal Health, Leawood, KS) is becoming more routinely used in many health-care facilities because of the frequency of iodine sensitivity in patients. It is a one-step application using a commercially prepared swab or sponge (ChloraPrep). The venipuncture site is scrubbed for 30 to 60 seconds in a back-and-forth motion creating a friction on the skin, which is effective in skin antisepsis. Chlorhexidine gluconate is not recommended for infants younger than 2 months.

▶ *Technical Tip 11-8.* Follow the manufacturer's instructions when using commercially packaged venipuncture site blood culture prep kits.

▶ *Technical Tip 11-9.* Phlebotomists should take every precaution not to retouch the puncture site after it has been cleaned. If the vein must be repalpated, the gloved finger must be cleaned in the same manner as the puncture site.

The tops of the blood culture bottles also must be cleaned before inoculating them with blood. The rubber stoppers can be cleaned using alcohol and allowed to dry before use or as recommended by the manufacturer. The alcohol pad remains on the bottles until inoculation. Iodine should not be used on the stoppers because it can enter the culture during sample inoculation and may cause deterioration of some stoppers during incubation.

Sample Collection

Two samples are routinely collected for each blood culture set, one to be incubated aerobically and the other anaerobically. When a syringe is used, the *anaerobic* bottle should be inoculated first to prevent possible exposure to air. When the sample is collected using a winged blood collection set, the *aerobic* bottle is inoculated first so that the air in the tubing does not enter the anaerobic bottle. Filling bottles directly through an evacuated tube needle and holder system is not recommended because of the possibility of broth media refluxing back into the vein. It also is difficult to ensure that the correct volume of blood has been collected.

Pediatric blood culture volume requirements are based on the child's weight and pediatric bottles are inoculated. Draw 1 mL of blood for every 5 kg (approximately 10 pounds) of patient weight. The sample of a child heavier than 45 kg is treated as that of an adult. Draw 1 mL of blood on babies weighing less than 5 kg, and place all of the blood in one pediatric bottle.

Because the number of organisms present in the blood is often small, the amount of blood inoculated into each container is critical. There should be at least a 1:10 ratio of blood to media. Adult blood culture bottles usually require 8 to 10 mL for each and pediatric bottles require 1 to 3 mL for each. Read the bottle label for the volume of blood required. Phlebotomists should follow the instructions for the system being used. Overfilling of bottles should be avoided because this may cause false-positive results with automated systems. Underfilled blood culture bottles may cause false-negative results.

Preexamination Consideration 11-2.

Failure to follow the proper inoculation procedure for aerobic and anaerobic samples is most critical for the anaerobic sample because the addition of air to the anaerobic bottle will kill any anaerobic organisms present.

PROCEDURE 11-2 ✦ Blood Culture Sample Collection

EQUIPMENT:

- Requisition form
- Gloves
- Tourniquet
- Chlorhexidine gluconate (or other acceptable skin antiseptic)
- Alcohol pads
- Blood culture bottles
- Syringe
- Hypodermic needle with safety device or Point-Lok device
- Blood transfer device
- Winged blood collection set and tube holder
- 2 × 2 gauze
- Sharps container
- Indelible pen
- Bandage
- Biohazard bag

PROCEDURE:

Step 1. Obtain and examine the requisition form.

Step 2. Greet the patient and explain the procedure to be performed.

Step 3. Use two identifiers to correctly identify the patient.

Step 4. Prepare the patient and verify allergies.

PROCEDURE 11-2 ✦ **Blood Culture Sample Collection** (Continued)

Step 5. Select equipment.

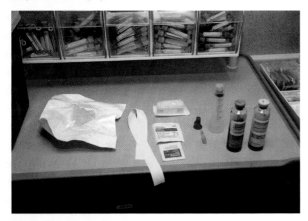

Step 6. Wash hands and don gloves.

Step 7. Apply the tourniquet and locate the venipuncture site.

Step 8. Release tourniquet.

Step 9. Sterilize the site using chlorhexidine gluconate. Creating a friction, rub for 30 to 60 seconds and allow to air dry for at least 30 seconds for antisepsis.

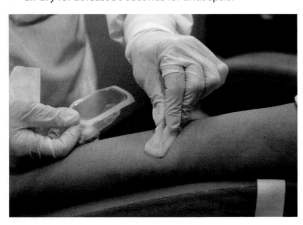

Step 10. Assemble equipment while the antiseptic is drying. Attach the needle to the syringe.

Step 11. Remove the plastic cap on the collection bottle. Confirm the volume of blood required from the label.

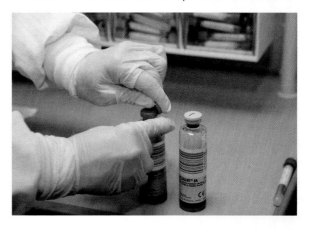

Step 12. Clean the top of the bottles with a 70 percent isopropyl alcohol pad and allow to dry.

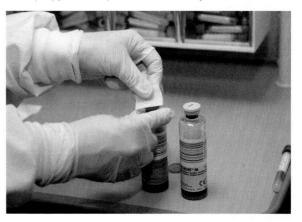

Continued

PROCEDURE 11-2 ✦ **Blood Culture Sample Collection** (Continued)

Step 13. Reapply the tourniquet and perform the venipuncture. Do not repalpate the site without cleansing the palpating finger in the same manner as the puncture site.

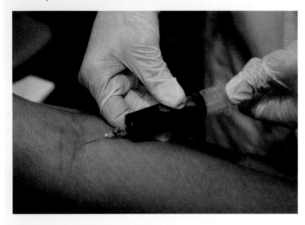

Step 14. Release the tourniquet. Place gauze over the puncture site, remove the needle, and apply pressure.

Step 15. Activate the safety device or remove the syringe needle with a Point-Lok device.

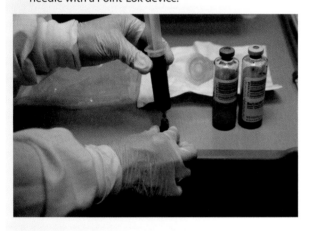

Step 16. Attach safety transfer device.

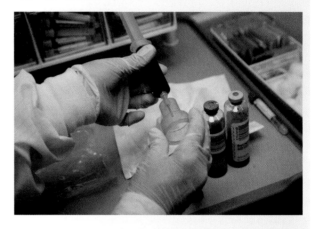

Step 17. Inoculate the anaerobic blood culture bottle first when using a syringe or second when using a winged blood collection set.

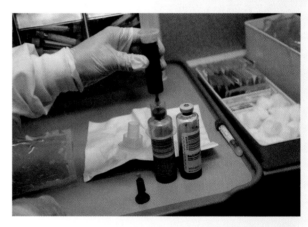

Step 18. Dispense the correct amount of blood into bottles. Some institutions require documenting the amount of blood dispensed.

PROCEDURE 11-2 ✦ **Blood Culture Sample Collection** (Continued)

Step 19. Mix the blood culture bottles by gentle inversion eight times.

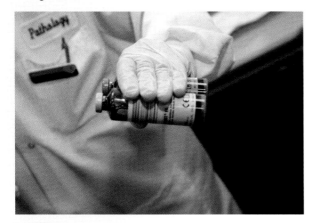

Step 20. Fill other collection tubes after the blood culture tubes.

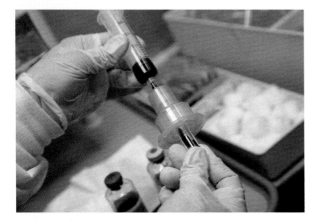

Step 21. Clean the iodine off the arm with alcohol if necessary.

Step 22. Label the samples appropriately and include the site of collection. Verify identification with the patient.

Step 23. Dispose of used equipment and supplies in a biohazard container.

Step 24. Check the venipuncture site for bleeding and bandage the patient's arm.

Step 25. Thank the patient, remove gloves, and wash hands.

BLOOD COLLECTION FROM CENTRAL VENOUS CATHETERS

Blood samples may be obtained from indwelling lines called central venous catheters (CVCs). However, this procedure must be performed by specially trained personnel and physician authorization is required. CVCs are a special type of catheter that is inserted by a physician or a certified health-care professional either as an internal catheter or external catheter into a large blood vessel. It can be used for administration of fluids, drugs, blood products, and nutritional solutions and to obtain blood. There are numerous types of CVCs and specific procedures must be followed for flushing the catheters with saline, and possibly heparin to prevent thrombosis, when blood collection is completed. Sterile technique procedures must be strictly adhered to when entering IV lines, because they provide a direct path for infectious organisms to enter the patient's bloodstream.

The four main types of CVCs used include the following:

1. Nontunneled, noncuffed CVC
   The nontunneled, noncuffed CVC is used for short-term dwell times and is inserted through the skin into the jugular, subclavian, or femoral vein and threaded to the superior vena cava by a physician during surgery or in a hospital room with local anesthetic. It can be a single-, double-, or triple-lumen catheter. When using multilumen catheters, the proximal lumen is the preferred lumen from which to obtain a blood sample. The lumens not being used should be clamped when drawing blood to avoid contamination of the blood sample. An occlusive waterproof dressing covers the insertion site, and flushes are necessary to maintain patency of the CVC.

2. Tunneled/cuffed
   The tunneled CVC is considered more permanent and is used for long-term dwell times, such as administration of chemotherapy. The Broviac, Hickman, and Groshong catheters are examples of this single-, double-, or triple-lumen type of external catheter. A surgeon performs a cut-down of the vein with local or IV sedation and tunnels the catheter in subcutaneous tissue under the skin with the catheter tip in the superior vena cava and some of the capped catheter tubing protruding from the exit site on the outside of the body. A sterile dressing is applied over the insertion site. Dressing changes and flushing with heparin or saline are required maintenance for this type of catheter (Fig. 11-1).

3. Implanted port
   The implanted port is a small chamber attached to a catheter that is also considered more permanent. It is used for long-term access to the central venous system for a patient requiring frequent IVs or receiving chemotherapy. Using local or IV sedation, a surgeon implants the port in subcutaneous tissue under the skin, usually at the collar bone with the catheter tip placed in the superior vena cava. It consists of a self-sealing septum housed in a metal or plastic case. The port is palpated to locate the septum. The self-sealing septum of the port withstands 1,000 to 2,000 needle punctures; however, only specially designed noncoring needles can be used. This needle has a deflected tip and is configured at a 90-degree angle. This type of port may be a single- or double-lumen catheter. The

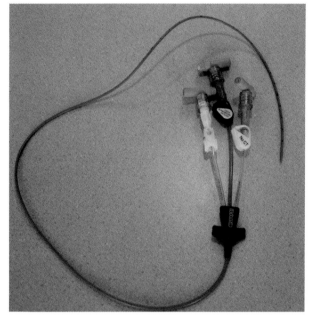

FIGURE 11-1 Triple-lumen catheter.

advantages of this CVC are that there is no visible catheter tubing and no site care is needed when it is not being used. It is flushed monthly with heparin or saline (Fig. 11-2).

4. Peripherally inserted central catheters (PICCs)
   The PICC is placed in the basilic or cephalic vein in the antecubital area of the arm, with the tip threaded to the superior vena cava. PICCs can be placed by IV team nurses or physicians and can be used for weeks to months. The

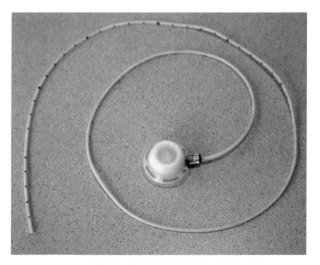

FIGURE 11-2 Implanted port.

catheter is threaded through an introducer needle with about 6 to 10 inches of catheter exposed and covered by an occlusive dressing. There is an antireflux valve connector device attached to the end of the catheter, where the IV is connected or blood samples are removed. The advantage of a PICC is that it has few risks and causes minimal discomfort to the patient. A disadvantage of blood collection from a PICC is that the catheter walls are easily collapsed.

Blood Sample Collection

Blood sample collection for laboratory testing can be routinely drawn from certain **central venous access devices** (CVADs). A health-care provider's order is required for the first time access of a newly inserted CVAD. Blood sample collection may be drawn from peripheral venous access devices only at the time of insertion. Blood samples are not collected from indwelling peripheral or midline catheters.

When IV fluids are being administered through the CVC, the flow should be stopped for 5 minutes before collecting the blood sample. Syringes larger than 20 mL should not be used because the high negative pressure produced may collapse the catheter wall. At all times, the first 5 mL of blood (or two times the dead space volume of the catheter) must be discarded or conserved and a new syringe must be used to collect the sample. Drawing coagulation tests from a venous catheter is not recommended, but if this is necessary, they should be collected after 20 mL (or five to six times the dead space volume of the catheter) of blood has been discarded or used for other tests.

Reinfusion of blood (instead of discarding blood) from CVADs for laboratory draws is an alternate procedure for patients in hospitals on the Blood Conservation Program. This procedure uses a three-way stopcock device with a sterile syringe attached to reinfuse the blood/saline back to the patient.

The order of tube fill may vary slightly to accommodate the amount of blood that must be drawn before a coagulation test. As with other procedures, blood cultures are always collected first. Blood cultures are drawn from CVCs primarily to detect infection of the catheter tip and should be compared with results from blood cultures drawn from a peripheral vein. If these are ordered, the draw will satisfy the additional discard needed for coagulation tests. Therefore, the order of fill is as follows:

1. First syringe—5 mL, discard or conserve
2. Second syringe—blood cultures
3. Third syringe—anticoagulated tubes (light blue, lavender, green, and gray)
4. Clotted tubes (red and serum separator tube [SST])

If blood cultures are not ordered, the coagulation tests (light blue stopper tube) can be collected with a new syringe after the other samples have been collected using the order shown earlier. Phlebotomists are frequently responsible for assisting the nurse who is collecting blood from the CVC and should understand these sample collection requirements. The source of the sample should be noted on the requisition form. Under no circumstances should a person without specialized training collect samples from a CVC. Institutional policy must be followed.

 Technical Tip 11-10. When blood is collected from a central venous access device (CVAD), blood should not be left in the syringe while extensive flushing of the CVAD is performed. Anticoagulation of the sample also is important.

 Technical Tip 11-11. Flushing central venous catheters is performed to ensure and maintain patency of the catheter and to prevent mixing of medications and solutions that are incompatible. Follow manufacturer's instructions for correct use and institutional policy and procedure for flushing.

PROCEDURE 11-3 ✦ **Blood Sample Collection from Central Venous Access Device**

EQUIPMENT:

Requisition form
Sterile gloves
Alcohol wipes or chlorhexidine gluconate sponge
Two 10-mL syringes filled with normal saline, for flush
Two 5-mL syringes
3-way stopcock
Blood collection tubes
Syringes for blood collection
Blood transfer device

PROCEDURE:

Step 1. Verify patient's identity using two identifiers.

Step 2. Explain the procedure and position the patient in a supine position.

Step 3. Assemble the supplies.

Step 4. Wash hands and don sterile gloves. Maintain aseptic technique throughout the procedure.

Step 5. Discontinue administration of all infusates into the CVAD (all lumens) prior to obtaining blood samples. If the lumen to be used for laboratory draws has an infusion, cap the tubing with a male/female cap when disconnecting.

Step 6. When drawing from multilumen catheters, the proximal lumen is the preferred lumen from which to obtain the sample. Use clamp on lumen to control blood flow and to help eliminate confusion with the stopcock.

Step 7. Attach a 10-mL prefilled saline syringe to a three-way stopcock. Prime the stopcock with saline.

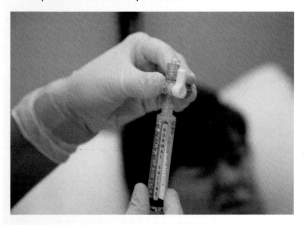

Step 8. Disinfect injection cap with alcohol wipe. Using vigorous friction, scrub on the top and in the grooves for 15 seconds. If laboratory draw is for a blood culture, scrub the injection cap with an alcohol wipe for 30 seconds.

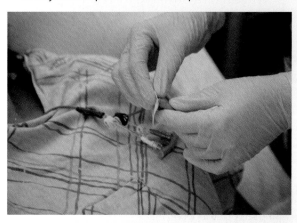

Step 9. Attach stopcock with syringe to injection cap.

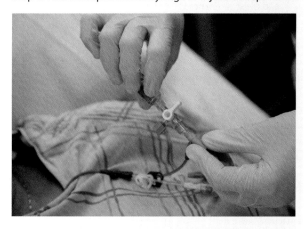

Step 10. Unclamp lumen and flush with remainder of saline. If the only lumen available to draw blood has total parenteral nutrition (TPN) infusing, flush with 18 to 19 mL of saline.

PROCEDURE 11-3 ✦ **Blood Sample Collection from Central Venous Access Device** (Continued)

Step 11. Clamp lumen and/or turn stopcock to "off" position to syringe port.

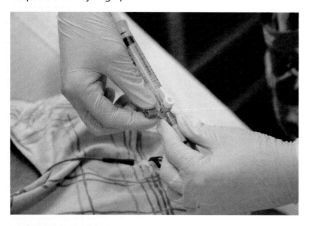

Step 12. Remove syringe and apply a new empty syringe to the same stopcock port (the inside of the first syringe is now contaminated by the plunger you have just touched and must be changed to keep the blood clean to reinfuse).

Step 13. Turn stopcock to "off" position to the unaccessed port. Unclamp lumen. Aspirate 5 mL blood into the empty syringe. Leave attached.

Step 14. Attach another empty syringe to the second stopcock port.

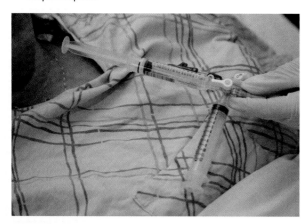

Step 15. Turn stopcock to "off" position to the blood-filled syringe.

Step 16. Draw blood sample into empty syringe.

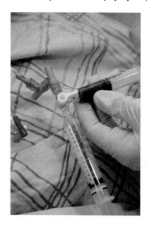

Step 17. Reinfuse blood from previously filled syringe.

Step 18. Remove stopcock and syringe. Cleanse injection cap with alcohol pad.

Step 19. Attach prefilled saline syringe and flush with 18 to 19 mL saline.

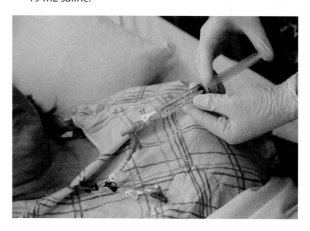

Step 20. If IV infusion has been disconnected, remove protective cap from tubing and reconnect infusion tubing.

Step 21. Resume all infusions in all lumens.

Continued

PROCEDURE 11-3 ✦ **Blood Sample Collection from Central Venous Access Device** (Continued)

Step 22. Connect a blood transfer device to the collection syringe and insert into evacuated tubes. Allow each tube to fill completely and according to the order of fill.

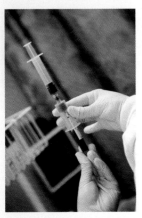

Step 23. Label each tube appropriately and confirm with patient.

Step 24. Prepare sample and requisition for transport to the laboratory.

Step 25. Dispose of used supplies in biohazard container.

Step 26. Remove gloves, wash hands, and thank the patient.

▶ *Technical Tip 11-12.* If there is any uncertainty about the integrity of the blood to be reinfused (contaminated or clotted), the blood must be discarded.

▶ *Technical Tip 11-13.* Potential test error can occur when blood is obtained from central venous access devices due to hemolysis caused by air leaks when using incompatible blood collection components and incomplete flushing of the collection site causing contamination or dilution of the sample.

PROCEDURE 11-4 ✦ **Blood Collection From an Implanted Port**

EQUIPMENT:

Sterile drape, gloves
Noncoring needle
Two 10-mL syringes
Two 10-mL syringes filled with saline
One 10-mL syringe filled with heparinized flush solution (follow institutional protocol)
Chlorhexidine gluconate sponge or alcohol and iodine pads
One 5-mL syringe
2 × 2 gauze pads
Dressing to cover insertion site

PROCEDURE:

Step 1. Identify patient using two identifiers.

Step 2. Assemble equipment.

Step 3. Palpate the shoulder area to locate and identify the septum of the access port.

Step 4. Prepare the area with a vigorous scrub using a chlorhexidine gluconate applicator. If using alcohol and iodine pads, prep in a circular motion from within to outward, approximately 4 to 6 inches. Allow iodine to dry completely.

Step 5. Connect the noncoring needle tubing on the end of one 10-mL saline flush syringe and prime the needle with saline until it is expelled.

Step 6. Locate the septum of the port with the nondominant hand; firmly anchor the port between the thumb and the forefinger.

Step 7. Holding the noncoring needle with the other hand, puncture the skin and insert the needle at a 90-degree angle into the septum using firm pressure. Advance the needle until resistance is met and the needle touches the back wall of the port.

Step 8. Inject 1 to 2 mL of saline, observe the area for swelling and ease of flow; if swelling occurs, reposition

---

PROCEDURE 11-4 ✦ **Blood Collection From an Implanted Port** (Continued)

the needle in the port without withdrawing it from the skin. If there is not swelling, aspirate for blood return. If blood return is observed, continue to flush with saline.

Step 9. Using the same syringe, aspirate 10 mL of blood and discard or conserve it. If samples will be collected for coagulation studies, discard 20 mL.

Step 10. Attach the syringe or the evacuated tube holder to the needle tubing and collect the blood necessary for ordered laboratory tests. Dispense the blood into the appropriate blood sample tubes using a blood transfer device if a syringe is used. Mix the blood by gentle inversion three to eight times.

Step 11. Flush the needle and the port with 10 mL of saline.

Step 12. Change syringes and flush with 3 mL of heparinized saline or follow your facility's policy.

Step 13. Remove the needle and apply a sterile dressing over the site.

Step 14. Label samples appropriately, confirm label with patient, remove gloves, and wash hands.

Step 15. Prepare sample and requisition form for transport to the laboratory. Dispose of used supplies.

Step 16. Thank the patient.

SPECIAL SAMPLE HANDLING PROCEDURES

Instructions for the collection, transportation, and storage of all laboratory samples are available from the laboratory and should be strictly followed to maintain sample integrity. Some tests require that the sample be kept warm, chilled, frozen, or protected from light.

Cold Agglutinins

Cold agglutinins are autoantibodies produced by persons infected with *Mycoplasma pneumoniae* (atypical pneumonia) or with autoimmune hemolytic anemias. The autoantibodies react with red blood cells at temperatures below body temperature.

Because the cold agglutinins in the serum attach to red blood cells when the blood cools to below body temperature, the sample must be kept warm until the serum can be separated from the cells. Samples are collected in tubes that have been warmed in an incubator at 37°C for 30 minutes and that contain no additives or gels that could interfere with the test. The phlebotomist can carry the warmed tube to the patient's room in a warm container or possibly a tightly closed fist, collect the sample as quickly as possible, return the sample to the laboratory in the same manner, and place it back in the incubator. Small portable heat blocks that have been warmed to 37°C are available for transporting samples that must be maintained at body

temperature. Failure to keep a sample warm before serum separation will produce falsely decreased test results. Cryofibrinogen and cryoglobulin are two proteins that precipitate when cold and must be collected and handled in the same manner as cold agglutinins.

Chilled Samples

Chilling a sample inhibits metabolic processes that continue after blood collection and can adversely affect laboratory results. Examples of samples that require chilling to prevent deterioration are shown in Box 11-4. Chilling is contraindicated for some analytes. Potassium levels will be falsely increased if the sample is chilled; therefore, whole blood samples collected for electrolytes must be collected in a separate tube when ordered with other tests that require chilling. Chilling blood samples for prothrombin time (PT) (international normalized ratio [INR]) testing is unacceptable as it may cause activation of Factor VII and alter the results. The Clinical and Laboratory Standards Institute (CLSI) recommends not chilling arterial blood gases (ABGs) unless collecting them in conjunction with lactic acid, when they have been collected in plastic syringes and analyzed within 30 minutes (see Chapter 14).

For adequate chilling, the sample must be placed in either crushed ice or a mixture of ice and water, or in a uniform ice block at the bedside (Fig. 11-3). Placing a sample in or on large ice cubes is not acceptable because uniform chilling will not occur and may

BOX 11-4 Examples of Analytes That May Require Chilling
Ammonia
Lactic acid
Acetone
Free fatty acids
Pyruvate
Glucagons
Gastrin
Adrenocorticotropic hormone (ACTH)
Parathyroid hormone (PTH)
Renin
Angiotensin-converting enzyme (ACE)
Catecholamines
Homocysteine
Some coagulation studies
Arterial blood gases (if indicated)

BOX 11-5 Samples Sensitive to Light
Bilirubin
Beta-carotene
Vitamin A
Vitamin B_6
Vitamin B_{12}
Folate
Porphyrins

tubes in aluminum foil or using an amber sample container or the equivalent can protect samples (Fig. 11-4).

▶ *Technical Tip 11-14.* Bilirubin is rapidly destroyed in samples exposed to light and can decrease up to 50% after 1 hour of exposure to light.

Legal (*Forensic*) Samples

When drawing samples for test results that may be used as evidence in legal proceedings, phlebotomists must use extreme care to follow the stated policies exactly. Documentation of sample handling, called the ***chain of custody***, is essential. It begins with patient identification and continues until testing is completed and results reported. Special forms are provided for this documentation, and special containers and seals may be required (Fig. 11-5). For each person handling the sample, documentation must include the date, the time, and the identification of the handler. Patient identification and sample collection should be done

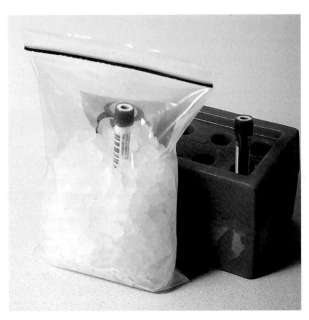

FIGURE 11-3 Sample placed in crushed ice and a uniform ice block.

cause part of the sample to freeze, resulting in hemolysis. It is important that these samples be immediately delivered to the laboratory for processing.

Samples Sensitive to Light

Exposure to artificial light or sunlight (ultraviolet) for any length of time may decrease the concentration of various analytes that are listed in Box 11-5. Wrapping the

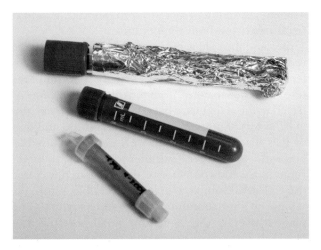

FIGURE 11-4 Samples protected from light.

Saint Joseph Hospital Toxicology Laboratory
601 N. 30th Street
Omaha, NE 68131-2197
(402) 449-4940

Drug Testing Custody & Control Form
NON-DOT/NON-HHS (NON-NIDA)

SPECIMEN ID NO. _____

LABORATORY ACCESSION NO. _____

▶ **STEP 1: TO BE COMPLETED BY COLLECTOR OR EMPLOYER REPRESENTATIVE**

A. Name, Address and I.D. No.

B. MRO Name and Address

C. Tests to be Performed: ☐ DS1   ☐ DS2   ☐ NON-NIDA5   ☐ URINE ALCOHOL   ☐ BLOOD ALCOHOL

D. Reason for Test: ☐ pre-employment ☐ current employment ☐ periodic ☐ reasonable susp/cause ☐ post accident ☐ other _____ specify

E. Donor I.D. _____

▶ **STEP 2: TO BE COMPLETED BY COLLECTOR** - Specimen temperature must be read within 4 minutes of collection.

Specimen temperature within range: ☐ Yes, 90.5° - 99.8°F/32.5° - 37.7°C   ☐ No, Record specimen temperature here _____

▶ **STEP 3: TO BE COMPLETED BY COLLECTOR AND DONOR** - Collector affixes bottle seal(s) to bottle(s). Collector dates seal(s). Donor initials seal(s).

▶ **STEP 4: TO BE COMPLETED BY DONOR** - Go to copy 2 (pink page); STEP 4.

▶ **STEP 5: TO BE COMPLETED BY COLLECTOR**

COLLECTION SITE LOCATION:

_____   (_____) _____
Collection Facility   Collector's Business Phone No.

_____   _____ _____ _____
Address   City   State   Zip

REMARKS: _____

I certify that the specimen identified on this form is the specimen presented to me by the donor providing the certification on Copy 2 of this form, that it bears the same specimen identification number as that set forth above, and that it has been collected, labeled and sealed.

X _____   ☐ AM
                                                                              ☐ PM
_____   _____   _____/_____/_____
(PRINT) Collector's Name (First, MI, Last)   Signature of Collector   Date (Mo./Day/Yr.)   Time

▶ **STEP 6: TO BE INITIATED BY THE COLLECTOR AND COMPLETED AS NECESSARY THEREAFTER**

DATE MO. DAY YR.	SPECIMEN RELEASED BY	SPECIMEN RECEIVED BY	PURPOSE OF CHANGE
__/__/__	DONOR - NO SIGNATURE	Signature _____ Name _____	PROVIDE SPECIMEN FOR TESTING
__/__/__	Signature _____ Name _____	Signature _____ *Courier* Name _____	TRANSPORT TO LABORATORY
__/__/__	Signature _____ *Courier* Name _____	Signature _____ Name _____	

– INTENTIONALLY LEFT BLANK –

_____
Date (Mo. Day. Yr.)

_____
Donor's Initials

PLACE OVER CAP

SPECIMEN ID NO. _____

_____
Date (Mo. Day. Yr.)

_____
Donor's Initials

PLACE OVER CAP

SPECIMEN ID NO. _____

TRANSPORT BOX CUSTODY SEAL

COLLECTOR'S INITIALS _____ DATE _____

COPY 1 - ORIGINAL - MUST ACCOMPANY SPECIMEN TO LABORATORY

FIGURE 11-5 Sample chain-of-custody form. *(Courtesy of Creighton University Medical Center, Omaha, NE.)*

in the presence of a witness, frequently a law enforcement officer. Identification may include fingerprinting or heel printing in paternity cases. Tests most frequently requested are alcohol and drug levels and DNA analysis.

Blood Alcohol Samples

Blood alcohol levels may be requested on a patient for medical reasons, legal reasons, or as part of employee drug screening. The chain of custody protocol must be strictly followed. When collecting blood alcohol levels, the site should be cleansed with soap and water or a nonalcoholic antiseptic solution such as benzalkonium chloride (Zephiran Chloride) to prevent compromising the results.

 Technical Tip 11-15. Skin disinfectants such as tincture of iodine and chlorhexidine gluconate contain alcohol and should not be used to clean the site for a blood alcohol level.

To prevent the escape of the volatile alcohol into the atmosphere, tubes should be completely filled and not uncapped for longer than necessary. Blood alcohol levels are frequently collected in gray stopper tubes with sodium fluoride; however, laboratory protocol should be strictly followed.

Molecular Diagnostics

The field of molecular diagnostic testing is rapidly expanding from the original blood testing of DNA primarily to determine paternity and body fluid DNA in criminal cases. In addition to samples collected by swabs for the identification of microorganisms, blood samples are collected for HIV and hepatitis C virus (HCV) viral loads, diagnosis of hematological disorders, coagulation disorders, management of warfarin (Coumadin) therapy, and identification of genetic disorders. More tests are rapidly being developed.

Depending on the test requested and the laboratory performing the test, the type of evacuated tubes collected will vary. Yellow stopper tubes containing acid-citrate-dextrose (ACD) are commonly used for DNA paternity testing. Two concentrations of ACD tubes are available and the sample must be collected in the tube with the required concentration. Other procedures may require ethylenediaminetetraacetic acid (EDTA) or sodium citrate as the anticoagulant. A variety of specialized tubes is also available.

 Technical Tip 11-16. Yellow stopper tubes containing sodium polyanethol sulfonate used for blood cultures are not acceptable for molecular diagnostic testing.

Drug Screening

Health-care systems, work places, universities and colleges may require scheduled or random drug screening. Urine is the sample of choice because of the ease of collection and because the substance remains in the urine for a longer period of time.

Phlebotomists may be involved in the collection of urine samples that are part of a screening process for the use of illegal drugs. Following and documenting the chain of custody procedures are again essential. Sample substitution, contamination, or dilution must also be prevented (see Chapter 16).

 Technical Tip 11-17. Technical errors and failure to follow chain-of-custody protocol are primary targets of the defense in legal proceedings.

SPECIAL PATIENT POPULATIONS

Phlebotomists encounter patients of all ages, which will require different technical and communication skills appropriate for each age group. The Joint Commission recommends that phlebotomists be proficient with all age groups and that age-specific competencies be demonstrated and evaluated. Sometimes modifications to blood collection techniques and equipment are necessary to successfully accommodate the challenges of blood collection for the pediatric and *geriatric* populations. Phlebotomists must develop and increase their knowledge and skills in working with all age groups of patients while performing blood collection procedures. An example of a phlebotomy department checklist for age-specific competency is shown in Figure 11-6.

Geriatric Population

Blood collection in the older patient population presents a unique challenge for the phlebotomist. Physical and emotional factors related to the aging process can cause difficulty with the blood collection procedure and sample integrity. The goal is to perform an atraumatic

EMPLOYEE: Write examples of care you have provided specific to your job, department, and patient population. Please give one example for each category for all of the age groups you have identified.

1. Provide care to **infant and toddler patients** through utilization of the following:
   a. Communication: Recognize and respond to communication cues.
   b. Health: Assist in creating an environment so infants are able to get ample sleep.
   c. Safety: Limit number of strangers.

2. Provide care to **young children** through utilization of the following:
   a. Communication: Explain procedure and equipment.
   b. Health: Provide rest periods.
   c. Safety: Provide safety habits.

3. Provide care to **older children** through utilization of the following:
   a. Communication: Involve patient whenever possible to help them feel useful.
   b. Health: Promote good nutrition and hygiene.
   c. Safety: Promote safety habits.

4. Provide care to **adolescent patients** through utilization of the following:
   a. Communication: Explain procedure and equipment supplementing explanations with reasons.
   b. Health: Encourage discussions and listen to issues on sexual responsibility and substance abuse without being judgmental.
   c. Safety: Prevent sports accidents.

5. Provide care to **young adults** through utilization of the following:
   a. Communication: Provide privacy.
   b. Health: Encourage decision-making regarding personal healthcare.
   c. Safety: Assist in adjustment to physical/psychosocial changes related to illness

6. Provide care to **middle adults** through utilization of the following:
   a. Communication: Realize need for self-reflection.
   b. Health: Encourage discussion and actively listen to issues regarding active retirement without being judgmental.
   c. Safety: Encourage preventative practice in relation to injuries.

7. Provide care to **older patients** through utilization of the following:
   a. Communication: Recognize need for some control due to multiple losses.
   b. Health: Plan for a balance between activity and rest during the day.
   c. Safety: Focus object directly in line of vision if patient experiences decreased visual acuity.

8. Provide care to **adults ages 80 and older** through utilization of the following:
   a. Communication: Encourage discussion and listen to end-of-life concerns without being judgmental.
   b. Health: Plan for a balance between activity and rest during the day.
   c. Safety: Orient patient well to surroundings, remind patient to use call button, if assistance is needed.

_____   _____
Employee's Signature   Date

_____   _____
Supervisor's Signature   **Date**

FIGURE 11-6 Department-specific checklist for age-specific competency. *(Adapted from Nebraska Methodist Hospital, courtesy of Diane Wolff, MLT [ASCP] Phlebotomy Team Leader, Omaha, NE.)*

venipuncture without bruising or excessive bleeding and provide a quality sample for analysis.

Physical Factors

Physical changes that occur in the geriatric patient that have an effect on blood collection are the following:

- Normal aging often results in gradual hearing loss. The phlebotomist may have to speak louder or repeat instructions while facing the patient. The phlebotomist must confirm that the patient thoroughly understands the instruction and identification procedures. Use of nonverbal methods or paper and pencil to explain the procedure or obtain permission may be required before performing the venipuncture.
- Failing eyesight is common in the older patient. The patient may have to be guided to the blood-drawing chair and have help being seated.
- The senses of taste, smell, and feeling also are affected. Malnourishment or dehydration may result from a lack of appetite. Malnutrition or dehydration because of not eating or drinking adequately can make locating veins for venipuncture difficult because of decreased plasma volume and can affect laboratory test results, with inherent higher potassium levels.
- Muscle weakness may cause the patient to drop things or be unable to make a fist before venipuncture or to hold the gauze after the venipuncture.
- Memory loss may cause the older patient to not remember medications he or she may have taken that can affect laboratory test results. A patient's inability to remember when he or she has last eaten can affect a test requiring fasting.
- With aging, the epithelium and subcutaneous tissues become thinner, causing veins to be less stable and harder to anchor. The phlebotomist must firmly anchor the vein below the site so that the vein does not move when punctured.
- Muscles become smaller. The angle of the needle may need to be decreased for venipuncture.
- Epidermal cell replacement in the aging patient is delayed, increasing the chance of infection. If the patient already has a weakened immune system, the patient may not heal as quickly or have the ability to fight bacteria that can be introduced during venipuncture. Extra care must be taken when preparing the site for venipuncture. Always wash hands before applying gloves and use gloves when palpating for the vein.

- Aging veins have decreased collagen and elasticity, making them less firm, more likely to collapse, more difficult to anchor and puncture, and more prone to hematoma formation.
- Older patients often feel cold because of the decreased fatty tissue layer, and warming of the site may be required.
- Arteries and veins often become sclerotic in the older patient, making them poor sites for venipuncture because of the compromised blood flow.

Disease States

Certain disease states found predominantly in the older patient contribute to the challenge of venipuncture and include the following:

- A patient with Alzheimer's disease may be confused or combative, which can cause problems with identification and performing the procedure. Assistance from a family member or the patient's caretaker may be necessary to calm the patient and hold the arm steady.
- Stroke patients may have paralysis or speech impairments requiring assistance in positioning and holding the arm and help with communication.
- Patients in a coma should be treated as if they can hear what is being said. Again, assistance will be required when holding the arm.
- Arthritic patients may be in pain or unable to straighten the arm and may require assistance gently positioning and holding the arm. Using a winged blood collection set with flexible tubing will allow the phlebotomist to access veins at awkward angles.
- Older patients may have tremors, as evidenced in Parkinson's disease, and may not be able to hold the arm still for the venipuncture procedure.

Emotional Factors

Patients are often embarrassed by these conditions, which may cause anxiety or fear of blood collection. As previously stated, emotional stress can alter blood composition and laboratory testing. In addition to the physical changes of aging, the older patient often faces the loss of career, spouse, family members, and friends. These life changes can bring about depression, sadness, and anger. The fear of pain or the expense associated with venipuncture may make the patient anxious or even tearful. All of these physical and emotional factors can alter test results, and the phlebotomist must be sensitive to them. In preparing the patient for venipuncture, it is important to take more time than usual to assist and reassure the patient. Treat patients with respect and dignity, giving them a sense of control.

Blood Collection

The venipuncture procedure is basically the same for geriatric patients; however, unique preparation and sometimes modification to the blood collection technique are necessary to successfully accommodate the collection of blood.

Patient Identification

When identifying older patients without identification bands, be sure to have them state their names. An elderly patient who is confused or who has difficulty hearing is very likely to answer "yes" to any question. When identifying patients, address them by their rightful title and not by their first name. Always be considerate and thank the patient.

Equipment Selection

Because of the small, fragile veins frequently seen in the older patient, the evacuated tube system is usually not the best choice of equipment. The vacuum pressure in the collection tube may cause fragile veins to collapse. A better choice is a winged blood collection set with a 23-gauge needle attached to a syringe that will allow the phlebotomist to control the suction pressure on the vein. A small-gauge needle with a syringe also is an option. If an evacuated tube system is used, the smallest possible tubes should be filled. Because of the tendency to develop anemia by older patients, the volume of blood collected also should be kept to the minimum acceptable amount.

Tourniquet Application

Elderly patients are prone to bruising when applying the tourniquet. The tourniquet can be placed over the patient's sleeve and must not be applied too tight to avoid injury to the patient or collapsing the vein. Gently release the tourniquet after venipuncture without snapping it against the patient's skin to avoid bruising the area. Blood pressure cuffs can be used for the thin patient with small, hard-to-find veins.

Site Selection

Because of the difficulty in locating and anchoring veins and the presence of hematomas from previous venipunctures in the elderly patient, the antecubital fossa may not be the best site selection. The veins in the hand or forearm may be a better choice. It may require a little extra time and using techniques for making the veins more prominent. Applying heat compresses for 3 to 5 minutes and stimulating the area with alcohol can make the vein more prominent. To avoid bruising the patient, do not tap the vein. Other techniques used by phlebotomists to enhance the prominence of veins include massaging the arm upward from the wrist to the elbow and briefly hanging the arm down. Remember that when performing these techniques, the tourniquet should not remain tied for more than 1 minute at a time.

Performing the Venipuncture

Elderly patients' veins "roll" easily; therefore, the skin must be pulled taut, anchored firmly, and the vein punctured in a quick motion. Loose skin can be pulled taut by wrapping your hand around the arm from behind. The angle of the needle may need to be decreased for venipuncture because the veins are often close to the surface of the skin.

Bandages

Older patients may have increased sensitivities to adhesive bandages and an increased tendency to bruise. Therefore, it is preferable to use a self-adhering pressure-dressing bandage (e.g., Coban) because adhesive bandages on the fragile skin of older patients can actually take off a layer of skin when they are removed and leave a raw wound susceptible to infection. A better alternative is for the phlebotomist to hold pressure on the site for 3 to 5 minutes or until the bleeding has stopped. Older patients are often on anticoagulant therapy for heart problems or stroke. Extra time is necessary to hold pressure on the site until bleeding has stopped before bandaging the area to avoid excessive bleeding or hematoma formation. The bandage may not be applied until the bleeding has stopped. The extra time and consideration given to the patient is well spent.

 Technical Tip 11-18. Direct light on the venipuncture sight may help locate hard-to-find veins in the older patient.

Additional Considerations

Dermal puncture, when possible, should be performed on the older patient as a way of avoiding complications such as hematomas, bruising, collapsed veins, and anemia. The advances in point-of-care testing (see Chapter 15) have made it possible to perform many types of tests on a small amount of blood that can be obtained by a dermal puncture.

Pediatric Population

Ideally, children younger than 2 years should have blood collected by a dermal puncture procedure (see Chapter 12). However, special tests for coagulation, erythrocyte sedimentation rates, special diagnostic studies, or blood cultures require more blood than can be collected from a finger or heel stick and must be collected by venipuncture.

Patient/Parent Preparation

Pediatric blood collection involves preparing both the child and parent, using certain restraining procedures, and special equipment. Pediatric phlebotomy presents emotional as well technical difficulties and should be performed by only experienced phlebotomists. A negative experience can lead to a child's life-long fear of needles. Often, there is only one chance to attempt a venipuncture on a child.

The phlebotomist must develop interpersonal skills to successfully gain both the young patients' and parents' trust and cooperation as well as be skilled with the special types of equipment used for pediatric venipuncture. It is important to keep the patient as calm as possible during the procedure because, as previously discussed, emotional stress and crying can affect blood analytes and cause erroneous test results.

Techniques for Dealing with Children

Techniques for dealing with children vary depending on the child's age. It is best to establish guidelines and to be honest with both the patient and parent. Newborns and infants are totally dependent on their parents. The phlebotomist should introduce him or herself to the parents and explain the procedure. Ask the parents about the child's previous experiences with blood collection. If possible, have the parent hold the child and encourage the parent to use distraction and comforting techniques. The parents must identify the child if it is an outpatient setting. Hospitalized patients will have an identification band.

Toddlers

Toddlers have limited language skills and fear of strangers. It is important to talk to the child calmly and maintain eye contact. Demonstrate the procedure using toys. Allow children to have their comfort toys or blanket and develop strategies to distract or entertain

them. Again, it is helpful to have the parents assist with holding and comforting the child. Reward the child with praise and stickers. Thank the child and parent for their cooperation.

Older Children

Older children are more willing to participate. Explain the steps of the procedure and demonstrate the equipment. Demonstrate and allow the child to touch the tourniquet or other clean equipment. Answer their questions honestly. Never tell a child it will not hurt. Explain that "it will hurt a little bit, but if you hold very still, it will be over quickly." Enlist the child's help in holding the gauze. Give the child permission to cry.

Teenagers

Teenagers are more independent and often embarrassed to show their emotions. Use adult language with teenagers for identification and explanation of the procedure. Ask them if they have fainted or had any reaction to a previous venipuncture procedure. Encourage them to ask questions about the procedure. They may or may not want their parents present.

Methods of Restraint

Older children can usually sit in a drawing chair by themselves. An infant cradle pad (see Chapter 8) facilitates blood collection for infants. Never draw blood from a small child without some type of assistance. Physical restraint may be required to immobilize the young child and steady the arm for the venipuncture procedure. This can be accomplished by having someone hold the child or by using a papoose board. Either a vertical or horizontal restraint will work.

Vertical Restraint

In the vertical position, the parent holds the child in an upright position on the lap. The parent places an arm around the toddler to hold the arm not being used. The other arm holds the child's venipuncture arm firmly from behind, at the bend of the elbow, in a downward position.

Horizontal Restraint

In the horizontal restraint, the child lies down, with the parent on one side of the bed and the phlebotomist on the opposite side. The parent leans over the child holding the near arm and body securely while reaching over the body to hold the opposite venipuncture arm for the phlebotomist.

In some instances, a child may become extremely combative. The procedure should be discontinued to avoid the risk of injury to the patient or phlebotomist and the health-care provider notified.

Equipment Selection

The minimum amount of blood required for laboratory testing should be collected from infants and small children because drawing excessive amounts of blood can cause anemia. The amount of blood collected within a 24-hour period must be monitored owing to the small blood volume in newborns and small children. It is recommended that no more than 3% of a child's blood volume be collected at one time and no more than 10% in a month. To quickly estimate a child's blood volume, divide the child's weight in pounds by 2 to convert to kilograms and multiply the kilograms by 100 to get the estimated blood volume in milliliters.

When using an evacuated tube system, select the smallest evacuated pediatric tubes available to collect the least amount of blood and to avoid causing the vein to collapse. Evacuated tubes as small as 1.8 mL are available. A 23-gauge winged blood collection set needle with a syringe is recommended because of the small, fragile veins. If only a very small amount of blood is collected, use a microcollection tube rather than an evacuated tube. Using an evacuated tube system on older children is acceptable. Pediatric-sized tourniquets are also available. Assemble equipment out of view of the child and cover threatening-looking equipment when approaching the pediatric patient.

Pain Interventions

A local topical anesthetic, eutectic mixture of local anesthetics (EMLA) (Abraxis Pharmaceuticals) is ideal for use on an apprehensive child before venipuncture. This emulsion of lidocaine and prilocaine is applied directly to intact skin and covered with an occlusive dressing. EMLA penetrates to a depth of 5 mm through the epidermal and dermal layer of the skin. It takes 60 minutes to reach its optimal effect and lasts for 2 or 3 hours. Because of the length of time necessary to anesthetize the area, it is necessary that accurate vein selection is made or more than one site treated. EMLA should not be used on infants younger than 1 month or if the child is allergic to local anesthetics. One side effect of this emulsion may be pallor at the site or a slight redness because of the adhesive covering. It is a prescription medication and must be administered by a nurse, health-care provider, or parent. Other topical anesthetics include a nonprescription gel, L.M.X4 (4% lidocaine) (Ferndale Labs), which is effective 15 to 30 minutes after application

and Ametop gel (4% amethocaine) (Smith & Nephew Healthcare). Tetracaine, a topical anesthetic patch, has been shown to be effective when applied 30 minutes before venipuncture.

Research has shown that glucose, dextrose, and sucrose solutions have a calming effect on infants. When administered before or during venipuncture or heelsticks, pain was significantly reduced as opposed to a topical anesthetic. The duration of crying was lessened, which minimized the temporary increase in the white blood cell counts. Commercial sucrose pacifiers or nipples are available. A 24% solution of sucrose may be made by mixing 4 teaspoons of water with 1 teaspoon of sugar. This sucrose solution may be given to the infant using a syringe, dropper, nipple, or pacifier (Fig. 11-7) about 2 minutes before venipuncture and the effects last for about 5 minutes.

Other methods for reducing pain and calming a child include breastfeeding and holding a child tightly swaddled in a blanket during heelsticks or venipuncture. Iontophoresis, the application of an anesthetic by a low-voltage electrical current, is faster than the gel application and has been shown to be effective against venipuncture pain; however, it is not recommended for children younger than 5 years. Products that utilize this technology include Numby Stuff (Iomed), Lidosite (B. Braun), and Needle-Buster (Life-Tech).

Preexamination Consideration 11-3.
Utilizing techniques to calm an infant and reduce crying times will minimize the preexamination effect of transient elevated white blood cell counts.

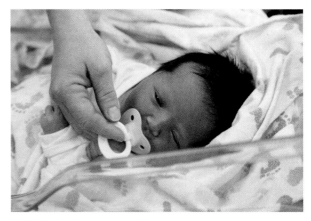
FIGURE 11-7 Sucrose pacifier.

Site Selection

The veins located in the antecubital fossa are the best choice for children older than 2 years. Do not use deep veins. Site selection and technique is similar to that used for adults (see Chapter 9).

Dorsal hand venipuncture can be used for children younger than 2 years of age. This technique can be used to collect samples from a superficial hand vein directly into appropriate microsample containers. The advantage of this technique is that more blood can be collected from the vein as compared with a heelstick and there is less chance of hemolyzing the sample or contaminating the sample with tissue fluid. Use of this technique requires additional training and is an institutional decision, because saving all veins for IV therapy may be preferred. Use extreme care when disposing of the contaminated needle.

PROCEDURE 11-5 ✦ Dorsal Hand Vein Technique

EQUIPMENT:

Requisition form
Gloves
Alcohol pads
Gauze
23- to 25-gauge hypodermic needle
Microtainers

PROCEDURE:

Step 1. Obtain and examine the requisition form.

Step 2. Greet the parent and explain the procedure.

Step 3. Wash hands and put on gloves.

Step 4. Identify the infant/child.

Step 5. Immobilize the infant/child.

Step 6. Select the vein by encircling the wrist and gently bending it downward. Bending the wrist too much may cause the vein to flatten out and be hard to see or may cause the vein to collapse.

Step 7. Do not use a tourniquet.

Step 8. Cleanse the site with alcohol and allow it to air dry.

Step 9. Select a 23- to 25-gauge hypodermic needle with a clear hub and appropriate Microtainers.

Step 10. Encircle the vein with the thumb underneath and the index and middle finger on top of the wrist and apply pressure with the index finger.

Step 11. Insert the needle with the bevel up into the vein at a 15-degree angle to the skin. Stop advancing the needle as soon as blood appears in the hub.

Step 12. Fill Microtainers directly from the blood that drips from the hub of the needle.

Step 13. Release the finger pressure intermittently to allow the blood to continue to flow.

Step 14. After collection of samples, place gauze over the needle but do not push down.

Step 15. Remove the needle and apply pressure for 2 to 3 minutes or until the bleeding stops.

Step 16. Do not apply a bandage.

Step 17. Label the tubes.

Step 18. Perform appropriate sample handling.

Step 19. Dispose of used supplies in biohazard containers.

Step 20. Remove gloves and wash hands.

Step 21. Enter blood collection volume in the infant's/child's chart or log book.

Step 22. Deliver samples promptly to the laboratory.

Key Points

- ✦ Test collection priorities determine how phlebotomists prioritize their workload to achieve maximum turnaround times. Routine samples are collected throughout the day or at scheduled "sweep" times. ASAPs are collected as soon as possible. Timed samples are drawn at a specific time. Stat samples have the highest priority are collected and analyzed immediately.

- ✦ A fasting sample is collected from a patient who has had nothing to eat or drink except water for 12 hours. Tests results affected in a nonfasting patient are glucose, cholesterol, triglycerides, and lipid profiles.

- ✦ Timed samples are requested to measure the body's ability to metabolize a substance, monitor changes in a patient's condition, determine blood levels of medications, measure analytes that exhibit diurnal variation, measure cardiac markers following a myocardial infarction, and monitor anticoagulant therapy.

- ✦ Methods to diagnose hyperglycemia include the 2-hour OGTT for diabetes mellitus and the one-step and two-step methods for diagnosing gestational diabetes. A sample for a fasting blood sugar measurement is collected and tested before a glucose solution is given to the patient. Blood samples are drawn at designated times.

- ✦ Substances that exhibit diurnal variation are at different levels in the blood at certain times of the day. For example, cortisol levels drawn between 0800 and 1000 will be twice as high as levels drawn at 1600.

- ✦ Therapeutic drug levels are tested to monitor the effectiveness and safety of a therapeutic drug. The trough level is drawn before the next dosage is given and the peak level is drawn at a specified time after the medication is given. Peak levels vary with the medication and the method of administration.

- ✦ Blood cultures are requested for a patient with suspected septicemia. Two samples are collected for each blood culture set, one to be incubated aerobically and the other anaerobically. Blood cultures are ordered as timed or stat collections and strict aseptic technique is required.

- ✦ Blood samples can be collected from central venous catheter devices by specially trained personnel. The phlebotomist must be familiar with the various types of catheters, the flush protocol, and order of fill for blood collection tubes.

- ✦ Samples for cold agglutinins are collected in tubes that have been warmed in a 37°C incubator for 30 minutes and contain no additive or gel. The blood is collected into the warmed tube, returned to the laboratory as soon as possible, and placed back into the incubator before testing.

- ✦ Chilling samples prevents deterioration of specific analytes such as ammonia, lactic acid, pyruvate, gastrin, adrenocorticotrophic hormone (ACTH), renins, catecholamines, and parathyroid hormone. Samples should be immediately placed into a crushed ice and water slurry or uniform ice block after blood collection.

- ✦ Exposure to light will destroy bilirubin; beta-carotene; vitamins A, B_6, and B_{12}, and folate; and porphyrins. Wrapping tubes in aluminum foil or using amber-colored tubes will protect the sample.

- ✦ *Forensic* studies are performed on samples for legal proceedings. The most common are blood alcohol tests, urine drug tests, and DNA analysis. Documentation of sample handling, the chain of custody, must be strictly followed.

- ✦ Molecular diagnostic tests are continuing to be developed for the identification of microorganisms, HIV and HCV viral loads, diagnosis of hematological disorders, coagulation disorders, management of warfarin (Coumadin) therapy, and identification of genetic disorders.

- ✦ Geriatric and pediatric patients may require modifications in the venipuncture technique. Phlebotomists must be proficient with all age groups and demonstrate age-specific competencies.

BIBLIOGRAPHY

American Diabetes Association: Diagnosis and Classification of Diabetes Mellitus. *Diabetes Care* 2008;31(suppl 1); 562-567.

CLSI. Procedures for the Collection of Diagnostic Blood Specimens by Venipuncture; Approved Standard-Sixth Edition. CLSI document H3-A6. Clinical and Laboratory Standards Institute, 2007, Wayne, PA.

CLSI. Procedures for the Handling and Processing Blood Specimens; Approved Guideline, ed. 3. CLSI document H18-A4. Clinical and Laboratory Standards Institute, 2010, Wayne, PA.

CLSI. Collection, Transport, and Processing for Testing Plasma-Based Coagulation Assays and Molecular Hemostasis Assays; Approved Standard H21-A5, ed. 5. CLSI document H21-A5. Clinical and Laboratory Standards Institute, 2008, Wayne, PA.

Ernst, DJ: Pain Reduction During Infant and Pediatric Phlebotomy. http://www.mlo-online.com. *Medical Laboratory Observer,* July 2007.

Methodist Hospital Nursing Service Policy and Procedure Manual: Intravenous Therapy: Blood Specimen Collection From Vascular Access Device. 2008, Omaha, NE.

 ## Study Questions

1. At 0730, the phlebotomist receives requests for a cortisol level on Unit 4B, a fasting blood sugar (FBS) on Unit 4A, and a stat crossmatch in the ER. In which order should the phlebotomist collect these samples?
   a. cortisol, FBS, crossmatch
   b. FBS, cortisol, crossmatch
   c. crossmatch, FBS, cortisol
   d. FBS, crossmatch, cortisol

2. The timing for a glucose tolerance test begins when:
   a. the fasting sample is drawn
   b. the test results are completed on the fasting sample
   c. the patient finishes drinking the glucose
   d. 30 minutes after the patient finishes drinking the glucose

3. Samples are scheduled for collection at specific times for all of the following reasons **EXCEPT:**
   a. measuring the body's metabolism of the test substance
   b. the substance exhibits diurnal variation
   c. patients must be tested 2 hours before meals
   d. to determine blood levels of medications prior to the next dose

4. The trough level for therapeutic drug monitoring is collected:
   a. 30 minutes after the medication is administered
   b. 30 minutes before the medication is administered
   c. at the time specified by the manufacturer
   d. after the patient has fasted for 8 hours

5. When blood is inoculated into blood culture bottles using a winged blood collection set, the:
   a. anaerobic bottle is inoculated first
   b. safety device is activated first
   c. aerobic bottle is inoculated first
   d. volume of blood inoculated is increased

6. Blood collected from CVADs is collected in evacuated tubes by attaching a/an:
   a. sterile 20-gauge needle to the collection syringe
   b. evacuated tube holder to the catheter line
   c. blood transfer device to the collection syringe
   d. Luer-Lok to the catheter line

7. Which of the following has a self-sealing septum that is accessed with a noncoring needle?
   a. implanted port
   b. PICC line
   c. Hickman
   d. peripheral IV

8. Samples that require chilling immediately after collection are placed in a:
   a. container of large ice cubes
   b. a container of crushed ice and water
   c. a bag of dry ice
   d. flask of cold water

9. Samples for cold agglutinins must be:
   a. transported on ice
   b. drawn in a green stopper tube
   c. processed in a refrigerated centrifuge
   d. kept warm

Study Questions—cont'd

10. A falsely decreased blood alcohol level may be obtained if:
   a. blood is collected in a gray stopper tube
   b. the site is cleansed with Zephiran chloride
   c. the tube is only partially filled
   d. the tube is overfilled

11. When performing venipuncture on a pediatric patient, the phlebotomist may require:
   a. assistance
   b. a pediatric requisition
   c. small evacuated tubes
   d. both A and C

12. Older patients are more prone to hematoma formation because:
   a. they have smaller veins
   b. tourniquets must be tied tighter
   c. their veins have decreased elasticity
   d. they have difficulty making a fist

Clinical Situations

1 An outpatient comes to the laboratory at 1300 with a requisition for a lipid profile.
   a. Before collecting the sample, what should the phlebotomist ask the patient?
   b. What specific tests requested for this patient are of concern to the phlebotomist?
   c. State the instructions that should have been given when the patient received the requisition.

2 Two sets of blood cultures, each consisting of an aerobic and an anaerobic bottle, are drawn from a patient 1 hour apart. The first set is drawn using a syringe and the second set using a winged blood collection set.
   a. Is this a common ordering pattern for blood cultures? Why or why not?
   b. What error in technique could cause a positive anaerobic culture from the first set and a negative anaerobic culture in the second set?
   c. What is the significance of a known skin contaminant growing in the aerobic bottle from the first set and not in the aerobic bottle from the second set?
   d. Would failure to mix the bottles after the blood is added most probably cause a false-positive or false-negative culture?

3 While collecting blood from an elderly patient using an evacuated tube, the phlebotomist notices that the puncture site is beginning to swell.
   a. Why is this happening?
   b. What should the phlebotomist do?
   c. How could the sample be collected?

Evaluation of Blood Culture Collection Competency

RATING SYSTEM
2 = Satisfactorily Performed,   **1** = Needs Improvement,   **0** = Incorrect/Did Not Perform

_____ **1.** Examines requisition and identifies patient

_____ **2.** Correctly assembles equipment

_____ **3.** Washes hands

_____ **4.** Puts on gloves

_____ **5.** Applies tourniquet

_____ **6.** Selects puncture site

_____ **7.** Releases tourniquet

_____ **8.** Scrubs site with alcohol for 1 minute

_____ **9.** Cleanses site with iodine

_____ **10.** Completes iodine cleaning using concentric circles

_____ **11.** Allows iodine to dry

_____ **12.** Cleanses tops of blood culture containers

_____ **13.** Cleanses palpating finger in the same manner as the puncture site if necessary

_____ **14.** Reapplies tourniquet

_____ **15.** Performs venipuncture

_____ **16.** Inoculates anaerobic container first from syringe or second from a winged blood collection set

_____ **17.** Dispenses correct amount of blood into containers

_____ **18.** Mixes containers

_____ **19.** Disposes of used equipment and supplies

_____ **20.** Removes iodine from patient's arm

_____ **21.** Bandages patient's arm

_____ **22.** Correctly labels blood culture containers and confirms with patient

_____ **23.** Overall aseptic technique

TOTAL POINTS _____

MAXIMUM POINTS = 46

Comments:

Evaluation of Blood Sample Collection From Central Venous Access Device Competency

RATING SYSTEM
2 = Satisfactorily Performed,   **1** = Needs Improvement,   **0** = Incorrect/Did Not Perform

_____ 1. Examines requisition and verifies patient

_____ 2. Correctly assembles equipment

_____ 3. Explains the procedure

_____ 4. Positions the patient in a supine position

_____ 5. Washes hands

_____ 6. Puts on sterile gloves

_____ 7. Discontinues administration of all infusates into the CVAD

_____ 8. Chooses the proximal lumen to obtain the sample

_____ 9. Attaches a 10-mL prefilled saline syringe to a three-way stopcock

_____ 10. Primes the stopcock with saline

_____ 11. Disinfects the injection cap with alcohol wipe with friction scrub for the correct amount of time

_____ 12. Attaches stopcock with syringe to injection cap

_____ 13. Unclamps lumen and flushes with remainder of saline

_____ 14. Clamps lumen and/or turns stopcock to "off" position to syringe port

_____ 15. Removes syringe and applies a new empty syringe to the same stopcock port

_____ 16. Turns stopcock to "off" posistion to the unaccessed port

_____ 17. Unclamps lumen

_____ 18. Aspirates 5 mL blood into the empty syringe, discards or conserves

_____ 19. Attaches another empty syringe to the second stopcock port

_____ 20. Turns stopcock to "off" position to the blood-filled syringe

_____ 21. Draws correct amount of blood sample into empty syringe

_____ 22. If using a blood conservation program, reinfuses blood from previously filled syringe

_____ 23. Removes stopcock and syringe

_____ 24. Cleanses injection cap with alcohol pad

_____ 25. Attaches prefilled saline syringe and flushes with 18 to 19 mL saline

_____ 26. Removes protective cap from tubing and reconnects infusion tubing, if IV infusion has been disconnected

_____ 27. Resumes infusions in all lumens

_____ 28. Connects a blood transfer device to the collection syringe and fills evacuated tubes completely and according to the order of fill

_____ 29. Labels each tube correctly and confirms identification with patient

Continued

Evaluation of Blood Sample Collection From Central Venous Access Device Competency (Continued)

_____ **30.** Prepares sample and requistion for delivery to the laboratory and send or delivers

_____ **31.** Disposes of used supplies in biohazard container

_____ **32.** Removes gloves, washes hands, and thanks the patient

_____ **33.** Overall asceptic technique

TOTAL POINTS _____

MAXIMUM POINTS = 66

Comments:

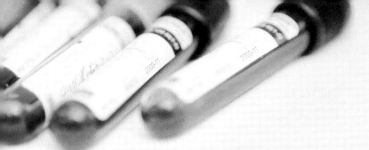

CHAPTER 12

Dermal Puncture

Learning Objectives

Upon completion of this chapter, the reader will be able to:

1. State the complications associated with puncture of the deep veins in infants.
2. List six reasons for performing dermal punctures on children and adults.
3. Describe the composition of capillary blood and name four test results that may differ between capillary and venous blood.
4. Describe the various types of equipment needed for dermal sample collection.
5. Discuss the purpose and methodology for warming the puncture site.
6. Identify the acceptable and unacceptable sites for performing heel and finger punctures and the conditions when each is performed.
7. State the complications produced by the presence of alcohol at the puncture site.
8. State the correct positioning of the lancet for dermal puncture.
9. Name the major cause of microsample contamination.
10. State the order of collection for dermal puncture samples.
11. Describe the correct labeling of microsamples.
12. Correctly perform dermal punctures on the heel and the finger.
13. Discuss the necessary precautions for collecting high-quality samples for newborn bilirubin tests.
14. Discuss why and how newborn filter paper screening tests are collected.
15. Describe the collection of capillary blood gases, including sources of technical error.
16. Explain the reason for thick and thin blood smears and describe how they are made.
17. State the purpose of the bleeding time and three reasons why it may be prolonged.

Key Terms

Calcaneus
Congenital hypothyroidism
Dermal
Ecchymoses
Feathered edge
Galactosemia
Jaundiced
Microsample
Osteochondritis
Osteomyelitis
Palmar
Phenylalanine
Phenylketonuria
Plantar
Platelet plug
Volar

Although venipuncture is the most frequently performed phlebotomy procedure, it is not appropriate in all circumstances. Advances in laboratory instrumentation and the popularity of point-of-care testing make it possible to perform a majority of laboratory tests on *microsamples* of blood obtained by *dermal* puncture on both pediatric and adult patients.

In most institutions, dermal (capillary or skin) puncture is the method of choice for collecting blood from infants and children younger than 2 years for the following reasons:

- Locating superficial veins that are large enough to accept even a small-gauge needle is difficult in these patients, and available veins may need to be reserved for intravenous therapy.
- Use of deep veins, such as the femoral vein, can be dangerous and may cause complications including cardiac arrest, venous thrombosis, hemorrhage, damage to surrounding tissue and organs, infection, reflex arteriospasm (that can possibly result in gangrene), and injury caused by restraining the child.
- Drawing excessive amounts of blood from premature and small infants can rapidly cause anemia, because a 2-pound infant may have a total blood volume of only 150 mL.
- Certain tests require capillary blood, such as newborn screening tests and capillary blood gases.

Dermal puncture may be required in many adult patients, including:

- Burned or scarred patients
- Patients receiving chemotherapy who require frequent tests and whose veins must be reserved for therapy
- Patients with thrombotic tendencies
- Geriatric or other patients with very fragile veins
- Patients with inaccessible veins
- Obese patients
- Apprehensive patients
- Patients requiring home glucose monitoring and point-of-care tests (see Chapter 15)

It may not be possible to obtain a satisfactory sample by dermal puncture from patients who are severely dehydrated or have poor peripheral circulation or have swollen fingers. Certain tests may not be collected by dermal puncture because of the larger amount of blood required such as some coagulation studies that require plasma, erythrocyte sedimentation rates, and blood cultures.

IMPORTANCE OF CORRECT COLLECTION

Correct collection techniques are critical because of the smaller amount of blood that is collected and the higher possibility of sample contamination, microclots, and hemolysis. Hemolysis is more frequently seen in samples collected by dermal puncture than it is in those collected by venipuncture. The presence of hemolysis may not be detected in samples containing bilirubin, but it interferes not only with the tests routinely affected by hemolysis but also with the frequently requested newborn bilirubin determination.

Hemolysis may occur in dermal puncture for the following reasons:

- Excessive squeezing of the puncture site ("milking")
- Newborns have increased numbers of red blood cells (RBCs) and increased RBC fragility
- Residual alcohol at the site
- Vigorous mixing of the microcollection tubes after collection

COMPOSITION OF CAPILLARY BLOOD

Blood collected by dermal puncture comes from the capillaries, arterioles, and venules. Therefore, it is a mixture of arterial and venous blood and may contain small amounts of interstitial and intracellular fluids. Because of arterial pressure, the composition of this blood more closely resembles arterial rather than venous blood. Warming the site before sample collection increases blood flow as much as sevenfold, thereby producing a sample that is very close to the composition of arterial blood.

With the exception of arterial blood gases (ABGs), very few chemical differences exist between arterial and venous blood. The concentration of glucose is higher in blood obtained by dermal puncture, and the concentrations of potassium, total protein, and calcium are lower. Therefore, when dermal punctures are performed, this factor should be noted on the requisition form. Alternating between dermal puncture and venipuncture should not be done when results are to be compared.

Technical Tip 12-1. By documenting that the sample was collected by dermal puncture, the health-care provider can consider the collection technique when interpreting results.

DERMAL PUNCTURE EQUIPMENT

In addition to the previously discussed venipuncture equipment, a phlebotomy collection tray or drawing station should contain skin puncture devices, microsample collection containers, glass slides, and possibly a heel warmer for use in performing dermal punctures.

Dermal Puncture Devices

As shown in Figure 12-1, a variety of skin puncture devices are commercially available, in varying lengths and depths. All devices must have Occupational Safety and Health Administration (OSHA) required safety devices that retract and lock after use to prevent reuse and accidental puncture. Many studies have been performed comparing the various devices with respect to efficiency of collection, sample hemolysis, and the formation of ***ecchymoses*** (bruising) at the collection site. No single method appears to be superior.

To prevent contact with bone, the depth of the puncture is critical. The Clinical and Laboratory Standards Institute (CLSI) recommends that the incision depth should not exceed 2.0 mm in a device used to perform heelsticks. There is concern that even this may be too deep in certain infants, particularly premature infants. The length of lancets and the spring release mechanisms control the puncture depth with automatic devices. Punctures should never be performed using an uncontrolled surgical blade. Manufacturers provide separate devices designed for heelsticks on premature infants, newborns, and babies; fingersticks on toddlers and older children; and fingersticks on adults.

To produce adequate blood flow, the depth of the puncture is actually much less important than the width of the incision. This is because the major vascular area of the skin is located at the dermal-subcutaneous junction, which in a newborn is only 0.35 to 1.6 mm below the skin and can range to 3.0 mm in a large adult (Fig. 12-2). Designated puncture devices can easily reach it. Therefore, the number of severed capillaries depends on the incision width. Incision widths vary from needle stabs to 2.5 mm. Sufficient blood flow should be obtained from incision widths no larger than 2.5 mm. Longer incisions should be avoided because they will produce unnecessary damage to the heel or finger.

As illustrated in the following examples, several color-coded lancets are available in varying depths and widths to accommodate low, medium, and high blood flow requirements. The type of device selected depends on the age of the patient, the amount of blood sample required, the collection site, and the puncture depth. The BD Microtainer Contact-Activated Lancet (Becton Dickinson) (Fig. 12-3) is designed to activate only when the blade or needle is positioned and pressed against the skin. The lancets are color-coded to indicate lancet puncture depths. The BD Quikheel Lancets are color-coded heelstick lancets made specifically for premature infants, newborns, and babies (Fig. 12-4). International Technidyne Corporation (Edison, NJ) provides a range of color-coded, fully

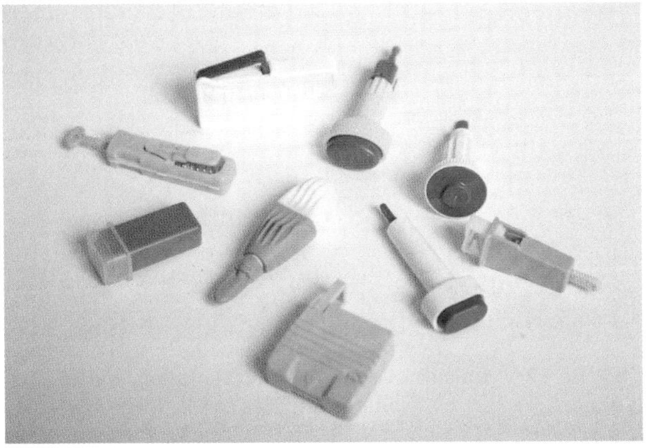

FIGURE 12-1 Dermal puncture devices.

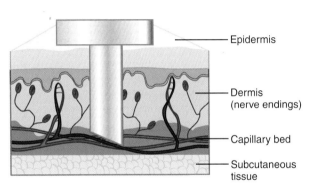

FIGURE 12-2 Vascular area of the skin, at the juncture between the dermis and the subcutaneous tissue.

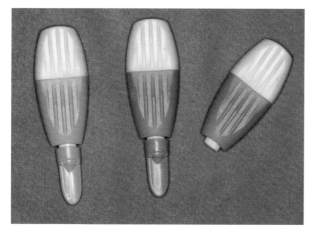

FIGURE 12-3 BD Microtainer Contact-Activated Lancet.

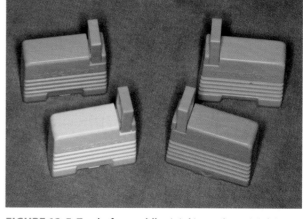

FIGURE 12-5 Tenderfoot toddler (pink), newborn (pink/blue), preemie (white), and micro-preemie (blue) heel incision devices (ITC, Edison, NJ).

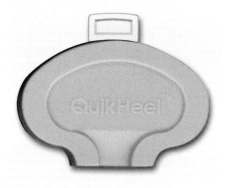

FIGURE 12-4 QuikHeel lancet. *(Courtesy of Becton, Dickinson, Franklin Lakes, NJ.)*

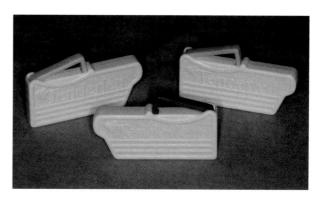

FIGURE 12-6 Tenderlett Toddler, Junior, and Adult lancets (ITC, Edison, NJ).

automated, single-use, retractable, disposable devices in varying depths. Tenderfoot and Tenderlett devices are designed for heel and finger punctures, respectively. Models are available ranging from the Tenderfoot for preemies (Fig. 12-5) to the Tenderlett for toddlers, juniors, and adults (Fig. 12-6).

Unistik 2 (Owen Mumford, Inc, Marietta, GA) safety lancets are available in five versions with varying needle gauges and penetration depths. The lancet used depends on the type of skin and amount of blood required for testing. The lancets range from a Unistik 2 Comfort for delicate skin, to Unistik 2 Normal for normal skin/general use, Unistik 2 Extra for tougher skin/larger sample, Unistik 2 Super for multitest situations and optimal blood flow, Unistik 2 Neonatal for heelsticks on newborns (Fig. 12-7).

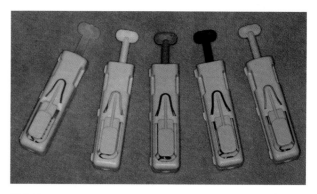

FIGURE 12-7 Unistik 2 Capillary blood sampling devices (Comfort, Normal, Extra, Super, and Neonatal). *(Owen Mumford, Inc., Marietta, GA).*

Laser lancets (Lasette Plus, Cell Robotics International, Inc., Albuquerque, NM) are available for clinical and home use, and are approved by the Food and Drug Administration (FDA) for adults and children older than 5 years. The lightweight, portable, battery-operated device eliminates the risks of accidental punctures and the need for sharps containers. The laser light penetrates the skin 1 to 2 mm, producing a small hole by vaporizing water in the skin. This creates a smaller wound, reduces the pain and soreness associated with capillary puncture, and allows up to 100 μL of blood to be collected (Fig. 12-8).

 Technical Tip 12-2. Select the puncture device that will safely provide the appropriate volume of blood to perform the required tests.

Microsample Containers

Figure 12-9 illustrates some of the major sample containers available for collection of microsamples. Microcollection tubes have largely replaced the large-bore glass Caraway and Natelson micropipettes. Some containers are designated for a specific test, and others serve multiple purposes. The type of container chosen is usually related to laboratory preference, because advantages and disadvantages can be associated with each system.

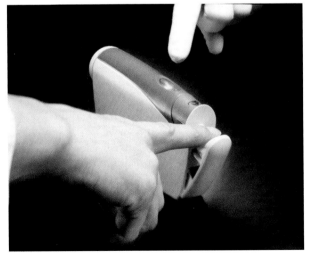

FIGURE 12-8 Laser lancet, the Lasette Plus. *(Courtesy of Cell Robotics, Inc., Albuquerque, NM.)*

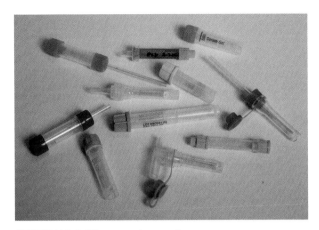

FIGURE 12-9 Microsample containers.

Capillary Tubes

Capillary tubes, which are frequently referred to as microhematocrit tubes, are small tubes used to collect approximately 50 to 75 μL of blood for the primary purpose of performing a microhematocrit test. The tubes are designed to fit into a hematocrit centrifuge and its corresponding hematocrit reader. Tubes are available plain or coated with ammonium heparin, and they are color coded, with a red band for heparinized tubes and a blue band for plain tubes. Heparinized tubes should be used for hematocrits collected by dermal puncture, and plain tubes are used when the test is being performed on blood from a lavender stopper ethylenediaminetetraacetic acid (EDTA) tube. When sufficient blood has been collected, the end of the capillary tube that has not been used to collect the sample is closed with clay sealant or a plastic plug. Phlebotomists should use extreme care to prevent breakage when collecting samples and sealing the tubes. Tubes protected by plastic sleeves and self-sealing tubes are available to prevent breakage when collecting samples and sealing the microhematocrit tubes (Fig. 12-10).

 Technical Tip 12-3. Use of glass capillary tubes is not recommended.

Microcollection Tubes

Plastic collection tubes such as the Microtainer (Becton, Dickinson, Franklin Lakes, NJ) provide a larger collection volume and present no danger

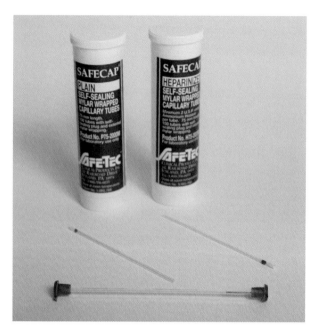

FIGURE 12-10 Microhematocrit capillary tubes and a micropipette for capillary blood gases with metal filing called a "flea."

from broken glass. A variety of anticoagulants and additives, including separator gel, are available, and the tubes are color coded in the same way as evacuated tubes. Some tubes are supplied with a capillary scoop collector top that is replaced by a color-coded plastic sealer top after the sample is collected. Microtainer tubes are designed to hold approximately 600 μL of blood.

BD Microtainer tubes with BD Microgard closures are designed to reduce the risk of blood splatter and blood leakage. The Microgard closure is removed by twisting and lifting. Tubes have a wider diameter, textured interior, and integrated blood collection scoop to enhance blood flow into the tube and eliminate the need to assemble the equipment. After completion of the blood collection, the cap is placed on the container, and anticoagulated tubes are gently inverted 5 to 10 times to ensure complete mixing. Tubes have markings to indicate minimum and maximum collection amounts to prevent underfilling or overfilling that could cause erroneous results. Tube extenders are available for this system to facilitate labeling and handling.

Other capillary blood collection devices have plastic capillary tubes inserted into the collection container (SAFE-T-FILL capillary blood collection system, RAM Scientific Co., Needham, MA). After blood has

been collected, the capillary tube is removed and the appropriate color-coded cap closes the tube.

Mixing of anticoagulated samples is enhanced by the presence of small plastic beads in some collection tube systems. Separation of serum or plasma is achieved by centrifugation in specifically designed centrifuges. Figure 12-11 shows the various manufacturers' microcollection containers.

> ◀ *Technical Tip 12-4.* Microcollection containers are color-coded to match evacuated tube colors and include amber containers for light-sensitive analyte testing.

Additional Dermal Puncture Supplies

Alcohol pads, gauze, and sharps containers are required for the dermal puncture just as they are for the venipuncture. Blood smears used for the white blood cell differential and the examination of RBC morphology may be made during the dermal puncture procedure and require a supply of glass slides.

As discussed previously, warming the puncture site increases blood flow to the area. This can be accomplished by using warm washcloths or towels, or a commercial heel warmer. A heel warmer is a packet containing sodium thiosulfate and glycerin that produces heat when the chemicals are mixed together by gentle squeezing of the packet (Fig. 12-12). The packet should be wrapped in a towel and held away from the face during the initial activation.

DERMAL PUNCTURE PROCEDURE

Many of the procedures associated with the venipuncture also apply to the dermal puncture. Therefore, major emphasis in this chapter is placed on the techniques and complications that are unique to the dermal puncture.

Phlebotomist Preparation

Before performing a dermal puncture, the phlebotomist must have a requisition form containing the same information required for the venipuncture. When a sample is collected by dermal puncture, this must be noted on the requisition form because, as discussed previously, the concentration of some analytes differs between venous and capillary blood.

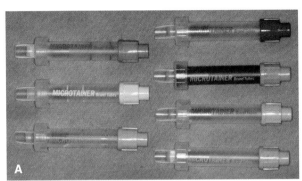

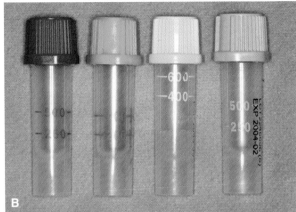

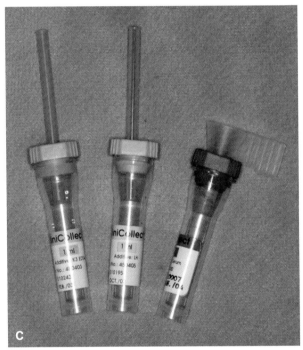

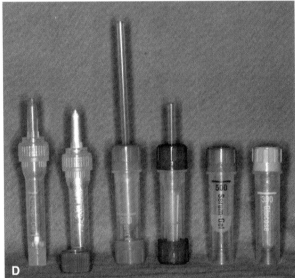

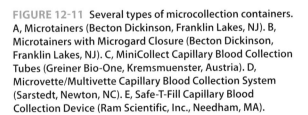

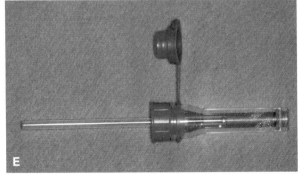

FIGURE 12-11 Several types of microcollection containers. A, Microtainers (Becton Dickinson, Franklin Lakes, NJ). B, Microtainers with Microgard Closure (Becton Dickinson, Franklin Lakes, NJ). C, MiniCollect Capillary Blood Collection Tubes (Greiner Bio-One, Kremsmuenster, Austria). D, Microvette/Multivette Capillary Blood Collection System (Sarstedt, Newton, NC). E, Safe-T-Fill Capillary Blood Collection Device (Ram Scientific, Inc., Needham, MA).

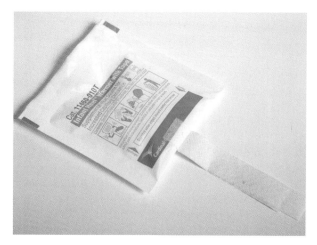

FIGURE 12-12 **Commercial heel warmer.**

Because of the variety of puncture devices and collection containers available for dermal puncture, phlebotomists should carefully examine the information on the requisition form to ensure that they have the appropriate equipment to collect all required samples as well as the skin puncture device that corresponds to the age of the patient.

Phlebotomists frequently perform dermal punctures in the nursery and must observe its specified protective isolation procedures, such as the wearing of gowns and gloves, extensive hand washing, and carrying only the necessary equipment to the patient area. Equipment should be kept out of reach of the patient at all times.

Patient Identification and Preparation

Patients for dermal puncture must be identified using the same procedures as those used for venipuncture (requisition form, verbal identification, and ID band). In the nursery, an identification band must be present on the infant and not just on the bassinet. Verbal identification of pediatric outpatients may have to be obtained from the parents.

Approaching pediatric patients can be difficult, and the phlebotomist must present a friendly, confident appearance while explaining the procedure to the child and the parents. Do not say the procedure will not hurt, and explain the necessity of remaining very still.

Parents should be given the choice of staying with the child or leaving the room. If they choose to stay, they may be asked to assist in holding and comforting the child . Very agitated children may need to have their legs and free hand restrained, as discussed in Chapter 11. This can be accomplished by a parent or coworker, or by confining the child in a blanket or commercially available papoose-style wrap. If a restraint is used, parental consent must be obtained and documented in the patient's medical record.

 Technical Tip 12-5. Having the parents present can provide emotional support and help enlist the child's cooperation.

 Preexamination Consideration 12-1. Excessive crying may affect the concentration of white blood cells and capillary blood gases. This condition should be noted on the requisition.

Patient Position

The patient must be seated or lying down with the hand supported on a firm surface, palm up, and fingers pointed downward for fingersticks. For heelsticks, infants should be lying on the back with the heel in a downward position.

Site Selection

As mentioned in the discussion of skin puncture devices, a primary danger in dermal puncture is accidental contact with the bone, followed by infection or inflammation (*osteomyelitis* or *osteochondritis*). This problem can be avoided by selection of puncture sites that provide sufficient distance between the skin and the bone. The primary dermal puncture sites are the heel and the distal segments of the third and fourth fingers. Performing dermal punctures on earlobes is not recommended. The choice of a puncture area is based on the age and size of the patient.

Areas selected for dermal puncture should not be callused, scarred, bruised, edematous, cold or cyanotic, or infected. Punctures should never be made through previous puncture sites because this practice can easily introduce microorganisms into the puncture and allow them to reach the bone. Do not collect blood from the fingers on the side of a mastectomy without a health-care provider's order.

Heel Puncture Sites

The heel is used for dermal punctures on infants younger than 1 year because it contains more tissue than the fingers and has not yet become callused from walking.

Acceptable areas for heel puncture are shown in Figure 12-13 and are described as the medial and lateral areas of the *plantar* (bottom) surface of the heel. These areas can be determined by drawing imaginary lines extending back from the middle of the large toe to the heel and from between the fourth and fifth toes to the heel. It is in these areas that the distance between the skin and the *calcaneus* (heel bone) is greatest. Notice the short distance between the back (posterior curvature) of the heel and the calcaneus (see Fig. 12-13). This is the reason why this area is never acceptable for heel puncture.

Punctures should not be performed in other areas of the foot, and particularly not in the arch, where they may cause damage to nerves, tendons, and cartilage.

Finger Puncture Sites

Finger punctures are performed on adults and children over 1 year of age. Fingers of infants younger than 1 year may not contain enough tissue to prevent contact with the bone.

The fleshy areas located near the center of the third and fourth fingers on the *palmar* side of the nondominant hand are the sites of choice for finger puncture (Fig. 12-14). Because the tip and sides of the finger contain only about half the tissue mass of the central area, the possibility of bone injury is increased in these areas. Problems associated with use of the other fingers include possible calluses on the thumb, increased nerve endings in the index finger, and decreased tissue in the fifth finger. A swollen or previously punctured site is unacceptable because the increased tissue fluid will contaminate the blood sample. Patients who routinely perform home glucose monitoring may request a specific finger, and their wishes should be accommodated. Box 12-1 summarizes dermal puncture selection sites.

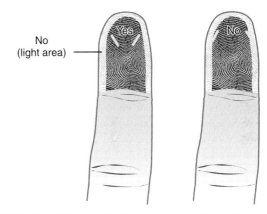

FIGURE 12-14 Acceptable finger puncture sites and correct puncture angle.

Heel Puncture Sites

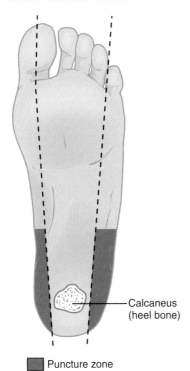

FIGURE 12-13 Acceptable heel puncture sites.

BOX 12-1 Summary of Dermal Puncture Site Selection

- Use the medial and lateral areas of the plantar surface of the heel.
- Use the central fleshy area of the third or fourth finger.
- Do not use the back of the heel.
- Do not use the arch of the foot.
- Do not puncture through old sites.
- Do not use areas with visible damage.
- Do not use fingers on newborns or children younger than 1 year.
- Do not use swollen sites.
- Do not use earlobes.
- Do not use fingers on the side of a mastectomy.

Warming the Site

For optimal blood flow, the finger or heel from which the sample is to be taken may be warmed. This is primarily required for patients with very cold or cyanotic fingers, for heelsticks to collect multiple samples, and for the collection of capillary blood gases. Warming dilates the blood vessels and increases arterial blood flow. Moistening a towel with warm water (42°C) or activating a commercial heel warmer and covering the site for 3 to 5 minutes effectively warms the site. Use caution in moistening the towel to ensure the water temperature is not greater than 42°C to avoid burning the patient. The site should not be warmed for longer than 10 minutes or test results may be altered.

Cleansing the Site

The selected site is cleansed with 70% isopropyl alcohol, using a circular motion. The alcohol should be allowed to dry on the skin for maximum antiseptic action, and the residue may be removed with gauze to prevent interference with certain tests. Failure to allow the alcohol to dry

1. Causes a stinging sensation for the patient
2. Contaminates the sample
3. Hemolyzes RBCs
4. Prevents formation of a rounded blood drop because blood will mix with the alcohol and run down the finger

Use of povidone-iodine is not recommended for dermal punctures because sample contamination may elevate some test results, including bilirubin, phosphorus, uric acid, and potassium.

 Preexamination Consideration 12-2.
Residual alcohol causes rapid hemolysis that can alter test results for certain analytes.

Performing the Puncture

While the puncture is performed, the heel or finger should be well supported and held firmly, without squeezing the puncture area. Massaging the area before the puncture may increase blood flow to the area.

Heel Puncture

The heel is held between the thumb and index finger of the nondominant hand, with the index finger held over the heel and the thumb below the heel (Fig. 12-15).

Finger Puncture

The finger is held between the nondominant thumb and index finger, with the palmar surface facing up and the finger pointing downward to increase blood flow.

Puncture Device Position

Choose a puncture device that corresponds to the size of the patient. Remove the trigger lock if necessary. Place the puncture device firmly on the puncture site. Do not indent the skin when placing the lancet on the puncture site. The blade of the puncture device should be aligned to cut across (perpendicular to) the grooves of the fingerprint or heel print. This aids in the formation of a rounded drop because the blood will not have a tendency to run into the grooves.

Depress the lancet release mechanism and hold for a moment, then release. Pressure must be maintained because the elasticity of the skin naturally inhibits penetration of the blade. Removal of the lancet before the puncture is complete will yield a low blood flow.

 Technical Tip 12-6. Failure to place puncture devices firmly on the skin is the primary cause of insufficient blood flow. One firm puncture is less painful for the patient than two "mini" punctures.

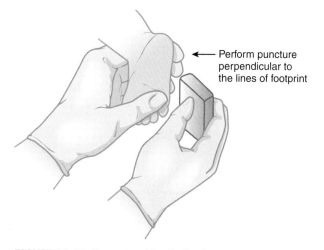

← Perform puncture perpendicular to the lines of footprint

FIGURE 12-15 Correct position for heel puncture.

Puncture Device Disposal

After completing the puncture, the puncture device should be placed in an appropriate sharps container. A new puncture device must be used if an additional puncture is required.

Sample Collection

Before beginning the blood collection, the first drop of blood must be wiped away with a clean gauze (unless testing the first drop of blood is required by the manufacturer of a point-of-care instrument). This will prevent contamination of the sample with residual alcohol and tissue fluid released during the puncture. When collecting microsamples, even a minute amount of contamination can severely affect the sample quality. Therefore, blood should be freely flowing from the puncture site as a result of firm pressure and should not be obtained by milking of the surrounding tissue, which will release tissue fluid. Alternately applying pressure to the area and releasing it will produce the most satisfactory blood flow. Tightly squeezing the area with no relaxation cuts off blood flow to the puncture site.

 Technical Tip 12-7. Applying pressure about ½ inch away from the puncture site frequently produces better blood flow than pressure very close to the site.

Because collection containers fill by capillary action, the collection tip can be lightly touched to the drop of blood and the blood will be drawn into the container. Collection devices should not touch the puncture site and should not be scraped over the skin because this will produce sample contamination and hemolysis. As stated previously fingers are positioned slightly downward with the palmar surface facing up during the collection procedure.

 Technical Tip 12-8. While the sample is being collected, the patient's hand does not have to be completely turned over. Rotating the hand 90 degrees allows the phlebotomist to clearly see the blood drops without placing himself or herself in an awkward position and produces adequate blood flow.

 Technical Tip 12-9. Using a scooping motion to collect the blood must be avoided as it can hemolyze the sample.

Capillary Tubes and Micropipettes

To prevent the introduction of air bubbles, capillary tubes and micropipettes are held horizontally while being filled. Place the end of the tube into the drop of blood and maintain the tube in a horizontal position to fill by capillary action during the entire collection. Removing the microhematocrit tube from the drop of blood causes air bubbles in the sample. The presence of air bubbles limits the amount of blood that can be collected per tube and will interfere with blood gas determinations. When the tubes are filled, they are sealed with sealant clay or designated plastic caps. Recommended tubes are plastic or coated with a puncture-resistant film. When using a sealant tray, place the end that has not been contaminated with blood into the clay taking care to not break the tube. Remove the tube with a slight twisting action to firmly plug the microhematocrit tube.

Microcollection Tubes

Microcollection tubes are slanted down during the collection, and blood is allowed to run through the capillary collection scoop and down the side of the tube. The tip of the collection container is placed beneath the puncture site and touches the underside of the drop. The first three drops of blood provide the channel to allow blood to freely flow into the container. Gently tapping the bottom of the tube may be necessary to force blood to the bottom. When a tube is filled, the color-coded top is attached. Tubes with anticoagulants should be inverted 5 to 10 times or per manufacturer's instructions. If blood flow is slow, it may be necessary to mix the tube while the collection is in progress. It is important to work quickly, because blood that takes more than 2 minutes to collect may form microclots in an anticoagulated microcollection container. Adequate amounts of blood must be collected. An overfilled tube may clot, whereas an underfilled tube can cause morphological changes in cells.

 Technical Tip 12-10. Fast collection and mixing ensure more accurate test results.

Technical Tip 12-11. Clotting is triggered immediately on skin puncture and represents the greatest obstacle in collecting quality samples.

Order of Collection

The order of draw for collecting multiple samples from a dermal puncture is important because of the tendency of platelets to accumulate at the site of a wound. Blood to be used for tests for the evaluation of platelets, such as the blood smear, platelet count, and complete blood count (CBC), must be collected first. The blood smear should be made first, followed by the lavender EDTA tube. The order of collection for multiple tubes is

- Capillary blood gases
- Blood smear
- EDTA tubes
- Other anticoagulated tubes
- Serum tubes

Bandaging the Patient

When sufficient blood has been collected, pressure is applied to the puncture site with gauze. The finger or heel is elevated and pressure is applied until the bleeding stops. Confirm that bleeding has stopped before removing the pressure.

Bandages are not used for children younger than 2 years because the children may remove the bandages, place them in their mouth, and possibly aspirate the bandages. Adhesive may also cause irritation to or tear sensitive skin, particularly the fragile skin of a newborn or older adult patient.

Labeling the Sample

Microsamples must be labeled with the same information required for venipuncture samples. Labels can be wrapped around microcollection tubes or groups of capillary pipettes. For transport, capillary pipettes are then placed in a large tube because the outside of the capillary pipettes may be contaminated with blood. This procedure also helps to prevent breakage.

BD Microtainer tubes have extenders that can be attached to the container. This allows the computer label to be applied vertically.

Completion of the Procedure

The dermal puncture procedure is completed in the same manner as the venipuncture by disposing of all used materials in appropriate containers, removing gloves, washing hands, and thanking the patient and/or the parents for their cooperation.

All special handling procedures associated with venipuncture samples also apply to microsamples. Observe test collection priorities.

To prevent excessive removal of blood from small infants, a log sheet for documenting the amount of blood collected each time a procedure is requested for a patient must be completed. The phlebotomist should record the amount of blood collected on the log sheet before leaving the area.

As with venipuncture, it is recommended that only two punctures be attempted to collect blood. When a second puncture must be made to collect the sufficient amount of blood, the blood should not be added to the previously collected tube. This can cause erroneous results as a result of microclots and hemolysis. The puncture also must be performed at a different site using a new puncture device.

Procedure 12-1 shows the technique unique to the finger puncture and Procedure 12-2 shows the heelstick technique.

 PROCEDURE 12-1 ✦ **Collection of Blood from a Fingerstick**

EQUIPMENT:

Gloves
70% isopropyl alcohol pad
Finger puncture device
Microcollection container

Gauze
Warming device
Sharps container
Indelible pen
Bandage

PROCEDURE 12-1 ✦ **Collection of Blood from a Fingerstick** (Continued)

PROCEDURE:

Step 1. Obtain and examine the requisition form.

Step 2. Greet the patient and explain the procedure to be performed.

Step 3. Identify the patient verbally by having him or her state both the first name and last name and compare the information on the patient's ID band with the requisition form. A parent or guardian may do this for a child.

Step 4. Prepare the patient and/or parents and verify diet restrictions, as appropriate, allergies to latex, or previous problems with blood collection.

Step 5. Position the patient's arm on a firm surface with the hand palm up. The child may have to be held in either the vertical or horizontal restraint.

Step 6. Select equipment according to the age of patient, the type of test ordered, and the amount of blood to be collected.

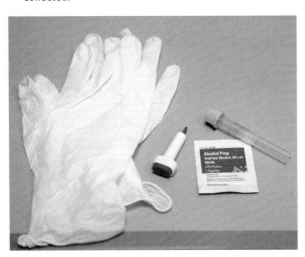

Step 7. Wash hands and put on gloves.

Step 8. Select the puncture site in the fleshy areas located off the center of the third or fourth fingers on the palmar side of the nondominant hand. Do not use the side or tip of the finger.

Step 9. Warm the puncture site if necessary.

Step 10. Cleanse and dry the puncture site with 70% isopropyl alcohol in concentric circles and allow to air dry.

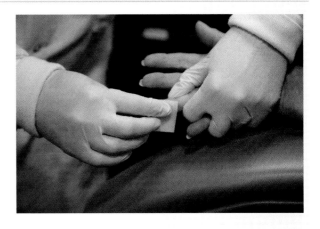

Step 11. Prepare the lancet by removing the lancet locking device and open the cap to the microcollection container.

Step 12. Hold the finger between the nondominant thumb and index finger, with the palmar surface facing up and the finger pointing downward.

Step 13. Place the lancet firmly on the fleshy area of the finger perpendicular to the fingerprint and depress the lancet trigger.

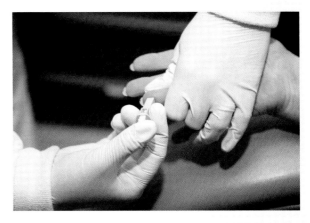

Step 14. Discard lancet in the approved sharps container.

Continued

PROCEDURE 12-1 ✦ **Collection of Blood from a Fingerstick** (Continued)

Step 15. Gently squeeze the finger and wipe away the first drop of blood that may contain alcohol residue and tissue fluid.

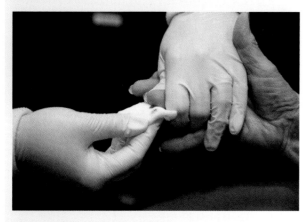

Step 16. Collect rounded drops into microcollection containers in the correct order of draw without scraping the skin. Do not milk the site. Collect the sample within 2 minutes to prevent clotting.

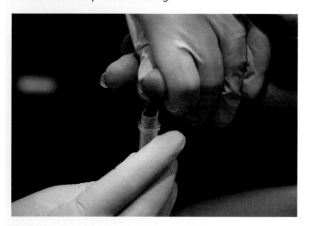

Step 17. Cap the microcollection container when the correct amount of blood has been collected.

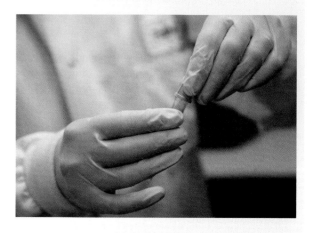

Step 18. Mix tubes 5 to 10 times by gentle inversion as recommended by the manufacturer. They may have to be gently tapped throughout the procedure to mix the blood with the anticoagulant.

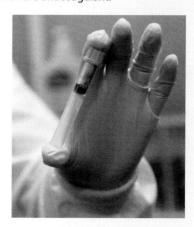

PROCEDURE 12-1 ✦ **Collection of Blood from a Fingerstick** (Continued)

Step 19. Place gauze on the site and ask the patient or parent to apply pressure until bleeding stops.

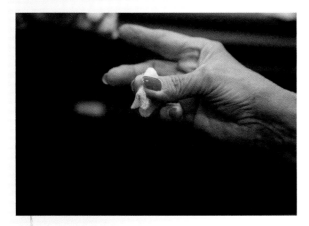

Step 20. Label the tubes before leaving the patient and verify identification with the patient ID band or verbally with an outpatient. Observe any special handling procedures.

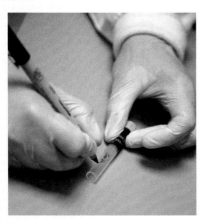

Step 21. Examine the site for stoppage of bleeding and apply bandage if the patient is older than 2 years.

Step 22. Dispose of used supplies in biohazard containers.

Step 23. Thank the patient.

Step 24. Remove gloves and wash hands.

Step 25. Complete paperwork.

Step 26. Deliver sample to the laboratory.

PROCEDURE 12-2 ✦ **Collection of Blood by Heelstick**

EQUIPMENT:

Gloves
70% isopropyl alcohol pad
Heel puncture device
Microcollection container
Gauze
Warming device
Sharps container
Indelible pen

PROCEDURE:

Step 1. Obtain and examine the requisition form.

Step 2. Place collection tray in a designated area.

Step 3. Check requisition and select necessary equipment.

Step 4. Wash hands and apply gloves. Put on a gown if it is a nursery requirement.

Step 5. Identify patient by comparing the ID band that is attached to the baby with the requisition form.

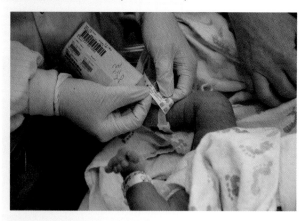

Step 6. Position the baby lying on his or her back with the foot lower than the body.

Step 7. Warm the heel for 3 to 5 minutes by wrapping the heel with a warm washcloth or using a commercial heel-warming device.

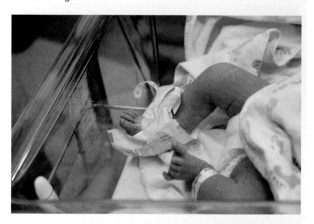

Step 8. Select the puncture site on the medial or lateral plantar surface of the heel. Do not use the arch or back of the heel.

Step 9. Cleanse the puncture site with 70% isopropyl alcohol and allow it to air dry.

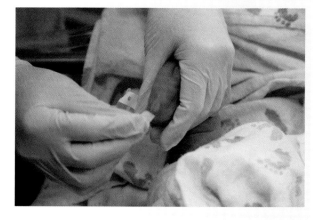

PROCEDURE 12-2 ✦ **Collection of Blood by Heelstick** (Continued)

Step 10. Prepare the lancet by removing the lancet locking device and open the cap to the microcollection container.

Step 11. Hold the heel firmly by wrapping the heel with the nondominant hand.

Step 12. Place the lancet perpendicular to the heel print and depress the lancet trigger.

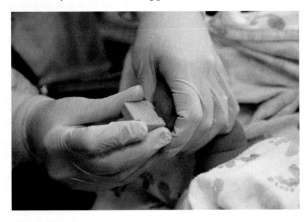

Step 13. Discard the lancet in an approved sharps container.

Step 14. Wipe away the first drop of blood.

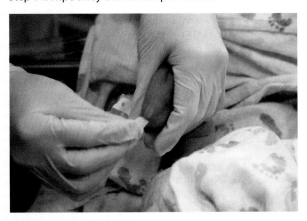

Step 15. Collect rounded drops of blood into microcollection containers without scraping the skin. Do not milk the site.

Step 16. Collect the proper amount of blood in the correct order of draw.

Step 17. Mix microcollection containers 5 to 10 times and/or seal microhematocrit tubes.

Step 18. Place gauze on site and apply pressure until bleeding stops.

Step 19. Label tubes and observe any special handling procedures.

Step 20. Check the site for bleeding. Do not place a bandage on an infant younger than 2 years.

Step 21. Dispose of used supplies and remove all collection equipment from the area.

Step 22. Remove gloves (and gown if wearing one) and wash hands.

Step 23. Complete patient log sheet.

Step 24. Deliver samples to the laboratory.

SPECIAL DERMAL PUNCTURE

Collection of Newborn Bilirubin

One of the most frequently performed tests on newborns measures bilirubin levels, and samples for this determination are often collected at timed intervals over several days. Bilirubin is a very light-sensitive chemical and is rapidly destroyed when exposed to light.

Increased serum bilirubin (hyperbilirubinemia) in newborns may be caused by the presence of hemolytic disease of the newborn, or it may simply occur because the liver of newborns (particularly premature infants) is often not developed enough to process the bilirubin produced from the normal breakdown of red blood cells. Bilirubin test results are critical to infant survival and mental health because the blood-brain barrier is not fully developed in neonates, a condition that allows bilirubin to accumulate in the brain and cause permanent or lethal damage. The decision to perform an exchange transfusion is based on the bilirubin levels and the newborn's age and condition. Phlebotomy technique is critical to the determination of accurate bilirubin results, and samples must be collected quickly and protected from excess light during and after the collection. Infants who appear *jaundiced* are frequently placed under an ultraviolet light (UV) to lower the level of circulating bilirubin. This light must be turned off during sample collection. Amber-colored microcollection tubes are available for collecting bilirubin (Fig. 12-16), or if multiple capillary pipettes are used, the filled tubes should be shielded from light. Hemolysis must be avoided; it will falsely lower bilirubin results in some procedures and must be corrected for in others. Also, samples must be collected at the specified time so that the rate of bilirubin increase can be determined. Noninvasive transcutaneous bilirubin measurements in neonates are discussed in Chapter 15.

 Technical Tip 12-12. When collecting samples for neonatal bilirubin tests, turn off the ultraviolet light during collection unless it is a newer model that is strapped directly to the infant.

 Preexamination Consideration 12-3. Bilirubin levels may decrease as much as 50% in a blood sample that has been exposed to light for 2 hours.

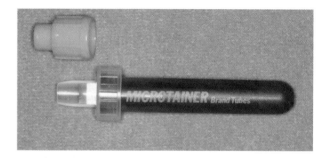

FIGURE 12-16 Amber-colored Microtainer for the collection of neonatal bilirubins.

Newborn Screening

Newborn screening is the testing of newborn babies for genetic, metabolic, hormonal, and functional disorders that can cause physical disabilities, mental retardation, or even death, if not detected and treated early. Screening of newborns for 50 inherited metabolic disorders can currently be performed from blood collected by heelstick and placed on specially designed filter paper. Each state has its own laws requiring specific test screening of newborns; however, all states screen newborns for the presence of the most prevalent disorders. Many of these disorders can be prevented by early changes in the newborn's diet or early administration of a missing hormone. Examples of the common disorders *phenylketonuria* (PKU), *congenital hypothyroidism,* and *galactosemia* are shown in Box 12-2.

Blood Collection

Newborn screening tests are performed on blood collected by dermal puncture, except for the hearing test. Ideally blood is collected between 24 and 72 hours after birth, before the baby is released from the hospital. Correct collection of the blood sample is critical for accurate test results. It is recommended that the newborn screening samples should be collected separately, after prewarming and puncturing a second site when additional blood tests are requested.

Special collection kits are used, consisting of a patient information form attached to specifically designed filter paper that has been preprinted with an appropriate number of circles that are part of the requisition (Fig. 12-17). The phlebotomist must be careful not to touch or contaminate the area inside the circles or to touch the dried blood spots. Care must be taken to avoid contaminating the sample with water, formula, alcohol, urine, lotions, or powder.

BOX 12-2 Mandatory Newborn Screening Disorders

Phenylketonuria

Phenylketonuria (PKU) is caused by the lack of the enzyme needed to metabolize the amino acid ***phenylalanine*** to tyrosine, which accumulates and causes problems with brain development and mental retardation. Early detection is crucial because the damage is irreversible but can be treated with a diet low in phenylalanine and high in tyrosine.

Congenital Hypothyroidism

Congenital hypothyroidism is a thyroid hormone deficiency present at birth. Delays in growth and brain development that produce mental retardation can be avoided by the use of oral doses of thyroid hormone within the first few weeks after birth.

Galactosemia

Galactosemia is a genetic metabolic disorder caused by the lack of the liver enzyme needed to convert galactose (sugar in milk) into glucose. Galactose accumulates in the blood and can cause liver disease, renal failure, cataracts, blindness, mental retardation, and death. Treatment is the elimination of all milk and dairy products from the infant for life.

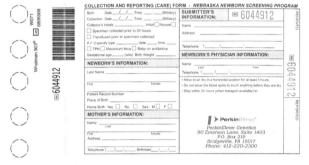

FIGURE 12-17 Newborn screening sample form.

Causes for invalid newborn screening samples are listed in Table 12-1.

The heelstick is performed in the routine manner, and the first drop of blood is wiped away. A large drop of blood is then applied directly onto a filter paper circle. Do not touch the filter paper to the heel. To obtain an even layer of blood, only one large free-falling drop should be used to fill a circle. Blood is applied to only one side of the filter paper, and there must be enough to soak through the paper and be visible on the other side. Each circle must be filled

TABLE 12-1 • Causes for Invalid Newborn Screening Samples

INVALID SAMPLE	POSSIBLE CAUSES
Quantity insufficient for testing	Filter paper is removed before blood has completely filled circle or before blood has soaked through to other side
	Filter paper touches gloves, powder, or lotion
Appears scratched	Blood applied with capillary pipette
Not dry before mailing	Sample mailed before drying a minimum of 3 hours
Appears supersaturated	Excess blood applied to filter paper using an alternate device
	Blood applied to both sides of filter paper
Appears diluted, discolored, or contaminated	"Milking" area surrounding puncture site
	Filter paper contaminated with powder, alcohol, formula, water, lotion
	Blood spots exposed to direct heat

Continued

TABLE 12-1 • Causes for Invalid Newborn Screening Samples—cont'd	
INVALID SAMPLE	**POSSIBLE CAUSES**
Exhibits serum rings	Alcohol not dry before puncture
	Filter paper contaminated with powder, alcohol, formula, water, lotion
	"Milking" the puncture site
	Sample dried improperly
	Using a capillary pipette to fill the spots
Appears clotted or layered	Several drops of blood used to fill the circle
	Blood applied to both sides of filter paper

for testing. As shown in Figure 12-18, if a circle is not evenly or completely filled, a new circle and a larger drop of blood should be used. The collected sample must be allowed to air dry in a suspended horizontal position, at room temperature, and away from direct sunlight. To prevent cross-contamination, samples should not be hung to dry or stacked during or after the drying process. When dry, the sample is placed in a special envelope and sent to the appropriate laboratory for testing. Procedure 12-3 describes the technique for collecting blood for newborn screening tests.

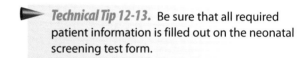
Technical Tip 12-13. Be sure that all required patient information is filled out on the neonatal screening test form.

Technical Tip 12-14. Specific state mandates for newborn screening can be found at the U.S. National Newborn Screening and Genetics Resource Center website. http://genes-r-us.uthscsa.edu/

Technical Tip 12-15. Uneven or incomplete saturation of filter paper circles because of layering from multidrop application will yield an unacceptable sample for testing.

Technical Tip 12-16. Blood spots must be thoroughly dry before the attached fold-over flap is closed over the spots.

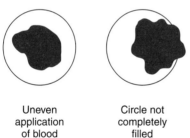

Acceptable specimen	Uneven application of blood	Circle not completely filled

FIGURE 12-18 Correct and incorrect blood collection with filter paper.

PROCEDURE 12-3 ✦ Newborn Screening Blood Collection

EQUIPMENT:

Newborn screening filter paper form
Gloves
70% isopropyl alcohol pad
Heel puncture device
Gauze
Warming device
Sharps container
Indelible pen

PROCEDURE:

Step 1. Perform Steps 1 to 14 of Procedure 12-2: Collection of Blood by Heelstick.

PROCEDURE 12-3 ✦ **Newborn Screening Blood Collection** (Continued)

Step 2. Touch the filter paper to a large drop of blood.

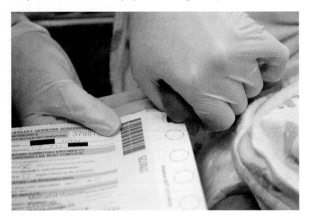

Step 3. Evenly fill the circle on one side of the filter paper, allowing the blood to soak through the paper to be visible on the other side.

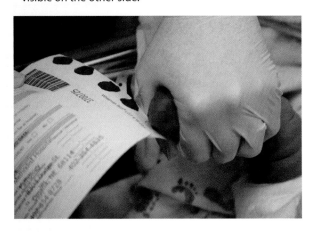

Step 4. Fill all required circles correctly.

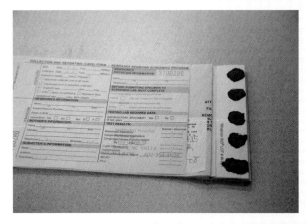

Step 5. Place gauze on site and apply pressure until bleeding stops.

Step 6. Place the filter paper in a suspended horizontal position to dry. Do not stack multiple filter papers.

Step 7. Label the sample and place it in the special envelope when dry.

Step 8. Check the site for bleeding. Do not place a bandage on an infant.

Step 9. Dispose of used supplies and remove all collection equipment from the area.

Step 10. Remove gloves (and gown if wearing one) and wash hands.

Step 11. Complete patient log sheet.

Step 12. Deliver sample to laboratory for mailing to the reference testing agency.

Capillary Blood Gases

Arterial blood is the preferred sample for blood gases (oxygen and carbon dioxide content) and pH levels in adults (see Chapter 14). Performing deep arterial punctures in newborns and young children is usually not recommended; therefore, unless blood can be obtained from umbilical or scalp arteries, blood gases are performed on capillary blood. Blood is collected from the plantar area of the heel or big toe and the palmar area of the fingers.

As discussed in Chapter 7, capillary blood is actually a mixture of venous and arterial blood, with a higher concentration of arterial blood. The concentration of arterial blood is also increased when the collection site is warmed. Therefore, when collecting capillary blood gases, it is essential to warm the collection site to arterialize the sample using a commercial heel warmer or warm, moist washcloth.

 Technical Tip 12-17. Do not forget to wipe away the first drop of blood before collecting a capillary sample.

Samples are collected in heparinized blood gas pipettes designed to correspond with the volume and sampling requirements of the blood gas analyzer being used. Plugs or clay sealants are needed for both ends of the pipettes, and a magnetic stirrer "flea" and circular magnet are used to mix the sample with heparin to prevent clotting.

After warming the site to 40°C to 42°C for 3 to 5 minutes to increase the flow of arterial blood, blood is collected using routine dermal puncture. Pipettes must be completely filled and must not contain air bubbles. The pipette should fill in less than 30 seconds. When the pipette is full, both ends are immediately sealed to prevent exposure to room air that could affect the blood gas composition. The round magnet is slipped over the tube. The blood is mixed by moving the magnet up and down the tube several times. The tubes are labeled and placed horizontally in an ice slurry to slow white blood cell metabolism and changes in the pH and blood gas concentrations. The sample is immediately transported to the laboratory. Procedure 12-4 describes the technique for collecting capillary blood gas by heel puncture.

 Technical Tip 12-18. To avoid air bubbles, hold the tube in a horizontal position and be sure that blood flows easily from the puncture site.

PROCEDURE 12-4 ✦ Capillary Blood Gas Collection by Heel Puncture

EQUIPMENT:

Gloves
70% isopropyl alcohol pad
Heel puncture device
Heparinized capillary pipettes with seals (caps)
Metal stirrer "flea"
Round magnet
Warming device
Gauze
Sharps container
Indelible pen
Ice slurry

PROCEDURE:

Step 1. Perform Steps 1 to 14 of Procedure 12-2: Collection of Blood by Heelstick.

Step 2. Place the magnetic "flea" in the capillary pipette.

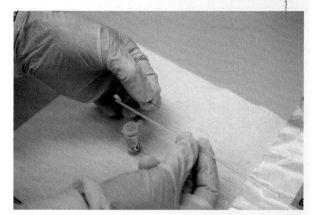

PROCEDURE 12-4 ✦ **Capillary Blood Gas Collection by Heel Puncture** (Continued)

Step 3. Hold the capillary pipette horizontal to the drop of blood and fill the capillary pipette in less than 30 seconds to avoid exposure to air in the blood.

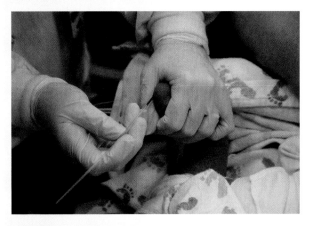

Step 4. Completely fill the pipette without any air spaces.

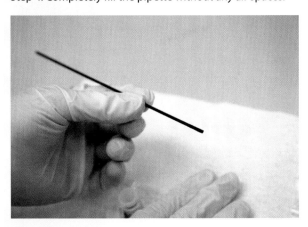

Step 5. Immediately seal both ends of the capillary pipette.

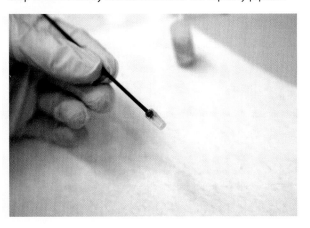

Step 6. Mix the sample with the heparin by moving the magnet up and down the tube several times.

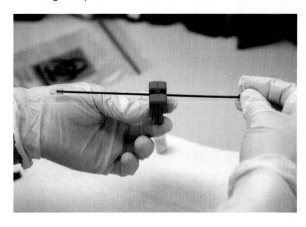

Step 7. Place gauze on site and apply pressure until bleeding stops.

Step 8. Label tubes and place in an ice/water slurry.

Step 9. Check the site for bleeding. Do not place a bandage on an infant younger than 2 years.

Step 10. Dispose of used supplies and remove all collection equipment from the area.

Step 11. Remove gloves (and gown if wearing one) and wash hands.

Step 12. Complete patient log sheet.

Step 13. Deliver samples to the laboratory.

Preparation of Blood Smears

Blood smears are needed for the microscopic examination of blood cells that is performed for the differential blood cell count, for special staining procedures, and for nonautomated reticulocyte counts. Phlebotomists may make smears when one of these tests is ordered and a dermal puncture is performed. Blood smears should be collected before other samples to avoid platelet clumping.

When samples are collected by venipuncture, the smear is usually made in the laboratory from the EDTA tube. Blood smears should be made within 1 hour of collection to avoid cell distortion caused by the EDTA anticoagulant. The EDTA tube must be mixed for 2 minutes. A plain capillary pipette or a device called DIFF-SAFE is used to dispense a drop of blood onto the slide (Fig. 12-19). Blood smears may be made manually (Fig. 12-20) or using an automated instrument (Fig. 12-21).

Performing smears at the bedside after a venipuncture may sometimes be necessary to be sure there is no anticoagulant interference. This practice can be dangerous, however, because blood must be forced from the needle onto the slide and the needle cannot be disposed of until the smear has been made. In addition, blood smears must be considered infectious until they have been fixed with alcohol in the laboratory, and gloves must be worn when handling them. Carrying numerous smears in a crowded collection tray can cause contamination of equipment and ungloved hands.

Learning to prepare an acceptable blood smear requires considerable practice and can be a source of frustration for beginning phlebotomists. Once the technique is mastered, however, it is seldom that an acceptable smear is not achieved on the first attempt. The technique for preparing a blood smear is described in Procedure 12-5.

A properly prepared blood smear has a smooth film of blood that covers approximately one-half to two-thirds of the slide, does not contain ridges or holes, and has a lightly *feathered edge* without streaks. The microscopic examination is performed in the area of the feathered edge because here the cells have been spread into a single layer. An uneven smear indicates that the cells are not evenly distributed; therefore, test results will not be truly representative of the patient's blood. Errors in technique that result in an unacceptable sample are summarized in Table 12-2.

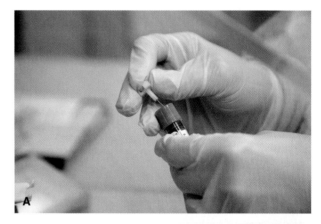

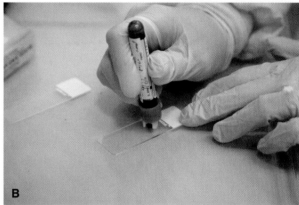

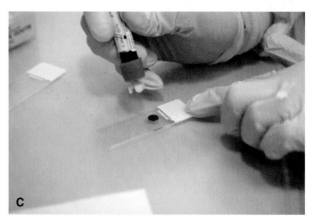

FIGURE 12-19 A, Inserting Diff-Safe device. B, Applying blood drop to slide. C, Blood drop on slide.

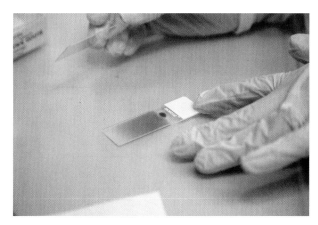

FIGURE 12-20 Manually made blood smear.

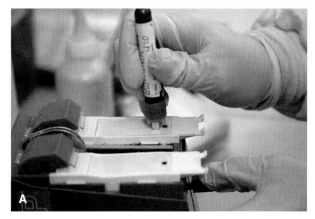

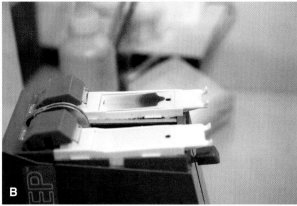

FIGURE 12-21 A, Placing drop of blood on automated instrument. B, Blood smear.

TABLE 12-2 • **Effects of Technical Errors on Blood Smears**	
DISCREPANCY	**POSSIBLE CAUSES**
Uneven distribution of blood (ridges)	Increased pressure on the spreader slide
	Movement of the spreader slide not continuous
	Delay in making slide after drop is placed on slide
Holes in the smear	Dirty slide
	Contamination with glove powder
No feathered edge	Spreader slide not pushed the entire length of the smear slide
Streaks in the feathered edge	Chipped or dirty spreader slide
	Spreader slide not placed flush against the smear slide
	Pulling the spreader slide into the drop of blood so that the blood is pushed instead of pulled
	Drop of blood starts to dry out owing to delay in making smear
Smear too thick and short	Drop of blood is too big
	Angle of spreader slide is greater than 40 degrees
Smear too thin and long	Drop of blood is too small
	Angle of spreader slide is less than 30 degrees
	Spreader slide pushed too slowly

PROCEDURE 12-5 ✦ **Preparing a Blood Smear from a Dermal Puncture**

EQUIPMENT:

Gloves
70% isopropyl alcohol pad
Finger or heel puncture device
3 plain or frosted glass slides
Gauze
Warming device
Sharps container
Pencil
Bandage

PROCEDURE:

Step 1. Perform dermal puncture on finger or heel.

Step 2. Obtain three clean glass slides.

Step 3. Wipe away the first drop of blood.

Step 4. Place the second drop of blood in the center of a glass slide approximately ½ to 1 inch from the end or just below the frosted end by lightly touching the drop with the slide. The drop should be 1 to 2 mm in diameter.

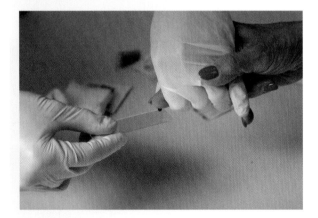

Step 5. Place a second slide (spreader slide) with a clean, smooth edge in front of the drop at a 30- to 40-degree angle inclined over the blood.

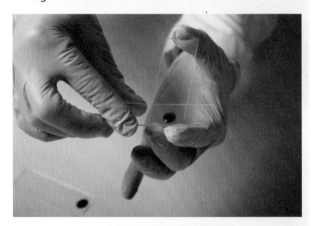

Step 6. Draw the spreader slide back to the edge of the drop of blood, allowing the blood to spread across the end. Choose the slide position that works best for you.

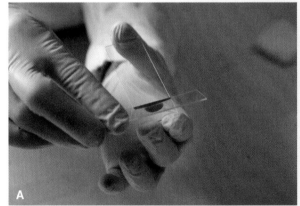

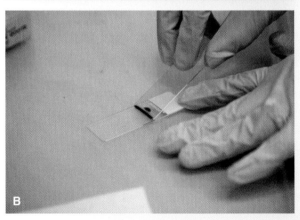

PROCEDURE 12-5 ✦ **Preparing a Blood Smear from a Dermal Puncture** (Continued)

Step 7. When blood is evenly distributed across the spreader slide, lightly push the spreader slide forward with a continuous movement all the way past the end of the smear slide. Be sure to maintain the 30- to 40-degree angle, and do not apply pressure to the spreader slide.

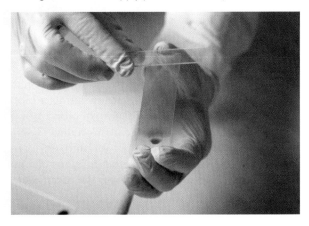

Step 8. Place the slide in an area where it can dry undisturbed and repeat the procedure for the second smear using the clean side or end of the spreader slide.

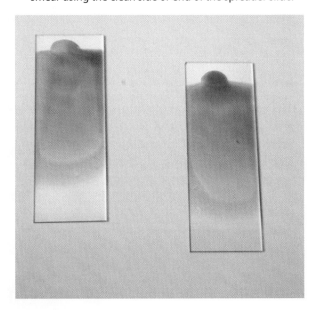

Step 9. Place gauze on site and apply pressure until bleeding stops.

Step 10. Smears collected on slides with frosted ends are labeled by writing the patient information on the frosted area with a pencil. Labels containing the appropriate information are attached to the thick end of smear slides that do not have frosted ends.

Step 11. Place slides in a biohazard container.

Step 12. Remove gloves and wash hands.

Step 13. Deliver slides to the laboratory.

Blood Smears for Malaria

The parasites (*Plasmodium* species) that cause malaria invade the RBCs, and their presence is detected by microscopic examination of thick and thin blood smears. Patients with malaria exhibit periodic episodes of fever and chills related to the multiplication of the parasites within the RBCs. Therefore, sample collection is frequently requested on a timed basis similar to that of stat blood cultures. Smears may be prepared from EDTA anticoagulated blood unless a dermal puncture is requested.

Thin smears (two or three) are prepared in the manner previously described. Thick smears are made by placing a large drop of blood in the center of a glass slide and then using a wooden applicator stick to spread the blood into a circle about the size of a dime. The smear must be allowed to dry for at least 2 hours before staining. Thick smears concentrate the sample for detection of the parasites, and thin smears are then examined for parasitic morphology and identification.

Bleeding Time

The bleeding time (BT) is performed to measure the time required for platelets to form a plug strong enough to stop bleeding from an incision. The length of the BT is increased when the platelet count is low, when platelet disorders affect the ability of the platelets to stick to each other to form a plug, and in persons taking aspirin and certain other medications and herbs. Test results can also be affected by the type and condition of the patient's skin, vascularity, and temperature and the phlebotomist's technique. Therefore, the BT is considered a screening test, and abnormal results are followed by additional testing. BTs may be ordered as part of a presurgical workup or evaluation of a bleeding disorder; however, the BT has essentially been replaced by other platelet function tests.

The BT is performed by making an incision on the *volar* surface of the forearm, and inflating a blood pressure cuff to 40 mm Hg to control blood flow to the area. Automated disposable incision devices, such as the Surgicutt (International Technidyne Corp., Edison, NJ), produce standardized incisions of 1 mm in depth and 5 mm in length. The BT procedure is shown in Procedure 12-6.

PROCEDURE 12-6 ✦ Bleeding Time

EQUIPMENT:

Gloves
70% isopropyl alcohol pad
Automated bleeding time incision device
Blood pressure cuff
Filter paper (No. 1 Whatman)
Stopwatch
Butterfly bandage
Bandages
Sharps container
Indelible pen

PROCEDURE:

Step 1. Identify the patient following routine protocol.

Step 2. Explain the procedure to the patient, including the possibility of leaving a small scar, and obtain information about any prescribed or over-the-counter medications, particularly aspirin, that may have been taken in the last 7 to 10 days. Many medications contain salicylate (aspirin); therefore, the contents of any medication mentioned by the patient should be checked before performing the test, and if salicylate has been taken, the physician should be notified.

Step 3. Assemble required materials, filter paper, stopwatch, and bandages.

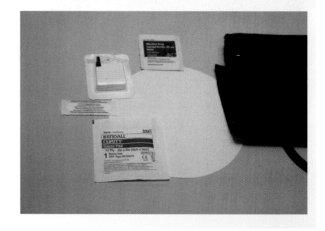

PROCEDURE 12-6 ✦ **Bleeding Time** (Continued)

Step 4. Wash hands and put on gloves.

Step 5. Place the patient's arm on a steady surface with the volar surface facing up.

Step 6. Place a blood pressure cuff on the upper arm.

Step 7. Select an area, approximately 5 cm below the antecubital crease and in the middle of the arm, that is free of surface veins, scars, bruises, and edema.

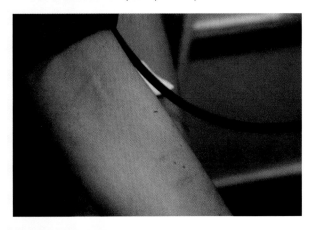

Step 8. Cleanse the area with alcohol and allow it to dry.

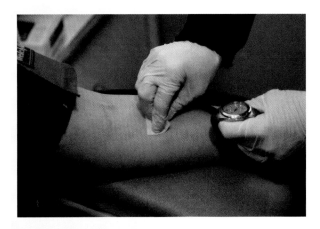

Step 9. Inflate the blood pressure cuff to 40 mm Hg. This pressure must be maintained throughout the procedure. The time between inflation of the blood pressure cuff and making the incision should be between 30 and 60 seconds.

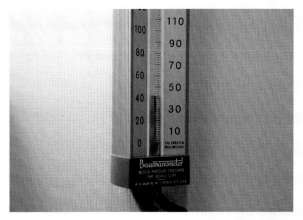

Step 10. Remove the incision device from its package and release the safety lock, being careful not to touch the blade area.

Step 11. Place the incision device firmly, but without making an indentation, on the arm and position it so that the incision will be horizontal (parallel to the antecubital crease). In adults, horizontal incisions are slightly more sensitive to hemorrhagic disorders and are less likely to leave a scar, whereas in newborns, a vertical incision is preferable for the same reasons.

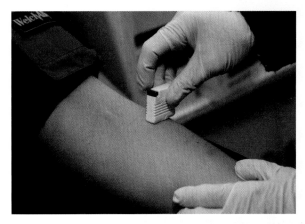

Continued

PROCEDURE 12-6 ✦ **Bleeding Time** (Continued)

Step 12. Depress the trigger, simultaneously start the stopwatch, and then remove the incision device. Place incision device in sharps container.

Step 13. After 30 seconds, remove the blood that has accumulated on the incision by gently "wicking" it onto a circle of Whatman No. 1 filter paper or Surgicutt Bleeding Time Blotting Paper (International Technidyne Corp., Edison, NJ). Do not touch the incision because this disturbs formation of the *platelet plug* and prolongs the BT.

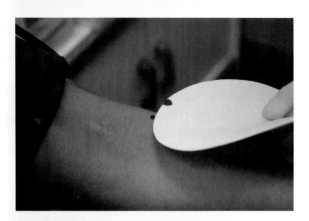

Step 14. Continue to remove blood from the incision every 30 seconds in the manner described previously until the bleeding stops.

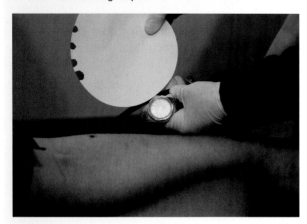

Step 15. When the bleeding has stopped, record the time to the nearest 30 seconds.

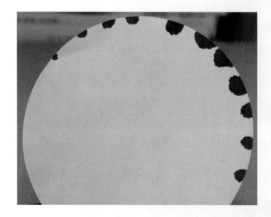

PROCEDURE 12-6 ✦ **Bleeding Time** (Continued)

Step 16. Deflate the blood pressure cuff.

Step 17. Clean the patient's arm and apply a butterfly bandage to hold the edges of the incision together tightly. Cover this bandage with a regular bandage. Instruct the patient to leave the bandages on for 24 hours.

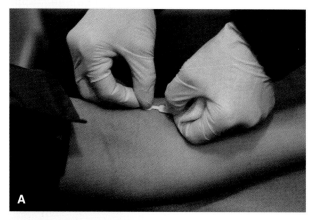

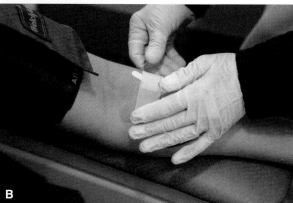

Step 18. Depending on the method and device used, normal BTs range from 2 to 10 minutes. The test can be discontinued after 15 minutes and reported as greater than 15 minutes following hospital protocol. It is important to follow the manufacturer's procedure exactly for reproducible results.

Step 19. Dispose of used supplies. Remove the blood pressure cuff.

Step 20. Thank the patient, remove gloves, and wash hands.

 Technical Tip 12-19. Consideration should be given to documenting that the patient understands the possibility of a scar.

Technical Tip 12-20. Often patients do not consider aspirin and herbal medication and will not offer that specific information unless asked.

Technical Tip 12-21. Never instruct a patient to stop taking prescribed medication. The health-care provider must be notified and will make this decision before the bleeding time test is repeated.

Preexamination Consideration 12–4.

Ingestion of aspirin, medications containing salicylate (aspirin), and drugs such as ethanol, dextran, streptokinase, streptodornase, and various herbs within the last 7 to 10 days of the test may cause a prolonged bleeding time.

POINT-OF-CARE TESTING

The development of portable hand-held instruments capable of performing a variety of routine laboratory procedures has increased the efficiency of patient testing. Samples can be collected by dermal puncture and tested by phlebotomists or other health-care personnel in the patient area. Test results are available quickly and transportation of samples to the laboratory is avoided. Dermal punctures are performed following routine dermal puncture, unless modifications are recommended by the instrument manufacturers. Phlebotomists performing point-of-care testing (POCT) should follow all manufacturer recommendations. The most routinely performed POCTs are discussed in Chapter 15.

Key Points

◆ Dermal puncture is the method of choice for blood collection on children younger than 2 years to avoid causing anemia because smaller amounts of blood can be collected. Deep vein puncture in children is dangerous and may cause complications.

◆ Dermal puncture in adults is advantageous for patients who are burned or scarred, are receiving chemotherapy, have thrombotic tendencies, are geriatric with fragile veins, are obese, are apprehensive, have inaccessible veins, or are diabetic.

◆ Capillary blood is a mixture of arterial and venous blood and may contain small amounts of interstitial and intracellular fluids. Potassium, total protein, and calcium have lower concentrations in capillary blood and glucose is higher. Note on the requistion when capillary blood is collected.

◆ A variety of automated retractable puncture devices are available. The type of device selected depends on the age of the patient, the amount of blood sample required, the collection site, and the puncture depth. The incision depth should not exceed 2.0 mm in a device used to perform heelsticks.

◆ Sample collection containers available include microhematocrit tubes and microcollection containers that are color coded to match the evacuated tube system indicating the type of additive in the tube.

◆ Recommended sites for dermal puncture include the medial and lateral plantar surface of the heel and the fleshy areas near the center of the palmar surface of the third and fourth finger.

◆ Unacceptable areas for puncture include the back or the arch of the foot, the tips or sides of the finger, previous puncture sites, areas with visible damage, and fingers on the side of a mastectomy.

◆ Warming the site increases the blood flow sevenfold. The site can be warmed with a commercial heel warmer or by covering the site with a warm towel at a temperature no higher than 42°C for 3 to 5 minutes.

◆ Failure to allow the alcohol to dry after cleansing the site will cause a stinging sensation for the patient, contaminate the sample, hemolyze the RBCs, and prevent the formation of a rounded blood drop because the blood will mix with the alcohol and run down the finger.

◆ The blade of the puncture device should be aligned to cut across (perpendicular to) the grooves of the finger or heel print.

◆ The order of collection for multiple tubes is capillary blood gases, EDTA tubes (blood smear first if required), other anticoagulated tubes, and serum tubes.

◆ Samples collected for newborn bilirubin levels must be collected at the correct time and protected from light during and after collection to prevent the bilirubin from breaking down. Hemolyis must be avoided.

◆ Mandatory newborn screening tests are performed by dermal puncture on the heel for genetic, metabolic, hormonal, and functional disorders that when not detected or treated at birth may cause physical and mental disorders. Blood is collected on filter paper and sent to a reference laboratory for testing.

◆ Capillary blood gases are collected in infants and small children from the heel or finger. Samples must be collected quickly and without air spaces in the pipette that would expose the sample to room air causing inaccurate results. Heparinized pipettes are mixed with a magnetic stirrer "flea" and round magnet that is moved up and down the tube.

◆ Blood smears are needed for the microscopic examination of blood cells that is performed for the differential blood cell count, special staining procedures, and nonautomated reticulocyte counts. A properly prepared blood smear covers approximately one-half to two-thirds of the slide, does not contain ridges or holes, and has a lightly feathered edge without streaks.

◆ Thick and thin smears are made to diagnose the presence of malaria. Thick smears concentrate the sample for detection of the parasites, and thin smears are then examined for parasitic morphology and identification.

◆ The bleeding time test is performed to evaluate platelet number and function. Factors such as the patient's vascular integrity, ingested medications (aspirin), and the phlebotomist technique influence the accuracy of the test. It is rapidly being replaced by platelet function tests.

BIBLIOGRAPHY

CLSI: Blood Collection on Filter Paper for Newborn Screening Programs; Approved Standard, ed. 5. CLSI document LA04-A5. Clinical and Laboratory Standards Institute, 2007, Wayne, PA.

CLSI: Procedures and Devices for the Collection of Diagnostic Capillary Blood Specimens; Approved Standard, ed. 6. CLSI document H04-A6. Clinical and Laboratory Standards Institute, 2008, Wayne, PA.

CLSI: Procedures for the Collection of Arterial Blood Specimens; Approved Standard, ed. 4. CLSI document H11-A4. Clinical & Laboratory Standards Institute, 2004, Wayne, PA.

Jones, PM: Newborn Screening: What's New? *Lab Medicine* 2008;39(12);737-741.

March of Dimes: Recommended Newborn Screening Tests: 29 Disorders. http://www.marchofdimes.com/professionals/14332_15455.asp.

Study Questions

1. When selecting a dermal puncture device, the most critical consideration is the:
   a. width of the incision
   b. amount of blood needed
   c. depth of the incision
   d. tests requested

2. Dermal punctures are often performed on:
   a. patients receiving chemotherapy
   b. geriatric patients
   c. diabetic patients
   d. all of the above

3. The concentration of this analyte is higher in blood collected by dermal puncture than in venipuncture:
   a. glucose
   b. potassium
   c. total protein
   d. calcium

4. Dermal punctures on newborns are performed on the:
   a. index finger
   b. medial or lateral plantar areas of the heel
   c. back of the heel
   d. earlobe

5. The maximum length of a puncture device used on the heel is:
   a. 1.0 mm
   b. 1.5 mm
   c. 2.0 mm
   d. 2.5 mm

6. Failure to puncture across the fingerprint will cause:
   a. blood to run down the finger
   b. hemolysis
   c. contamination of the sample
   d. additional patient discomfort

7. The order of draw for a bilirubin, blood smear, and CBC by dermal puncture is:
   a. CBC, blood smear, and bilirubin
   b. blood smear, CBC, and bilirubin
   c. bilirubin, blood smear, and CBC
   d. blood smear, bilirubin, and CBC

8. The blood sample for this test must be protected from light:
   a. capillary blood gases
   b. CBC
   c. PKU
   d. bilirubin

9. A test included in a newborn screen that is collected using filter paper is:
   a. PKU
   b. electrolytes
   c. bilirubin
   d. CBC

10. The proper angle of the spreader slide when preparing a blood smear is:
    a. 15°
    b. 25°
    c. 30°
    d. 45°

11. A laboratory test to detect platelet number and function is the:
    a. bilirubin
    b. capillary blood gases
    c. PKU
    d. bleeding time

Clinical Situations

1 The phlebotomy supervisor is informed that many of the samples collected by dermal puncture are hemolyzed. The supervisor schedules a continuing education in-service for the phlebotomy team.

a. Why should preparation of the collection site be stressed?
b. Why is it important for the phlebotomists to obtain rounded drops of blood to prevent hemolysis?
c. Should the in-service include the procedure to follow when a second puncture must be performed to obtain a full tube of blood? Why or why not?

2 A phlebotomist delivers a lavender-top Microtainer to hematology and two red-top Microtainers to the chemistry laboratory collected by dermal puncture from a newborn's heel. The hematology supervisor is concerned because the platelet count is much lower than the previous day's count and all other CBC parameters match the previous values. The serum in the red-top tubes appears hemolyzed.

a. Could the phlebotomy technique have caused this?
b. Why or why not?
c. What factors could cause hemolysis in the tubes?

3 A phlebotomist collects a sample for a serum bilirubin in a red Microtainer, labels the sample, and leaves the tube on the counter in chemistry while everyone is at lunch. The chemistry supervisor rejects the sample.

a. Why is this sample unacceptable?
b. How could this be avoided?
c. State a sample characteristic that made the sample unacceptable.

Evaluation of a Microtainer Collection by Heelstick Competency

RATING SYSTEM:
2 = Satisfactorily Performed,   **1** = Needs Improvement,   **0** = Incorrect/Did Not Perform

_____ 1. Places collection tray in designated area

_____ 2. Checks requisition and selects necessary equipment

_____ 3. Washes hands, puts on gown (if required) and gloves

_____ 4. Assembles equipment and carries it to patient

_____ 5. Identifies patient using ID band

_____ 6. Warms heel

_____ 7. Selects appropriate puncture site

_____ 8. Cleanses puncture site with alcohol and allows it to air dry

_____ 9. Does not contaminate puncture device

_____ 10. Performs puncture smoothly

_____ 11. Disposes of puncture device in sharps container

_____ 12. Wipes away first drop of blood

_____ 13. Collects rounded drops into Microtainer without scraping

_____ 14. Does not milk site

_____ 15. Collects adequate amount of blood

_____ 16. Mixes Microtainer 5 to 10 times

_____ 17. Cleanses site and applies pressure until bleeding stops

_____ 18. Removes all collection equipment from area

_____ 19. Disposes of used supplies

_____ 20. Labels tube and verifies identification

_____ 21. Removes and disposes of gloves and gown

_____ 22. Washes hands

_____ 23. Completes patient blood collection log sheet

TOTAL POINTS _____

MAXIMUM POINTS = 46

Comments:

Evaluation of Fingerstick on an Adult Patient Competency

RATING SYSTEM:
2 = Satisfactorily Performed,   **1** = Needs Improvement,   **0** = Incorrect/Did Not Perform

_____ 1. Greets patient and explains procedure

_____ 2. Examines requisition form

_____ 3. Asks patient to state full name

_____ 4. Compares requisition and patient's statement

_____ 5. Organizes and assembles equipment

_____ 6. Washes hands

_____ 7. Puts on gloves

_____ 8. Selects appropriate finger

_____ 9. Warms finger, if necessary

_____ 10. Gently massages finger

_____ 11. Cleanses site with alcohol and allows to air dry

_____ 12. Does not contaminate puncture device

_____ 13. Smoothly performs puncture across fingerprint

_____ 14. Disposes of puncture device in the sharps container

_____ 15. Wipes away first drop of blood

_____ 16. Collects two microhematocrit tubes without air bubbles

_____ 17. Seals tubes

_____ 18. Asks patient to apply pressure with gauze

_____ 19. Labels tubes and verifies identification

_____ 20. Examines site for stoppage of bleeding and applies bandage

_____ 21. Thanks patient

_____ 22. Disposes of used supplies

_____ 23. Removes gloves

_____ 24. Washes hands

TOTAL POINTS _____

MAXIMUM POINTS = 48

Comments:

Evaluation of Neonatal Filter Paper Collection Competency

RATING SYSTEM:
2 = Satisfactorily Performed,   **1** = Needs Improvement,   **0** = Incorrect/Did Not Perform

_____	1.	Obtains requisition
_____	2.	Washes hands and put on gloves
_____	3.	Identifies patient
_____	4.	Assembles equipment
_____	5.	Selects appropriate heel site
_____	6.	Warms heel
_____	7.	Cleanses site and allows it to air dry
_____	8.	Performs the puncture
_____	9.	Wipes away first blood drop
_____	10.	Evenly fills a circle
_____	11.	Fills all required circles correctly
_____	12.	Does not touch inside of circles or blood spots
_____	13.	Places filter paper in appropriate transport position
_____	14.	Applies pressure until bleeding stops
_____	15.	Disposes of equipment and supplies
_____	16.	Correctly completes all required paperwork
_____	17.	Removes gloves
_____	18.	Washes hands

TOTAL POINTS _____

MAXIMUM POINTS = 36

Comments:

Evaluation of Capillary Blood Gas Collection Competency

RATING SYSTEM:
2 = Satisfactorily Performed, **1** = Needs Improvement, **0** = Incorrect/Did Not Perform

_____ 1. Obtains requisition

_____ 2. Identifies patient

_____ 3. Washes hands and puts on gloves

_____ 4. Begins 3- to 5-minute heel warming

_____ 5. Assembles equipment

_____ 6. Adds magnetic flea

_____ 7. Selects appropriate heel site

_____ 8. Cleanses site and allows it to air dry

_____ 9. Performs puncture

_____ 10. Wipes away first drop of blood

_____ 11. Fills capillary pipette without bubbles

_____ 12. Seals both ends of capillary pipette

_____ 13. Mixes sample with magnet

_____ 14. Applies pressure to site until bleeding stops

_____ 15. Labels pipette

_____ 16. Places pipette in an ice-water slurry

_____ 17. Disposes of equipment and supplies

_____ 18. Removes gloves

_____ 19. Washes hands

_____ 20. Immediately transports sample to laboratory

TOTAL POINTS _____

MAXIMUM POINTS = 40

Comments:

Evaluation of Blood Smear Preparation Competency

RATING SYSTEM:
2 = Satisfactorily Performed,   **1** = Needs Improvement,   **0** = Incorrect/Did Not Perform

_____ 1. Obtains requisition form

_____ 2. Obtains three clean glass slides

_____ 3. Identifies patient

_____ 4. Washes hands and puts on gloves

_____ 5. Selects and cleanses an appropriate site and allows it to air dry

_____ 6. Performs puncture

_____ 7. Wipes away first drop

_____ 8. Puts correct size drop on appropriate area of slide

_____ 9. Positions slide

_____ 10. Places spreader slide at correct angle

_____ 11. Pulls spreader slide back to blood drop

_____ 12. Allows blood to spread across spreader slide

_____ 13. Pushes spreader slide evenly forward

_____ 14. Places smear to dry

_____ 15. Collects second smear using correct technique

_____ 16. Labels smears

_____ 17. Smear has feathered edge with no streaks

_____ 18. Blood is evenly distributed

_____ 19. Smear does not have holes

_____ 20. Smear is not too long or too thin

_____ 21. Smear is not too short or too thick

_____ 22. Disposes of equipment and supplies

_____ 23. Removes gloves and washes hands

TOTAL POINTS _____

MAXIMUM POINTS = 46

Comments:

Evaluation of Bleeding Time Technique Competency

RATING SYSTEM:
2 = Satisfactorily Performed,   **1** = Needs Improvement,   **0** = Incorrect/Did Not Perform

_____ 1. Obtains requisition form

_____ 2. Identifies patient

_____ 3. Explains procedure to patient

_____ 4. Asks patient about medications

_____ 5. Assembles equipment

_____ 6. Puts on gloves

_____ 7. Positions patient's arm

_____ 8. Places blood pressure cuff on the upper arm

_____ 9. Selects appropriate site

_____ 10. Cleanses site and allows it to air dry

_____ 11. Opens and does not contaminate puncture device

_____ 12. Inflates blood pressure cuff to 40 mm Hg

_____ 13. Correctly aligns puncture device on patient's arm

_____ 14. Simultaneously performs puncture and starts stopwatch

_____ 15. Quickly removes puncture device

_____ 16. Correctly wicks blood after 30 seconds

_____ 17. Continues wicking every 30 seconds

_____ 18. Recognizes endpoint and discontinues timing

_____ 19. Records stopwatch time

_____ 20. Deflates blood pressure cuff

_____ 21. Applies butterfly bandage

_____ 22. Applies regular bandage

_____ 23. Instructs patient when to remove bandages

_____ 24. Removes blood pressure cuff

_____ 25. Disposes of equipment and supplies

_____ 26. Removes gloves and washes hands

TOTAL POINTS _____

MAXIMUM POINTS = 52

Comments:

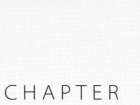

CHAPTER **13**

Quality Assessment and Management in Phlebotomy

Learning Objectives

Upon completion of this chapter, the reader will be able to:

1. Differentiate between quality control and quality assessment.
2. Discuss forms of documentation used in the phlebotomy department.
3. List the information contained in a procedure manual and describe how the manual is used by the phlebotomist.
4. Discuss the role of variables in the development of a quality management program.
5. Differentiate among preexamination, examination, and postexamination variables related to the phlebotomist's scope of practice.
6. For each step of the phlebotomy collection procedure state a quality control procedure failure that can affect the collection of a quality specimen.
7. Describe a quality management system.
8. State and describe the 12 quality essentials used in a quality management system.
9. Describe the purpose of quality indicators.
10. List the six areas of the Lean system and describe how Lean can benefit the phlebotomy department.
11. State the purpose of Six Sigma methodology in a management system.

Key Terms

Documentation
Examination variable
Incident report
Lean
Postexamination variable
Preexamination variable
Procedure manual
Quality assessment
Quality indicator
Quality management
  system
Quality system essentials
Six Sigma
Variable

In the previous chapters, many of the aspects of providing quality patient care have been discussed in relation to phlebotomy techniques. Following these procedures is needed to ensure that acceptable standards are being met while the procedures are being performed. This is called quality control (QC) and is a part of the laboratory's overall program of quality assessment (QA). In this chapter, it is appropriate to review these QC procedures, combine them with additional information, and discuss their interactions in laboratory QA, the institutional **quality management system,** and the prevention of medical errors. The actions of the phlebotomist in these programs are critical to their success.

 Technical Tip 13-1. Quality control includes not only using approved standardized procedures but also the use of standards, controls, and instrument calibrators when performing specimen testing (Chapter 15).

QUALITY ASSESSMENT

The term **quality assessment** (**QA**) refers to the overall process of guaranteeing quality patient care and is regulated throughout the total testing system. The Joint Commission (JC) requires a planned systematic process for the monitoring and evaluation of the quality and appropriateness of patient-care services and the resolving of identified problems.

DOCUMENTATION

Documentation required by the JC includes:

- A detailed procedure manual
- Identification of variables associated with the procedures
- Policies to control and monitor variables
- Reference manuals provided to nursing and other nonlaboratory staff who collect samples
- Competency assessments and continuing education (CE) records

The phlebotomy department is a central part of the laboratory QA program because of its close contact with patients and other hospital personnel. The quality of laboratory testing is absolutely dependent on the quality of the samples received.

 Technical Tip 13-2. Quality assessment is an essential part of preventing medical errors (Chapter 3).

PROCEDURE MANUALS

For each test or procedure performed, the **procedure manual** provides the principle and purpose, sample type and method of collection, equipment and supplies needed, standards and controls, step-by-step procedure, specific procedure notes, limitations of the method, corrective actions, method validation, normal values, and references. The procedure manual documents the intention of the laboratory to comply with the standards of good practice to achieve expected outcomes.

The procedure manual must be present in the department at all times. Phlebotomists should not hesitate to refer to the manual when unfamiliar requests are encountered. It is the responsibility of the phlebotomy supervisor to enter all policy and procedure changes into the manual, notify personnel of the changes, and document an annual review of the entire manual.

VARIABLES

A **variable** is defined as anything that can be changed or altered. Identification of variables throughout the testing process provides the basis for development of procedures and policies within the laboratory and its departments.

Variables can be divided into three groups:

1. **Preexamination variables:** Processes that occur before testing of the sample
2. **Examination variables:** Processes that occur during the testing of the specimen
3. **Postexamination variables:** Processes that affect the reporting and interpretation of test results

Phlebotomists are primarily involved with preexamination variables, which include the ordering, collection, transportation, and processing of samples. Their actions in these areas affect the quality of the examination results obtained in the various laboratory sections. They continue to be involved in the postexamination phase because the timeliness of collection affects the amount of time required to report the test results. Their duties may also include delivery of reports to the units and computer entry or retrieval of results.

▶ *Technical Tip 13-3.* Phlebotomists performing point-of-care testing (POCT) are involved in the examination processes (Chapter 15).

▶ *Technical Tip 13-4.* The goal of quality assessment is to develop procedures and policies to prevent variables from occurring and interfering with laboratory testing.

PREEXAMINATION VARIABLES

Ordering of Tests

This is a joint effort between the phlebotomy department and the personnel who generate the requests for laboratory tests. The laboratory must facilitate test ordering by providing a laboratory reference manual or a computerized medical information system. Information contained in the manual should include:

- Laboratory schedules for collection of routine samples. These may be called "sweeps" and are scheduled to correspond with the primary times that patient samples are requested. Examples of scheduled sweeps are the early morning, when patients are in a basal state, and late morning and afternoon, when physicians have completed their patient visits. Computerized medical information systems organize unit requisitions into scheduled times. The laboratory can then access the patient list (Fig. 13-1).
- A list of laboratory tests including the type of sample required, sample handling procedures, normal values, and any pertinent patient preparation or scheduling requirements. Instructions can also be included on computer-generated requisitions (Fig. 13-2).
- Any changes or additions to laboratory policies affecting personnel in the unit. These should be promptly added to the manual, and all personnel should be notified of the changes.
- Documentation of laboratory ordering required by the JC is shown in Box 13-1.

Errors in requisitioning include generation of duplicate requisitions and the missing of tests, either by the person transferring the health-care provider's orders to the requisition or by the phlebotomist when organizing or reading the requisitions.

▶ *Technical Tip 13-5.* The use of a hand-held computer system by phlebotomists can reduce the incidence of missed tests and requisitions. A barcode on the patient's identification band is scanned for the patient's identification and the test requests. A second scan of the barcode after the samples are collected prints out labels for the tubes collected.

▶ *Technical Tip 13-6.* The discovery of a missed test by personnel on the unit frequently causes a routine test to be ordered stat. A test overlooked by the phlebotomist may cause the patient to undergo a second, unnecessary venipuncture.

Monitoring of sample ordering can include records of:

- The number of incomplete requisitions
- The number of duplicate requisitions
- The number of missed tests
- Delays in the collection of timed tests
- The number of stat requests by hospital location
- The time between test requests and collection
- The number of unit collected samples rejected
- Turnaround time (TAT) (the amount of time between the ordering of a test and the reporting of the test results)
- Health-care provider complaints

Evaluation of these records may then be used to determine the need for additions or changes to the laboratory reference manual, for in-service continuing education presentations to personnel ordering tests in order to reduce the number of errors or decrease the number of stat requests, to justify additional phlebotomists or changes in staffing schedules to provide faster sample collection, and for additional training of phlebotomists who are missing tests or collecting samples inefficiently.

Patient Identification

Failure to identify a patient properly is the most serious error in phlebotomy and can result in injury or death

Preview of MH IP 0001-2300 2/11/2010 13:00
Preview as of: 2/11/2010 12:02

Patient	Location	Scheduled Date/Time	Orders	Collection priority	Specimen Type
Route: IP Unit R&T – mhph121					
ARTZ, KEVIN	7NORTH 0759 CC	2/11/2010 13:00	Glucose Point of Care	TI	Blood
JONES, SHAWN	7-FLR 0704 02	2/11/2010 13:00	Hemogram	RT	Blood
			Differential	RT	Blood
BAKER, GERRI	7-FLR 0720 01	2/11/2010 13:00	Glucose Point of Care	TI	Blood
FISCHER, ADAM	7-FLR 0721 02	2/11/2010 13:00	Heparin Anti Xa UFH	TI	Blood
SMITH, CALLIE	8-FLR 0811 01	2/11/2010 13:00	Glucose Point of Care	TI	Blood
DOSCH, NINA	8-FLR 0817 01	2/11/2010 13:00	Glucose Point of Care	TI	Blood
HARR, GEORGE	8-FLR 0821 01	2/11/2010 13:00	Calcium Level	TI	Blood
ADAMS, ALBERT	6-FLR 0635 -1	2/11/2010 13:00	Uric Acid	RT	Blood
			Hemogram	RT	Blood
			Differential	RT	Blood
			Comprehensive Metabolic Panel	RT	Blood
			hsCRP	RT	Blood
GUND, LOLA	1NORTH 0105 01	2/11/2010 13:58	Troponin T	TI	Blood
HARRY, DANIEL	6NORTH 0651 01	2/11/2010 13:00	Glucose Point of Care	TI	Blood

FIGURE 13-1 Computer collection list.

FIGURE 13-2 Requisitions with special instructions.

to the patient. Identification errors may be discovered in the laboratory, before the patient is harmed, through an QA procedure known as the delta check. A delta check is a comparison between a patient's previous test results and the current results. Variation of results outside of established parameters alerts laboratory personnel to the possibility of an error. Documentation of errors in patient identification can result in suspension or dismissal of a phlebotomist. Identification of patients using barcode technology could provide a solution to problems with patient identification.

 Technical Tip 13-7. Delta checks may be performed by the technologist who examines the results or reported by the instrument performing the testing. Autoverification is currently being programmed into many laboratory analyzers.

Phlebotomy Equipment

Ensuring the sterility of needles and puncture devices and the stability of evacuated tubes, anticoagulants, and additives is essential to patient safety and sample quality. Providing needle safety devices and needle disposal containers as specified by the Occupational Health and Safety Administration (OSHA) is essential for phlebotomist safety.

Technical Tip 13-8. Visual inspection of needles for nonpointed or barbed needles detects defects prior to inserting the needle.

Manufacturers of evacuated tubes must ensure that tubes, anticoagulants, and additives meet the standards established by the Clinical and Laboratory Standards Institute (CLSI). These standards specify the acceptable concentrations to provide quality samples. The expiration date of the evacuated tubes should be checked each time a new package of tubes is opened, and outdated tubes should not be used. For the most economical management of phlebotomy supplies, packages of tubes should be stored in groups by lot number, and lots with the shortest expiration dates should be placed in the front of the storage area. Box 13-2 describes procedures for performing QC on evacuated tubes.

Patient Preparation

Numerous variables in patient preparation can affect sample quality, and the phlebotomist cannot be expected to control and monitor all variables. However, phlebotomists should be aware of the most critical variables, such as fasting or abstaining from certain medications. Any discrepancies should be reported to the nursing staff or a supervisor.

 Technical Tip 13-9. Phlebotomists should also be alert for noticeable unusual circumstances occurring with the patient and report it to the nursing staff or a supervisor.

BOX 13-2 Quality Control (QC) Procedures on New Lots of Evacuated Tubes

1. Measure the amount of water drawn into a tube to QC the tube vacuum.
2. Check anticoagulant tubes for the presence of small clots.
3. Visually check the appearance of additives.
4. Check the stability of tubes and gel barriers following centrifugation.
5. Check stopper integrity and ease of stopper removal.
6. Document results of the checks.
7. Notify the manufacturer if defects are discovered.

Special patient preparation procedures must be included in the laboratory reference manual or floor book. Patient variables that may affect test results are discussed in Chapter 10 and inserted as preexamination variables throughout the text.

Monitoring and evaluation of QA in patient preparation must be done jointly by the laboratory, nursing staff, and health-care providers.

Tourniquet Application

Application of the tourniquet for longer than 1 minute increases the concentration of large molecules such as bilirubin, lipids, protein, and enzymes and may produce a slight hemolysis that affects potassium levels.

 Technical Tip 13-10. Investigation of an increase in unacceptable potassium results should include documentation of the length of tourniquet application time.

Site Selection

QA is affected by the choice of a puncture site. A site may be located in an area where sample contamination may occur or patient safety may be compromised.

Sites to be avoided because of the possibility of sample contamination include:

- Hematomas
- Edematous areas
- Arms adjacent to mastectomies
- Arms receiving intravenous fluids

Sites to be avoided to prevent injury to the patient include:

- Burned and scarred areas
- Arms adjacent to mastectomies
- Arms with fistulas and shunts
- The back of the heel
- Previous dermal puncture sites
- Arteries for routine testing

Errors in site selection are detected by delta checks, test results that are markedly affected by intravenous fluids, and reports from patients and nursing staff. Documentation of counseling, retraining, or dismissal of phlebotomists associated with poor choices in site selection should be available.

Cleansing the Site

Blood culture contamination is the most frequently encountered variable associated with improper cleansing of the puncture site. The microbiology department maintains records of contaminated blood cultures. Increases in contamination rates are investigated and documented. Corrective action documentation could include in-service training of personnel collecting blood cultures.

Performing the Puncture

Variables in phlebotomy technique affect both sample quality and patient safety. Errors affecting sample quality include collection in the wrong tube, failure to mix the sample adequately, failure to follow the correct order of draw or fill, and excessive dilution of dermal puncture samples with tissue fluid.

The patient's impression of the laboratory quality is heavily influenced by phlebotomy technique. Painful probing, hematomas, unsuccessful attempts, repeat draws because of poor sample quality, and excessive and inappropriately located heel punctures generate reports from patients, nursing staff, and health-care providers.

 Technical Tip 13-11. Phlebotomists should remember how often patients tell them about previous bad experiences and strive to not become another bad memory for the patient.

Documentation of poor technique affecting patients or sample quality is frequently made in the form of an *incident report* generated by a nursing or laboratory supervisor (Fig. 13-3). Incident reports describe the incident and the problem caused, document the corrective action taken, and become a part of an employee's permanent record.

Disposal of Puncture Equipment

The availability of and the proper use of sharps containers and activation of venipuncture safety devices is essential to quality performance by phlebotomists. Accidental punctures with contaminated sharps must be reported immediately to a supervisor. A protocol that includes immediate and follow-up testing and counseling for the affected employee must be in place and followed (see Chapter 4).

Documentation of excessive accidental punctures can lead to changes in the type of equipment used or to disciplinary action against employees who are not following acceptable disposal procedures.

 Technical Tip 13-12. Documentation of phlebotomist involvement in the selection of phlebotomy-related safety devices is required by Occupational Safety and Health Administration (see Chapter 4).

Transportation of Samples

Variables in the transportation of samples include the method and timing of delivery to the laboratory and the use of special handling procedures discussed in previous chapters.

Phlebotomists' duties include timely delivery of samples to the laboratory. This procedure requires the ability to organize the workload efficiently and to adapt to emergency situations. Documentation of the time between the delivery of a requisition to the laboratory and the arrival of the sample in the laboratory can be obtained by computer entry or by using a time-stamping machine.

Many hospitals have pneumatic tube systems running between the units and support areas. These systems increase the timeliness of sample delivery to the laboratory. However, they must be carefully monitored to ensure that samples are not hemolyzed or broken during transit. To transport laboratory samples, the system should be designed to avoid sharp turns, provide a soft landing, and use containers that can be equipped with shock-absorbent lining materials. Records of unacceptable samples must be maintained and evaluated to verify satisfactory performance of the pneumatic tube system.

Sample Processing

Variables associated with sample processing include the length of time between collection and processing or testing, centrifugation time and speed, contamination, evaporation, storage conditions, and labeling (see Appendix A).

Documentation of centrifuge calibration and maintenance is required for accreditation. Centrifuges are routinely calibrated every 3 months using a tachometer to confirm revolutions per minute at various settings. This information can then be converted into relative centrifugal force using nomograms provided by the centrifuge manufacturer. Marked changes in the calibration may indicate the need to replace the centrifuge brushes or problems with the bearings. Procedure manuals should include specifications for centrifuge speed, type, and time for each sample.

Quality Improvement Follow-up Report

CONFIDENTIAL

Instructions: Section I should be completed by the individual identifying the event.

Date of report: _____   Reported by: _____

Date of incident: _____   Date/time of discovery: _____

Patient MR# _____   Patient accession# _____

Section I

Summary of incident — *describe what happened* _____

_____

_____

What immediate corrective action was taken?_____

_____

_____

Provide the ORIGINAL to team leader/technical specialist within 24 hours of incident discovery

Date: _____

To: _____

Forwarded for follow-up:

Date: _____

To: _____

Section II. Management investigation: *Tracking #* _____

Instructions: Section II should be completed by laboratory management within 72 hours

Check appropriate problem category

☐ Unacceptable patient samples
   (Due to hemolysis, QNS, or contaminated)

☐ Equipment related event

☐ Standard operating procedure deviation

☐ Communication problem/complaint

☐ Accident

☐ Wrong tube type

☐ Misidentified sample

☐ Wrong location

☐ Other (explain)

Explain answers:

_____

_____

Preventive/corrective action recommendations:

_____

_____

Technical specialist/team leader: _____   Date: _____

Medical director review: _____   Date: _____

Quality assurance review: _____   Date: _____

FDA reportable: Yes or no _____   Date reported: _____

FIGURE 13-3 Incident report. *(From Strasinger, SK, and Di Lorenzo, MS: Urinalysis and Body Fluids, ed. 5. FA Davis, 2008, Philadelphia, with permission.)*

Failure to perform centrifuge calibration routinely or to follow the specifications stated in the procedure manual can affect specimen quality as a result of incomplete separation of liquid and formed elements, cellular damage caused by use of excessive speed or time, and deterioration of chemical elements if special requirements such as the use of a refrigerated centrifuge are needed.

 Technical Tip 13-13. Always check the centrifuge for proper balancing of tubes before operating.

Poor technique during sample processing can seriously alter sample composition by causing contamination or evaporation. All samples left uncovered for extended periods of time are subject to external contamination and fluid evaporation.

The temperatures of refrigerators and freezers used for specimen storage must be monitored, either continually with automatic temperature recorders or daily by recorded checks of thermometer readings. Documentation of temperature readings or recording charts and centrifuge calibration and maintenance must be available for accreditation reviews.

 Technical Tip 13-14. Specimens should not be stored in self-defrosting freezers because they may be thawed and refrozen during defrosting cycles.

When aliquoting specimens into different tubes, particular attention must be paid to labeling to ensure that sample numbers are correctly transferred. Computer-generated labels often include additional labels for this purpose.

Errors in sample processing can occur when personnel are not trained to prioritize samples. This can include:

- Failure to differentiate between tests designated stat and routine
- Rejection of samples because of minor paperwork discrepancies that could be easily resolved
- Rejection of critical samples such as cerebrospinal fluid without seeking assistance to resolve the problem
- General overestimation of one's knowledge and ability to make decisions.

Documentation in the sample processing area should include not only technical processing instructions but also instructions for contacting a designated supervisor when nontechnical situations arise. Records must be kept of any corrective actions taken.

 Technical Tip 13-15. A sample should never be rejected or arbitrarily classified as a lower priority than requested without consulting a supervisor.

EXAMINATION VARIABLES

Phlebotomists must be aware of examination variables when performing point-of-care testing (POCT). As discussed in Chapter 15, variables in the testing process are best controlled by strictly following the procedure and manufacturer's instructions, consistently using all available controls and performing all required instrument calibration.

POSTEXAMINATION VARIABLES

Reporting of test results to the appropriate health-care providers in an efficient and accurate manner is essential to quality patient care. Reports may be handwritten or instrument printouts and delivered, telephoned, or electronically transmitted to the requesting department. Phlebotomists can be involved in all forms of reporting.

Laboratory reports must be present in the patient's record. Required information includes:

- Patient's first and last name
- Patient's unique identification number
- Sample collection date and time (if pertinent to the test)
- Sample source (if pertinent to the test)
- Condition of unsatisfactory samples
- Tests performed, the results, and the reference ranges of the tests
- Date and time of the final results generation

Laboratories must maintain records of the personnel performing preexamination, examination, and postexamination duties.

 Technical Tip 13-16. Phlebotomist identification must be present on collected samples.

Written Reports

Computer capability has significantly reduced the use of handwritten results in the laboratory. However, phlebotomists may be involved with the physical delivery of reports to the patient area, which could include placement in the patient's chart. They also may be required to enter data from the written record into a computer system. The quality of patient care can be severely affected by a delay in delivery of results, failure to place the reports in the correct location, and errors in the transfer of written reports to the computer.

Electronic Results

Electronic transmission is now the most common method for reporting results. Many laboratory instruments, including those used for POCT, have the capability for the operator to generate and transmit reports directly from the instrument to the designated health-care provider. It is essential that the operator carefully review results before transmittal.

Documentation of the reporting of results is essential and required by accrediting agencies. Permanent records of all reported results must be available. A method to verify the actual reporting of results also must be available and used by all employees.

Telephone (Verbal) Results

The telephone is frequently used to transmit results of stat tests and critical values. Calls requesting additional results may be received from personnel on hospital units and health-care providers. When telephoning results, be sure that they are being reported to the appropriate person (ideally the actual health-care provider). Always document the time of the call and the name of the person receiving the results.

 Technical Tip 13-17. The Joint Commission Patient Safety Goals require that when verbally reporting test results the information must be repeated by the person receiving the information. This should be documented by the person giving the report.

Medical Records

Medical records must be kept on each patient to document a patient's medical history. The records include medications, prescriptions, diagnostic procedures, and test results. The primary purposes of a medical record are the following:

- To provide a plan for managing patient care
- To document communication between the health-care provider and others involved in patient care
- To provide documentation of patterns in the patient's illness and treatment
- To serve as a legal document for evidence in litigation and to protect the legal interests of the patient, hospital, and health-care workers
- To provide clinical data for peer review and medical research, education, and statistics
- To assist in billing, utilization review, and quality management system (QMS) review

A good medical record must be accurate, complete, and concise. The initials or name of every health-care worker that performed a diagnostic procedure, collected blood samples, or performed laboratory tests on a patient is documented in a patient's record. Without a medical record, it would be impossible for a phlebotomist to remember every patient from whom he or she had collected a blood sample. This is why it is important that the requisition or computer label be properly documented with the phlebotomist's initials, as well as the date and time. Document all actions completely on the patient's chart or in the computer stating unusual circumstances, such as deviations from standard practice, patient refusal to have blood collected, patient not fasting, or any other problems associated with the blood collection.

With the efficiency of computers, patient test results can be quickly transmitted to the patient's record. Before releasing results, always double-check that they have been entered into the computer accurately. If a result has been entered incorrectly and is on the patient's record, follow the institution's policy for correcting the result on the patient's chart or in the computer (Box 13-3).

QUALITY MANAGEMENT SYSTEMS

Phlebotomy QA is part of the laboratory and institutional QMS.

 Technical Tip 13-18. The term QMS has replaced the terms total quality management (TQM) and continuous quality improvement (CQI).

The QMS has incorporated many of the objectives of total quality management (TQM) and continuous quality improvement (CQI) to ensure quality results, staff competence, and efficiency within an organization. In addition, QMS also utilizes the concepts of the International Organization for Standardization (ISO 151189) and the Lean and Six Sigma methods. The requirements of the JC and the College of American Pathologists (CAP) accreditation organizations are included in QMS.

A QMS is designed to coordinate activities to direct and control an organization with regard to quality and the reduction of medical errors. The first step in a laboratory QMS is to determine the pathway of workflow through the laboratory as discussed previously under the preexamination, examination, and postexamination phases of testing (Fig.13-4). In each area of the pathway all the processes and procedures that occur are determined and analyzed so everyone knows what they are supposed to do, how they are supposed to do it, and when they are supposed to do it (Fig. 13-5). Instructions must be available for each activity.

Turnaround Time (TAT)

TAT is defined as the amount of time required from when a test is ordered by the health-care provider until the results are reported to the health-care provider. Laboratories determine the TAT for tests including both stat and routine tests as appropriate. The laboratory can then monitor the TATs to determine areas in the process that need improvement. This can be determined by creating a cause and effect diagram as shown in Figure 13-6 and can also be monitored as shown in Figure 13-7.

Quality System Essentials

Quality system essentials (QSEs) form the basis of a QMS. The 12 QSEs contain the management information needed for a laboratory to perform quality work. They were developed by the former National Committee for Clinical Laboratory Standards (NCCLS) and the current CLSI and include the methods to meet the requirements of regulatory, accreditation, and standard-setting organizations.

 Technical Tip 13-19. Although management is responsible for developing quality system essentials, it is the responsibility of all laboratory personnel to maintain them.

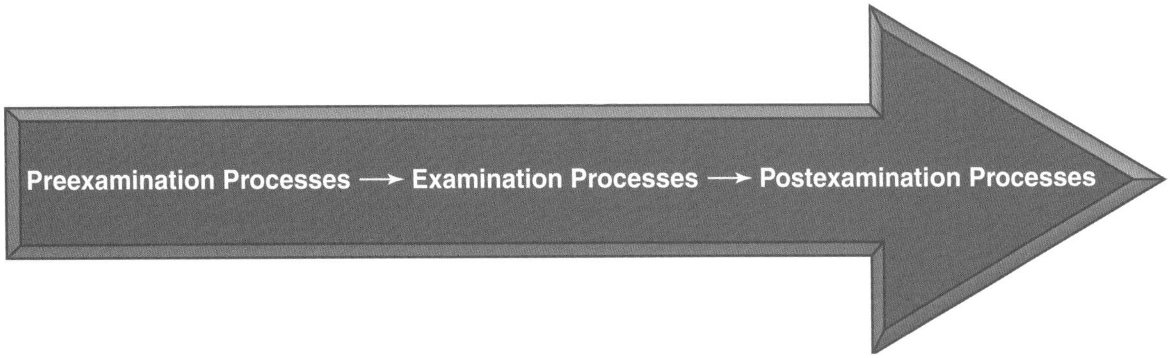

Preexamination Processes → Examination Processes → Postexamination Processes

FIGURE 13-4 **Workflow through laboratory flow chart.**

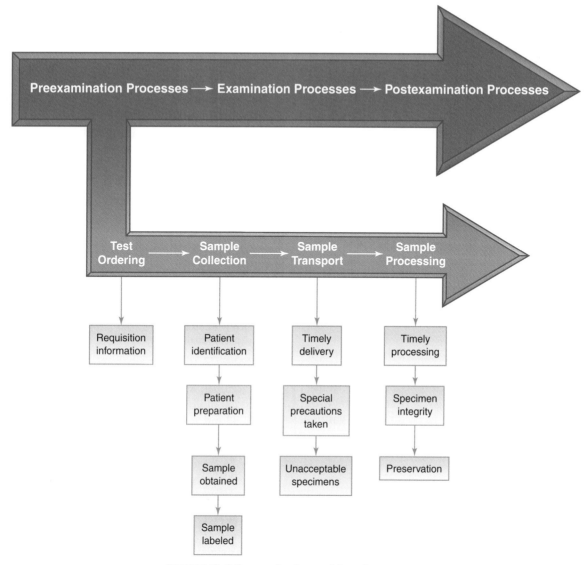

FIGURE 13-5 **Preexamination workflow chart.**

Description of the 12 Laboratory QSEs

A. The Laboratory
   1. Organization
      Personnel roles, responsibilities, and reporting
        relationships
      Quality planning and risk assessment
      Allocation of personnel and material re-
        sources
      Review and assessment of meeting goals
   2. Facilities and Safety
      Space designed for efficiency
      Adequate storage space
      Required safety precautions and equipment
        availability (Chapter 4)

   Housekeeping
   Safety training
   3. Personnel
      Qualifications
      Current job descriptions
      Orientation of new employees
      Competency assessment
      Continuing education
   4. Equipment
      Selection criteria
      Space needed and special instrument re-
        quirements
      Ongoing preventive maintenance
      Service and repair records

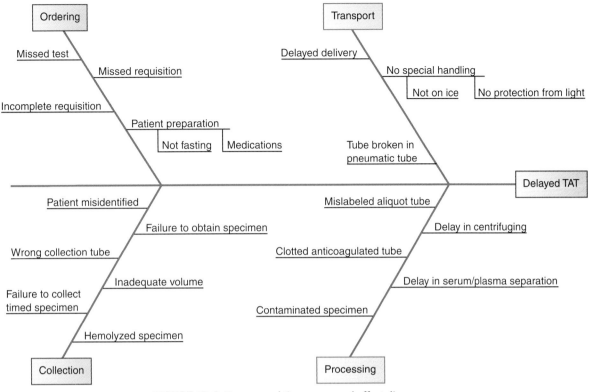

FIGURE 13-6 **Turnaround time cause and effect diagram.**

5. Purchasing and Inventory
   Inventory of initial materials and reagents
   Service contracts
   Availability of reagents, supplies, and service
B. The Work System QSEs
   6. Process Control
      Identification of all laboratory processes
      Procedure manuals/instructions for tasks
      Test method verification
      Verification that manufacturer specifications
        are in procedure manuals
      Quality control and statistics
   7. Documents and Records
      Availability of all process and procedure
        documents
      Periodic review of all process and procedure
        documents
      Access to quality control records
      Monitoring of record storage and reten-
        tion
   8. Information Management
      Availability of patient records
      Security of patient records

Methods for providing patient information
Processes to prevent Medicare and Medicaid
  fraud
C. Measurement QSEs
   9. Occurrence Management/Nonconforming
      Event management
      Identification and reporting of all events
      Remedial actions taken
      Plans to eliminate future events
      Initiation of changes
   10. Assessments: External and Internal
       Obtaining external licensing and accreditation
         (Chapter 3)
       Participation in external proficiency testing
       Periodic on-site auditing by accrediting agencies
       Development of *quality indicators* for each
         phase of testing (Box 13-4)
   11. Customer Service
       Feedback from customers including patients,
         patients' families, and health-care providers
       Feedback from employees
       Feedback from offsite referral laboratories
         and health-care providers

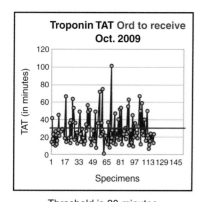
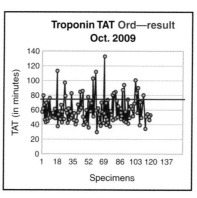
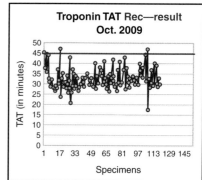

Threshold is 30 minutes	Threshold is 75 minutes	Threshold is 45 minutes
Average time for this data:	Average for this data:	Average for this data:
28.5 minutes	61.3 minutes	32.8 minutes

May	28.1	68.2	40.1
June	30.7	76.3	45.6
July	30.2	71.3	41.1
Aug.	33.2	69.3	38.1
Sept.	28.1	64.0	35.8
Oct.	28.5	61.3	32.8

Is the process in control (stable):	YES	**Assessment:**
If the process is not stable:		Best results ever! Still have large variance in
Is the data accurate?	n/a	Ord to Receive, which contributes to overall TAT.
Were there any unusual events during the period?	n/a	Only 2 data points above target in Rec to Result!
Were there any changes to machines, manpower,		**Action plan:**
methods, etc.?	n/a	Continue to monitor. Automate and autoverify
Is special cause effect desirable?	n/a	have made a huge improvement.
Does the process meet department/customer expectations?	NO	

FIGURE 13-7 Graphic monitoring of turnaround time.

12. Process Improvement
    Monitoring of the above QSE results
    Determination of the root cause of problems

    Utilize the **Lean** system tools
    Utilize **Six Sigma** methodology

 Technical Tip 13-20. Quality indicators are graphic measurements that monitor and track performance of work processes such as the identification process shown in Figure 13-8.

The Lean System

The Lean system originated with the automobile manufacturing industry in Japan. The concepts of Lean have been adopted by many American industries including the health-care industry. Lean focuses on the elimination of waste to allow a facility to do more with less and at the same time increase customer and employee satisfaction. In the current health-care environment, the ability to decrease costs while providing quality health-care is of primary importance.

BOX 13-4 Examples of Quality Indicators Related to Phlebotomy to Monitor

Requests for missing requisition information
Collection areas without current collection procedures
Inappropriate patient identification
Samples collected at an improper time
Samples received without special handling or preservation
Samples delayed in transport
Samples received without requisitions
The nature of problems with unacceptable samples
Needlestick injuries
Security violations

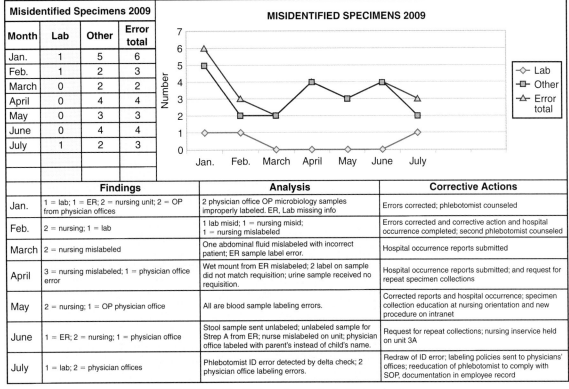

Misidentified Specimens 2009			
Month	Lab	Other	Error total
Jan.	1	5	6
Feb.	1	2	3
March	0	2	2
April	0	4	4
May	0	3	3
June	0	4	4
July	1	2	3

	Findings	Analysis	Corrective Actions
Jan.	1 = lab; 1 = ER; 2 = nursing unit; 2 = OP from physician offices	2 physician office OP microbiology samples improperly labeled. ER, Lab missing info	Errors corrected; phlebotomist counseled
Feb.	2 = nursing; 1 = lab	1 lab misid; 1 = nursing misid; 1 = nursing mislabeled	Errors corrected and corrective action and hospital occurrence completed; second phlebotomist counseled
March	2 = nursing mislabeled	One abdominal fluid mislabeled with incorrect patient; ER sample label error.	Hospital occurrence reports submitted
April	3 = nursing mislabeled; 1 = physician office error	Wet mount from ER mislabeled; 2 label on sample did not match requisition; urine sample received no requisition.	Hospital occurrence reports submitted; and request for repeat specimen collections
May	2 = nursing; 1 = OP physician office	All are blood sample labeling errors.	Corrected reports and hospital occurrence; specimen collection education at nursing orientation and new procedure on intranet
June	1 = ER; 2 = nursing; 1 = physician office	Stool sample sent unlabeled; unlabeled sample for Strep A from ER; nurse mislabeled on unit; physician office labeled with parent's instead of child's name.	Request for repeat collections; nursing inservice held on unit 3A
July	1 = lab; 2 = physician offices	Phlebotomist ID error detected by delta check; 2 physician office labeling errors.	Redraw of ID error; labeling policies sent to physicians' offices; reeducation of phlebotomist to comply with SOP, documentation in employee record

FIGURE 13-8 Monitoring of a quality indicator chart.

Lean utilizes a tool called "6S" that includes the words sort, straighten, scrub, safety, standardize, and sustain. In phlebotomy, use of the Lean tools enhances efficiency and proficiency as shown in Table 13-1. In addition, more time is available to focus on patient safety and satisfaction.

Six Sigma

Six Sigma is a statistical modification of the original Plan-Do-Check-Act (PDCA) method developed by Deming and adopted by the JC as a guideline for health-care organizations. The primary goal of

TABLE 13-1 • Lean 6S in Phlebotomy		
LEAN S	**TASK**	**BENEFIT**
Sort	Identify items in the department that can be discarded	More space and less clutter
Straighten	Identify designated areas for equipment and supplies	Time is not wasted hunting for supplies
Scrub	Maintain the work area on a daily basis	Less time is spent on major cleanups
Safety	Be alert for minor areas that can be fixed before they become major	Less chance of accidents
Standardize	All phlebotomy trays are stocked in the same manner	If necessary any tray can be used or restocked by anyone in the department
Sustain	Everyone maintains the five other S's on a daily basis	Less employee frustration and better outcomes

Six Sigma is to reduce variables and decrease errors to a level of 3.4 defects per 1 million opportunities. Attaining this goal indicates that the laboratory is addressing factors critical to customer satisfaction and quality care.

 Technical Tip 13-21. In statistics, 3.4 defects per 1 million opportunities is at the 6 Sigma (6σ) level. Therefore, the methodology is called Six Sigma.

The Six Sigma methodology utilizes the acronym DMAIC:

Define goals and current processes
Measure current processes and collect data
Analyze the data for cause and effect information
Improve the process using the data collected
Control the correction of concerns displayed in the data

Key Points

✦ Quality control involves performing individual procedures using acceptable standards. Quality assessment is the overall process of guaranteeing quality throughout the entire testing system.

✦ Documentation required in a phlebotomy department includes a procedure manual, reference manual for nonlaboratory personnel ordering and collecting samples, policies to control and monitor procedure variables, and records of competency assessment and continuing education.

✦ Procedure manuals include the principle, purpose, sample type, method of collection, equipment and supplies, standards and controls, step-by-step procedure, specific procedure notes, method limitations, corrective actions, normal values, and references for each procedure performed in the laboratory.

✦ Identification of variables in the testing process forms the basis for procedure and policy development.

✦ Preexamination variables occur before sample testing. Examination variables occur during the specimen testing. Postexamination variables occur during test results interpretation and reporting.

✦ Quality control failures in sample collection that affect sample quality include failure to collect an ordered test, improper patient identification, use of outdated evacuated tubes, collecting a fasting glucose from a nonfasting patient, leaving the tourniquet on too long, collecting blood from a hematoma, improper site selection, improper site cleansing when collecting a blood culture, excessive probing of the puncture site, delay in sample delivery, and failure to process samples in a timely manner.

✦ A quality management system coordinates activities within a department and an organization to better perform quality work and reduce medical errors.

✦ The 12 quality essentials provide the management documentation needed to demonstrate quality work.

✦ Quality indicators are developed to monitor each phase of testing.

✦ The Lean system utilizes the 6s tools (sort, straighten, scrub, safety, standardize, and sustain) to reduce increase efficiency and proficiency.

✦ The goal of the statistical Six Sigma method is to reduce variables and decrease errors to a level of 3.4 defects per one million opportunities. Six Sigma uses the define, measure, analyze, improve, and control (DMAIC) method.

BIBLIOGRAPHY

Berte, LM: Laboratory Quality Management: A Roadmap. *Clinics in Laboratory Medicine* 2007;27:771–779.

Ford, A: With Lean's Help, 14 Inspections Soon To Be One. *CAP Today* October 2008. Available at cap.org.

ISO 15189:2003. Medical Laboratories: Particular Requirements for Quality and Competence. 2003, International Organization for Standardization, Geneva, Switzerland.

Lusky, K: Laying Lean on the Line, One Change at a Time. *CAP Today* July 2009. Available at http://www.cap.org.

National Committee for Clinical Laboratory Standards: *A Quality Management System Model for Health Care.* HS1. NCCLS/CLSI, 2004, Wayne, PA.

National Committee for Clinical Laboratory Standards: Application of a Quality Management System Model for Laboratory Services; Approved Guideline, ed. 3. NCCLS/CLSI, 2004, Wayne, PA.

Six Sigma. http://isixsigma.com.

The Joint Commission: Lab Accreditation: Documentation and Process Control 2010. http://jointcommission.org/accreditationprograms.

Study Questions

1. Quality control includes all of the following **EXCEPT:**
   a. following standardized procedures
   b. using standards and controls
   c. Six Sigma methodologies
   d. instrument calibration

2. Documentation required in a phlebotomy department includes a/an:
   a. procedure manual
   b. evaluation of turnaround times
   c. reference manual
   d. both a and c

3. The principle and purpose of each test is included:
   a. on the requisition form
   b. in the laboratory report
   c. on the patient's wristband barcode
   d. in the procedure manual

4. When developing policies and procedures it is important to identify:
   a. qualifications of the persons performing the tests
   b. areas where the test is being performed
   c. variables that may affect the procedure
   d. the primary purpose of the procedure

5. An error in correctly reporting a patient's test result is considered a/an:
   a. preexamination variable
   b. examination variable
   c. postexamination variable
   d. all of the above

6. An error in properly identifying a patient whose hemoglobin is being monitored every 4 hours might be detected by:
   a. a delta check
   b. autoverification
   c. the chemistry supervisor
   d. both a and b

7. The primary goal of a QMS is to:
   a. increase laboratory efficiency
   b. reduce medical errors
   c. monitor laboratory productivity
   d. increase employee satisfaction

8. Documentation of the laboratory's overall quality of work is provided in the laboratory:
   a. quality control records
   b. quality essentials
   c. quality management system
   d. quality indicators

9. A recommended way to measure and assess the phlebotomy QSEs is to establish and monitor:
   a. quality indicators
   b. quality improvement
   c. quality control
   d. quality management

10. The basic principle of the Lean system is to increase efficiency and proficiency by:
    a. continuous quality improvement
    b. documentation of quality essentials
    c. elimination of waste
    d. rotation of duties

11. Which of the following does NOT pertain to the Lean system?
    a. sort
    b. sustain
    c. stabilize
    d. scrub

12. Six Sigma methodology is a:
    a. departmental assessment of variables
    b. statistical determination of variable and error reduction
    c. quality assessment method to control variables
    d. departmental assessment of errors and quality

Clinical Situations

1 The phlebotomy supervisor completes an assessment of sample ordering patterns initiated as a result of phlebotomy staff dissatisfaction with department organization and complaints about test TATs by the nursing units. State a reason and a corrective action that could be taken for each of the following problems identified by the study.

a. Increased requests for stat CBCs from the psychiatric unit.
b. Patient surveys reveal complaints that phlebotomists frequently return to perform a second venipuncture after a short period of time.
c. The hematology department is rejecting an increasing number of samples collected in the emergency department.
d. The medical unit reports delays in collecting timed samples.

2 The sample processing department is cited during an accreditation visit.

a. What daily equipment documentation could have been missing?
b. What documentation on preventive maintenance could have been missing?

3 The laboratory is accused of failure to report a critical result to the intensive care unit. What documentation is requested from the phlebotomist assigned to make the call?

Additional Techniques

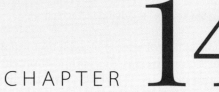

CHAPTER 14

Arterial Blood Collection

Learning Objectives

Upon completion of this chapter, the reader will be able to:

1. Describe the recommended requirements for personnel performing arterial punctures.
2. Define arterial blood gases and describe their diagnostic function.
3. List the equipment and materials needed to perform arterial punctures and discuss preparation of materials.
4. Define "steady state" and list additional patient information that must be recorded when performing blood gas determinations.
5. State four factors that are considered when selecting a site for arterial puncture and name the preferred site.
6. Perform and state the purpose of the modified Allen test.
7. Describe the steps in the performance of an arterial puncture.
8. State five technical errors associated with arterial puncture and their effect on the sample.
9. Discuss six complications of arterial puncture, including their effect on the patient and the precautions taken to avoid them.

Key Terms

Arteriospasm
Collateral circulation
Local anesthetic
Luer tip
Partial pressure
Respiration rate
Steady state
Thrombolytic therapy
Thrombosis
Vasovagal reaction
Ventilation device

The composition of arterial blood is uniform throughout the body, whereas the composition of venous blood varies because it receives waste products from different parts of the body. The normal values for most laboratory tests are based on venous blood. This is because arterial blood collection is more uncomfortable and dangerous for the patient and is more difficult to perform. Arterial blood is primarily requested for the evaluation of blood gases (oxygen and carbon dioxide) and may be requested for the measurement of lactic acid and ammonia in certain metabolic conditions.

Performing arterial punctures is not a routine duty for phlebotomists. The Clinical Laboratory Standards Institute (CLSI) recommends that all institutions require personnel performing arterial punctures to complete specialized training before performing the procedure. This training should include instruction on:

1. Complications associated with arterial punctures
2. Precautions taken to ensure a safe procedure
3. Sample handling procedures to prevent alteration of test results
4. Correct puncture technique
5. Supervised puncture performance

Personnel trained to perform arterial punctures include physicians, nurses, medical laboratory scientists, respiratory therapists, emergency medical personnel, and senior phlebotomists. In some institutions collecting and testing of arterial blood gases (ABGs) has become the responsibility of the respiratory therapy department. In institutions where the laboratory performs the testing, phlebotomists may be required to perform the puncture or to assist the person performing the puncture and delivering the sample to the laboratory following special procedures.

To provide phlebotomists with a thorough understanding of arterial punctures, whether or not they are required to perform them, this chapter covers the equipment, patient preparation, puncture technique, sample handling, and complications of the procedure. Collection of capillary blood gases (CBGs), a procedure routinely performed by phlebotomists, is covered in Chapter 12.

 Technical Tip 14-1. Phlebotomists should *not* perform arterial punctures until they complete specialized training in their place of employment.

ARTERIAL BLOOD GASES

Testing of ABGs measures the ability of the lungs to provide oxygen (O_2) to the blood and to remove carbon dioxide (CO_2) from the blood and exhale it.

Conditions requiring the measurement of blood gases may be of respiratory or metabolic origin and include chronic obstructive pulmonary disease (COPD), cardiac and respiratory failures, severe shock, lung cancer, diabetic coma, open heart surgery, and respiratory distress syndrome (RDS) in premature infants.

 Technical Tip 14-2. Patients requiring blood gas determinations are often critically ill.

ABGs are tested using specialized ABG instrumentation designed to measure the acidity (pH), the *partial pressure* of O_2 (P_{O_2}) and the partial pressure of CO_2 (P_{CO_2}). Using these measurements the bicarbonate (HCO_3), the oxygen content ($_{ct}O_2$) and the oxygen saturation (O_2Sat) are determined. See Table 14-1 for explanations and normal values for the tests performed.

 Technical Tip 14-3. Instrumentation is also available to perform arterial blood gases in addition to routine metabolic tests such as glucose, electrolytes, and hemoglobin from the same sample.

ARTERIAL PUNCTURE EQUIPMENT

Arterial blood is collected and transported in specially prepared syringes. Specimens are introduced directly into blood gas analyzers from the collection syringe as shown in Figure 14-1. This is necessary to protect the specimen from contact with room air.

Arterial Blood Collection Kits

Arterial blood collection kits contain preanticoagulated syringes with hypodermic needles containing a safety shield and a tightly fitting cap for the *Luer tip* of the syringe after the needle has been removed (Fig. 14-2).

Syringes and Needles

Syringes recommended by the CLSI for arterial punctures are plastic with freely moving plungers and contain

TABLE 14-1 • Arterial Blood Tests

ARTERIAL BLOOD TEST	DESCRIPTION/FUNCTION	NORMAL VALUES
Partial pressure of oxygen (P_{O_2})	Measures the pressure of O_2 dissolved in the blood. Tells how well O_2 moves from the lungs into the blood.	75–100 mm mercury (Hg)
Partial pressure of carbon dioxide (P_{CO_2})	Measures the pressure of CO_2 dissolved in the blood. Tells how well CO_2 moves out of the lungs.	35–45 mm Hg
pH	Measures the acidity or alkalinity of the blood. Indicates acidosis or alkalosis.	7.35–7.45
Bicarbonate (HCO_3)	Buffers the blood to prevent acidosis or alkalosis.	20–29 mEq/L
Oxygen content ($_{ct}O_2$)	Measures the amount of O_2 in the blood.	15–22 mL/100 mL of blood
Oxygen saturation (O_2Sat)	Measures how much of the hemoglobin in the red blood cells is carrying O_2.	95%–100%

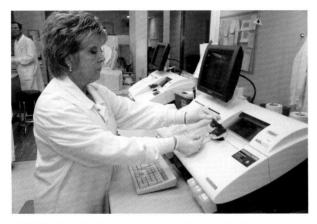

FIGURE 14-1 Technologist performing arterial blood gas determination.

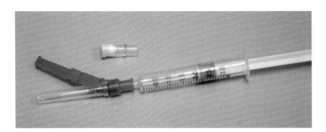

FIGURE 14-2 Arterial blood collection kit.

an appropriate anticoagulant. Based on the requirements of the testing instrument and the number of tests requested they may range in size from 1 to 5 mL. They should be no larger than the volume of sample required.

Based on the size and depth of the artery selected for puncture, acceptable needle sizes range from 20 to 25 gauge and are ⅝ to 1½ inches long. Ideally, the syringe should self-fill from the arterial pressure. When using 25-gauge needles it may be necessary to slowly pull the plunger.

 Technical Tip 14-4. Excessive pulling on the syringe plunger can cause air or capillary blood to enter the sample.

Heparin is the anticoagulant of choice for ABGs and must be present in the syringe when the sample is collected. The type of heparin used must not interfere with any additional tests being performed on the sample.

 Technical Tip 14-5. For example, sodium heparin would not be used if electrolytes were also requested.

Glass syringes must be available for use when samples cannot be tested within 30 minutes. They must be lubricated and heparinized prior to use. Liquid heparin can be used to prepare a glass syringe just before use. The procedure for lubrication and heparinizing a glass syringe is shown in Box 14-1.

A tightly fitting cap must be available to place on the Luer tip of the collection syringe after the needle has been removed. To prevent air from entering the sample, capping must be performed immediately after the safety needle has been removed from the syringe.

BOX 14-1 Heparin Preparation of a Lubricated and Heparinized Syringe

- Coat the plunger of the syringe with sterile mineral oil using a sterile cotton swab.
- Insert the plunger into the syringe with a circular motion to coat the inside of the syringe.
- Obtain a vial of heparin with a concentration of 1,000 IU/mL.
- Attach a 20-gauge needle to the collection syringe.
- Cleanse the top of the heparin vial with alcohol.
- Draw 0.5 mL of heparin into the syringe.
- Pull the plunger back to expose the area of the syringe that will be in contact with the blood and rotate the syringe so that the entire surface has been heparinized.

- Remove the 20-gauge needle and replace it with the needle to be used for performing the puncture.
- Hold the syringe with the needle pointing up and expel the air; then point the needle down, expel the excess heparin, carefully remove the needle, and attach a new sterile needle. (When the heparin is expelled with the needle pointing downward, the space in the needle that would normally contain air contains heparin, so that air cannot be introduced into the sample. It is important to expel the excess heparin from the syringe barrel because the presence of excess heparin will lower the pH value.)

Notice the device included with the collection kit in Figure 14-2. Capping devices are available that remove air bubbles already present in the syringe in addition to preventing the entry of air into the sample. Also available is the Point-Lok device (Sims Portex, Inc, Keene, NH), into which the needle can be inserted before removal.

Additional Supplies

A container of crushed ice, or ice and water, is required for maintaining sample integrity if the sample cannot be tested within 30 minutes. The container must be large enough to cover the entire blood sample with the ice and water. Materials used for sample labeling must be waterproof if the sample is placed in an ice bath. Materials for care of the puncture site include povidone-iodine or chlorhexidine for cleansing the site, alcohol pads to remove the iodine after the procedure is complete, gauze pads to apply pressure to the site, and bandages. Self-adhesive pressure dressing bandages such as Coban are used for additional pressure. A puncture-resistant needle disposal container must be present.

Some institutions administer a *local anesthetic* before performing arterial punctures. This requires a 1-mL hypodermic syringe with a 25- or 26-gauge needle containing 0.5 mL of an anesthetic such as lidocaine (Box 14-2).

ARTERIAL PUNCTURE PROCEDURE

As discussed previously for the venipuncture, when an arterial puncture is performed, a requisition containing appropriate information is required, patients must

BOX 14-2 Preparing and Administering the Local Anesthesia

- Obtain a 1-mL syringe with a 25- or 26-gauge needle and a vial of 1% lidocaine without epinephrine.
- Cleanse the vial top with alcohol.
- Withdraw 0.5 mL of lidocaine and recap the needle and place it horizontally on the table.
- Locate and cleanse the puncture site.
- Using the nondominant hand, raise the skin slightly above the artery, forming a wheal.
- Puncture the raised wheal subcutaneously.
- Slightly pull back on the syringe plunger before injecting the lidocaine to be sure that blood does not appear as that would indicate puncture of a blood vessel.
- Inject the lidocaine.
- Remove the needle and allow 2 to 3 minutes for the anesthesia to take effect.
- Proceed with the arterial puncture procedure when the patient has relaxed.

be properly identified, and samples must be labeled with required information.

Phlebotomist Preparation

After carefully examining the requisition form, the phlebotomist must collect all the required equipment, and if necessary, heparinize the collection syringe and prepare the syringe to administer the local anesthetic. All equipment must be conveniently accessible when the puncture is being performed.

Patient Assessment

Additional patient information concerning the conditions under which the sample was obtained should be provided on either the requisition form or a designated ABG form. This information includes the following:

1. Time of collection
2. Patient's temperature
3. Patient's *respiration rate*
4. Method of ventilation (room air or mechanical including the type of *ventilation device* in use)
5. The amount of oxygen the patient is receiving reported as either the fraction of inspired oxygen (FIO_2) or the rate of flow per minute shown on the oxygen monitor in liters per minute (L/M).

 Technical Tip 14-6. Patient assessment information may be included on the requisition form but should be rechecked at this time.

6. Patient activity, such as comatose, agitated, or anesthetized
7. Collection site and method (arterial puncture or cannula, capillary puncture)

Steady State

The patient should have been receiving the specified amount of oxygen and have refrained from exercise for at least 20 to 30 minutes before obtaining the sample. This is referred to as a ***steady state.***

Patients are often apprehensive about arterial punctures, and considerable time and care must be taken to reassure them because an agitated patient will not be in a steady state. Telling the patient that a local anesthetic will be administered after the site has been selected may aid in relaxing an apprehensive patient. The patient should be in a relaxed state with normal breathing for at least 5 minutes.

 Technical Tip 14-7. Keeping the patient calm is extremely important for patient safety and sample integrity. Agitated patients often have changed their breathing patterns such as hyperventilating that will change their partial pressure readings. Sample collection should not be performed hurriedly.

Site Selection (Fig. 14-3)

Arterial punctures can be hazardous, a situation that limits the number of acceptable sites. To be acceptable as a puncture site, an artery must be

1. Large enough to accept at least a 25-gauge needle
2. Located near the skin surface so that deep puncture is not required
3. In an area where injury to surrounding tissues will not be critical
4. Located in an area where other arteries are present to supply blood (***collateral circulation***) in case the punctured artery is damaged

The radial artery, located on the thumb side of the wrist, and sometimes the brachial artery, located near the basilic vein in the antecubital area, are the only arterial sites used by phlebotomists (Fig. 14-3A). Physicians and specially trained personnel must collect samples from sites such as the femoral artery, umbilical and scalp veins, and the foot artery (dorsalis pedis) (Fig. 14-3B). These are also the only personnel authorized to insert and collect samples from arterial cannulas. However, phlebotomists may be asked to assist in the collection of samples from cannulas.

Although it is smaller than the brachial artery, the radial artery is the arterial puncture site of choice because

1. The ulnar artery can provide collateral circulation to the hand.
2. It lies close to the surface of the wrist and is easily accessible.
3. It can be easily compressed against the wrist ligaments, so that pressure can be applied more effectively on the puncture site after removal of the needle and there is less chance of a hematoma.

In spite of its large size and the presence of adequate collateral circulation, the brachial artery is not routinely used. This is owing to its depth, its location near the basilic vein and median nerve, and the fact that it lies in soft tissue that does not provide adequate support for postpuncture pressure.

Modified Allen Test

Before performing a radial artery puncture, the Modified Allen Test is performed to determine if the ulnar artery is capable of providing collateral circulation to the hand. Lack of available circulation could result in loss of the hand or its function, and another site should be chosen.

The Modified Allen Test is shown in Procedure 14-1.

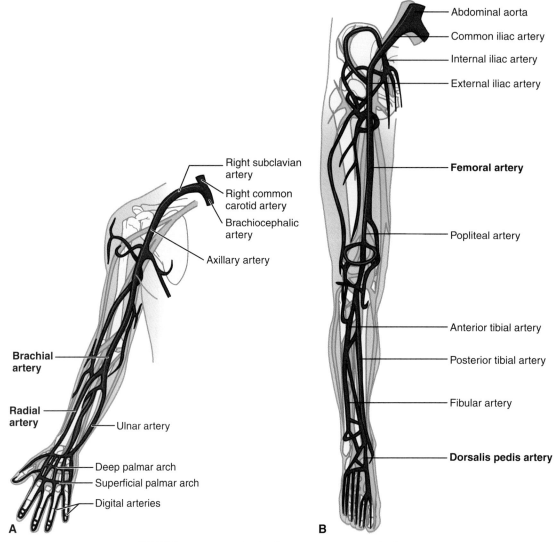

FIGURE 14-3 A, Arteries in the arm. B, Arteries in the leg.

PROCEDURE 14-1 ✦ **The Modified Allen Test**

EQUIPMENT: NONE

PROCEDURE:

Step 1. Extend the patient's wrist over a rolled towel and ask the patient to form a tight fist.

Step 2. Locate the pulses of the radial and ulnar arteries on the palmar surface of the wrist by palpating with the second and third fingers, not the thumb, which has a pulse.

Step 3. Compress both arteries.

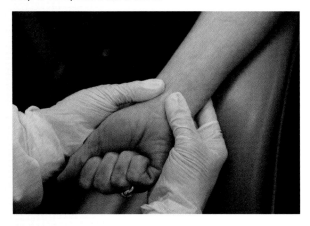

Step 4. Have the patient open the fist and observe that the palm has become pale (blanched).

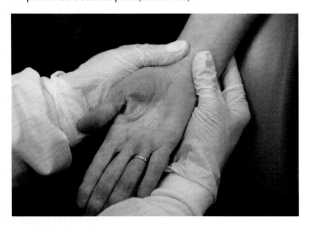

Step 5. Release pressure on the *ulnar artery only* and watch to see that color returns to the palm. This should occur within 5 seconds if the ulnar artery is functioning.

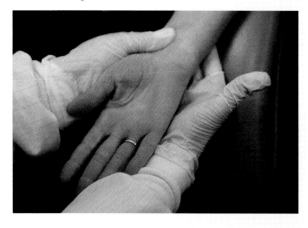

Step 6. If color does not appear (negative modified Allen test), the radial artery must not be used. If the modified Allen test is positive, proceed by palpating the radial artery to determine its depth, direction, and size.

Preparing the Site

The risk of infection is higher in arterial punctures than in venipunctures. Therefore, the puncture site is cleansed with povidone-iodine or chlorhexidine and the area is allowed to air dry. The gloved palpating fingers are cleansed in the same manner.

A local anesthetic may be administered at this time. This is done by injecting a small amount of anesthetic just under the skin, or into the surrounding tissue if the artery is deep. Before injecting the anesthetic, gently pull back on the plunger and check for the appearance of blood, which would indicate that a blood vessel—rather than tissue— has been entered. Should this happen, a new anesthetic syringe must be prepared and a slightly different injection site must be chosen. Allow 2 minutes for the anesthetic to take effect, and if the patient is apprehensive, allow him or her to relax for 5 minutes (Box 14-2).

 Safety Tip 14-1. Be sure to document that the patient does not have an allergy to local anesthesia.

 Technical Tip 14-8. The anesthesia begins to wear off in 15 to 20 minutes.

Performing the Puncture

Just before performing the puncture, the artery is relocated with the cleansed finger of the nondominant hand. The finger is placed directly over the area where the needle should enter the artery—not where the needle enters the skin.

The heparinized syringe is held like a dart in the dominant hand and the needle is inserted about 5 to 10 mm below the palpating finger at a 30- to 45-degree angle with the bevel up. The needle is slowly advanced into the artery until blood appears in the needle hub. At this time, arterial pressure should cause blood to pump into the syringe. The plunger may have to be very carefully pulled back when a plastic syringe and a small needle are used. If blood does not appear, the needle may be slightly redirected but must remain under the skin.

 Technical Tip 14-9. Blood that does not pulse into the syringe and appears dark rather than bright red may be venous blood and should not be used.

Needle Removal

When enough blood has been collected, remove the needle and apply firm pressure to the site with a gauze pad. Arterial punctures are often performed on patients receiving anticoagulant therapy (Coumadin or heparin) or ***thrombolytic therapy*** (tissue plasminogen activator [tPA], streptokinase, or urokinase). Application of pressure for longer than 5 minutes may be necessary for patients receiving this type of therapy.

 Technical Tip 14-10. The phlebotomist, not the patient, must apply firm pressure for a minimum of 3 to 5 minutes.

With the hand holding the syringe, immediately expel any air that has entered the sample. Activate the needle protection shield, remove the needle, and apply the Luer cap or insert the needle into a Point-Lok device. If a Point-Lok device is used, insert the needle into the device and apply the Luer cap when both hands are free. Immediately rotate the syringe to mix the anticoagulant with the entire sample. This can be done by rolling the syringe on a firm surface with the hand that has been holding the syringe.

 Technical Tip 14-11. One hand must hold pressure on the puncture site at all times.

After 3 to 5 minutes, check the puncture site and, if bleeding has stopped, discontinue the pressure. If bleeding has not stopped, reapply pressure for an additional 2 minutes. Repeat this procedure until the bleeding has stopped. Notify patient care personnel if the bleeding does not stop.

Completion of the Procedure

When both hands are free, the needle is discarded in an appropriate container and the Luer cap (Filter-Pro device) is applied to the hub of the syringe. The sample is labeled and, if using a glass syringe, placed in an ice-water bath.

After pressure has been removed for 2 minutes, the patient's arm is rechecked to be sure that a hematoma is not forming, in which case additional pressure is required.

The radial artery is checked for a pulse below the puncture site, and the nurse is notified if a pulse cannot be located. This would indicate a possible *arteriospasm.*

A pressure bandage is applied if no complications are discovered.

In the same manner as discussed with previous phlebotomy procedures, before leaving the room, the phlebotomist disposes of used materials in appropriate containers, removes gloves, washes hands, and thanks the patient. Procedure 14-2 describes the steps involved in performing the arterial puncture.

PROCEDURE 14-2 ✦ Radial Artery Puncture

EQUIPMENT:

Requisition form
Gloves
Antiseptic (iodine or chlorhexidine)
Alcohol pads
Heparinized syringe
Needle with safety device
Luer cap
Gauze pads
Self-adhesive pressure bandage
Ice slurry, if necessary
Indelible pen
Sharps container
Biohazard bag

PROCEDURE:

Step 1. Obtain a requisition form and check for completeness.

Step 2. Greet and identify the patient.

Step 3. Explain the procedure and reassure the patient.

Step 4. Obtain oxygen therapy information and ensure a steady state.

Step 5. Wash hands and put on gloves.

Step 6. Organize equipment.

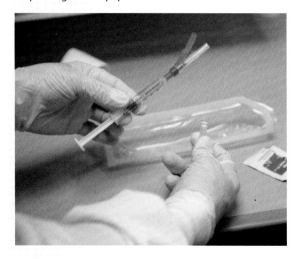

Step 7. Heparinize a glass syringe and prepare the local anesthesia syringe if necessary.

Step 8. Support and hyperextend the patient's wrist.

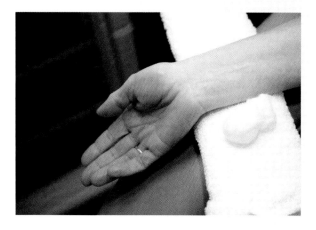

Step 9. Perform the Modified Allen Test.

Step 10. Locate and palpate the radial artery.

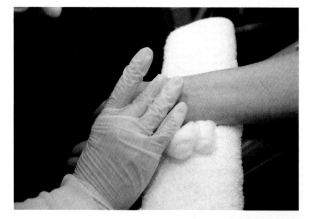

Step 11. Cleanse the site and the palpating finger.

Step 12. Administer anesthetic if necessary.

Continued

PROCEDURE 14-2 ✦ **Radial Artery Puncture** (Continued)

Step 13. Place a clean, gloved finger over the arterial puncture site.

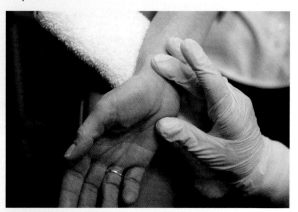

Step 14. Insert needle, bevel up at a 30-45-degree angle, 10 to 15 mm below the palpating finger.

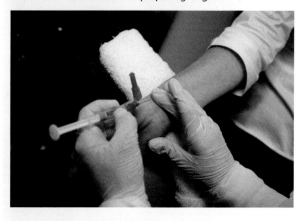

Step 15. Allow syringe to fill.

Step 16. Remove needle and apply pressure.

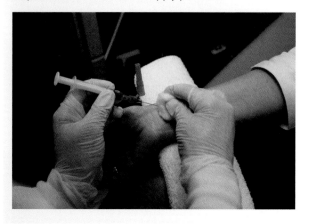

Step 17. Activate safety shield, maintaining pressure.

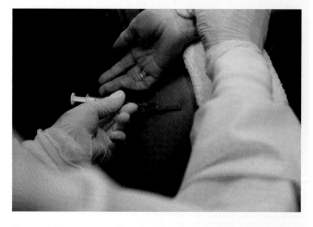

Step 18. Remove needle while retaining pressure.

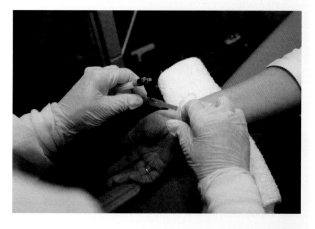

Step 19. Apply Luer device and mix syringe while retaining pressure.

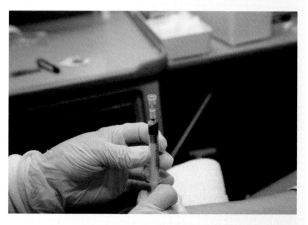

PROCEDURE 14-2 ✦ **Radial Artery Puncture** (Continued)

Step 20. Check puncture site for bleeding after 3-5 minutes. Maintain pressure if bleeding has not stopped.

Step 21. Label sample after bleeding has stopped.

Step 22. Reexamine puncture site.

Step 23. Check for radial pulse.

Step 24. Apply pressure bandage.

Step 25. Remove gloves, wash hands.

Step 26. Thank patient.

Step 27. Immediately deliver sample to the laboratory.

SAMPLE INTEGRITY

ABG test results can be noticeably affected by improper sample collection and handling. Of primary importance is maintaining the sample under strict anaerobic conditions. Sample integrity also is compromised by improper amount of anticoagulant, failure to analyze the sample in a timely manner, and collection of venous rather than arterial blood (Table 14-2).

PROCEDURAL ERRORS

Procedural errors include:

1. Introduction of air into the sample as a result of failure to firmly seat the plunger into the syringe, failure to immediately expel any bubbles from the syringe, or failure to seal the syringe or needle after collection
2. Excessive pulling of the syringe plunger resulting in increased suction may cause the aspiration of capillary blood into the sample
3. The presence of excess heparin in the syringe falsely lowers the blood pH (When preparing heparinized syringes, all excess heparin must be expelled from the syringe.)
4. An inadequate amount of heparin resulting in a clotted sample

Current CLSI recommendations state that samples that will be analyzed within 30 minutes should be collected in plastic syringes and not placed in an ice bath. The exception to this is when lactate (lactic acid) tests have been ordered with the ABG; these samples are iced immediately. Earlier recommendations to place all samples immediately in ice to prevent use of oxygen by leukocytes and platelets present in the sample have been amended as studies have shown that samples collected in plastic syringes and analyzed within 30 minutes are not affected. Samples that cannot be analyzed within 30 minutes are still collected in glass syringes and placed in ice and water.

 Technical Tip 14-12. Samples that will also have electrolytes performed cannot be placed on ice.

 Technical Tip 14-13. Every precaution should be taken to avoid the need to recollect an arterial sample because of improper handling.

TABLE 14-2 • **Effect of Technical Errors on Arterial Blood Gas Results**	
TECHNICAL ERROR	**EFFECT**
Air bubbles present	Atmospheric oxygen enters the sample, and carbon dioxide from the sample enters the air bubbles
Too much heparin	pH is lowered
Too little heparin/inadequate mixing	The presence of clots that will interfere with the analyzer
Delayed analysis	White blood cells and platelets in the sample continue their metabolism, utilizing oxygen and producing carbon dioxide
Venous rather than arterial sample	Falsely decreased Po_2 and increased Pco_2

ARTERIAL PUNCTURE COMPLICATIONS

As mentioned previously, the arterial puncture is more dangerous for the patient than the venipuncture. Possible complications include hematoma formation, arteriospasm, *vasovagal reaction, thrombosis,* hemorrhage, infection, and nerve damage (Table 14-3).

Hematoma

Hematomas are more common after arterial puncture because the increased pressure forces blood into the surrounding tissue. Failure of the phlebotomist to maintain pressure for at least 3 to 5 minutes and to check the site, use of arteries located in soft tissues where pressure is difficult to apply, and the decrease in elasticity in the arteries of older persons are frequent causes of hematomas.

Arteriospasm

An arteriospasm is a spontaneous, usually temporary constriction of an artery in response to a sensation such as pain. Closure of the artery prohibits collection of the sample and prevents oxygen from reaching the tissues so that tissue destruction and possible gangrene may result. This is why the presence of collateral circulation is essential when performing arterial punctures.

Vasovagal Reaction

Apprehensive patients may experience a vasovagal reaction resulting in a sudden loss of consciousness. Stimulation of the vagus nerve as a result of sudden stress or pain produces vascular dilation and a rapid drop in blood pressure (hypotension). Medical assistance should be summoned.

Thrombus Formation

Formation of a clot (thrombus) on the inside wall of an artery or vein in response to a puncture hole can produce occlusion of the vessel, particularly if the thrombus continues to grow. This is most frequently caused by irritation from the continued presence of a cannula. Collateral circulation again becomes important.

Hemorrhage

Patients with coagulation disorders or receiving anticoagulant or thrombolytic therapy have an increased risk of bleeding after arterial puncture. Puncture of a large artery, such as the femoral artery, using a large-gauge needle can produce considerable hemorrhaging in these patients.

Infection

Failure to cleanse the arterial puncture site adequately, resulting in the introduction of microorganisms into the arterial circulation, is more likely to cause infection than if microorganisms are introduced into the venous circulation. In the arterial circulation, the organisms are easily carried into many areas of the body without coming in contact with the protective capabilities of the lymphatic system, which runs in close proximity to the venous circulation.

Nerve Damage

The possibility of nerve damage is greater with arterial puncture because of the need to puncture more deeply into the tissue to reach the artery, thereby increasing

TABLE 14-3 • Arterial Puncture Complications		
COMPLICATION	**CAUSE**	**PREVENTION**
Hematoma	Arterial blood entering the tissue	Phlebotomist applies pressure until bleeding stops
Tissue destruction/gangrene	Arteriospasm	Evaluate collateral circulation
Vasovagal reaction	Apprehension/pain	Calming the patient, local anesthetic
Hemorrhage	Coagulation disorders and thrombolytic therapy	Increased pressure, smaller-gauge needles
Infection	Failure to adequately cleanse the site	Proper cleansing, sterile technique
Nerve damage	Deep punctures	Avoiding deep sites or additional training for deep sites

the possibility of encountering a nerve. Remember, the brachial artery is located very near the median nerve.

Considering these possible complications, it is easy to understand why phlebotomists should perform arterial punctures only after receiving specialized training and when the requisition form indicates an arterial puncture.

> **Safety Tip 14-2.** Phlebotomists should never perform an arterial puncture just because they have been unsuccessful with the venipuncture.

Accidental Arterial Puncture

Considering that the brachial artery is located near the basilic vein, it is possible for a phlebotomist to puncture this artery accidentally. Phlebotomists should be alert for the appearance of bright red blood that pulsates into the syringe. If an arterial puncture is suspected, the phlebotomist must apply pressure in the manner previously described for arterial punctures. The sample is submitted to the laboratory and the collection of arterial blood noted on the requisition form.

 Technical Tip 14-14. Never hesitate to report anything unusual observed while performing an arterial puncture.

Key Points

- ✦ Personnel performing arterial punctures must complete specialized training that includes complications, safety precautions, sample handling, puncture technique, and supervised puncture performance.
- ✦ ABGs measure the partial pressure of O_2 and CO_2 to determine the ability of the patient's lungs to supply O_2 to the blood and to exhale CO_2 removed from the blood. Additional tests include pH, bicarbonate, O_2 content, and O_2 saturation. Refer to Table 14-1.
- ✦ Specialized equipment needed for arterial puncture includes preheparinized 1- to 5-mL plastic syringes, 20- to 25-gauge 3/8- to 1.5-inch needles with safety shields, and Luer syringe caps. Glass syringes are used if the sample cannot be tested within 30 minutes. The procedure for heparinizing a glass syringe is shown in Box 14-1. To be in a steady state, the patient must have been receiving the same amount of ventilated oxygen and not exercised for 20 to 30 minutes. A steady state is important for accurate ABG results.
- ✦ Additional information required on a requisition for ABGs includes the time of collection, the patient's temperature and respiration rate, method of ventilation and the amount of oxygen the patient is receiving (L/M), patient activity, and the collection site.
- ✦ The preferred site for arterial puncture is the radial artery. Reasons for selection of an arterial puncture site include: the size of the artery, location of the artery in an area where injury to surrounding tissue would not be critical, proximity to the surface, and the presence of collateral circulation.
- ✦ The purpose for performing the Modified Allen Test before puncturing the radial artery is to ensure the presence of collateral circulation from the ulnar artery. Refer to Procedure 14-1.
- ✦ Radial artery puncture is made by holding the syringe like a dart and entering the artery at a 35- to 45-degree angle 3 to 10 mm below the palpating finger that is placed over the arterial puncture site. The phlebotomist must hold pressure on the puncture site for at least 3 to 5 minutes following needle removal. Refer to Procedure 14-2.
- ✦ Technical errors that affect ABG sample quality include the presence of air bubbles, excess heparin, not enough heparin, inadequate mixing, delayed analysis, and obtaining venous rather than arterial blood. Refer to Table 14-2.
- ✦ Complications from arterial puncture include hematomas, tissue destruction, vasovagal reactions, hemorrhage, infection, and nerve damage. Refer to Table 14-3.

BIBLIOGRAPHY

National Committee for Clinical Laboratory Standards Approved Standard H11-A4: Procedures for the Collection of Arterial Blood Specimens. NCCLS/CLSI, 2004, Wayne, PA.

Study Questions

1. To perform arterial punctures, a health-care worker must be:
   a. certified in his/her field
   b. licensed in his/her field
   c. trained in arterial punctures
   d. trained to insert IVs

2. The ABG test that measures the patient's ability to exhale is the:
   a. Po_2
   b. Pco_2
   c. HCO_3
   d. pH

3. The primary anticoagulant used for ABGs is:
   a. lithium heparin
   b. sodium citrate
   c. potassium oxalate
   d. ammonium citrate

4. ABG samples that cannot be tested within 30 minutes:
   a. are collected in glass syringes
   b. are collected in preheparinzed plastic syringes
   c. are placed in an ice slurry after collection
   d. both a and c

5. Which of the following patient information is NOT included on an ABG requisition form?
   a. collection site
   b. pulse rate
   c. respiration rate
   d. method of ventilation

6. The preferred site for arterial puncture is the:
   a. brachial artery
   b. ulnar artery
   c. femoral artery
   d. radial artery

7. A negative Modified Allen Test indicates:
   a. the ulnar artery can be punctured
   b. the radial artery can be punctured
   c. the radial artery cannot be punctured
   d. no collateral circulation by the radial artery

8. When performing an arterial puncture:
   a. the artery is entered below the palpating finger
   b. the artery is entered above the palpating finger
   c. a pressure bandage is immediately applied after puncture
   d. the needle is held at a 10- to 25-degree angle

9. All of the following are technical errors that affect the quality of an ABG sample **EXCEPT:**
   a. excess anticoagulant
   b. too little anticoagulant
   c. removing air bubbles from the syringe
   d. obtaining dark red blood

10. A complication of arterial puncture that can lead to tissue destruction is:
    a. an arteriospasm
    b. a lack of collateral circulation
    c. a vasovagal reaction
    d. both a and b

Clinical Situations

1 When entering a patient's room to collect an ABG sample, a phlebotomist learns that the patient has just returned from physical therapy and has been disconnected from a portable oxygen device and reconnected to the bedside oxygen system.

   a. When should the phlebotomist collect the sample? Why?
   b. What additional information related to the patient's status should the phlebotomist obtain?

2 When performing an arterial puncture, the phlebotomist notices that the blood is not pulsating into the syringe.

   a. What other observation should the phlebotomist make?
   b. Should the phlebotomist be concerned? Why or why not?
   c. Which ABG test result could be falsely decreased? Increased?

3 When performing a venipuncture in the antecubital area of an obese patient, the phlebotomist notices that blood is pulsating into the evacuated tube.

   a. What other observation should the phlebotomist make?
   b. What blood vessel may have been punctured?
   c. What additional precautions should the phlebotomist take to protect the patient?
   d. What is the most probable complication for this patient?

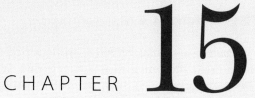

CHAPTER 15

Point-of-Care Testing

Learning Objectives

Upon completion of this chapter, the reader will be able to:

1. Define point-of-care testing (POCT) and state various locations where POCT is performed.
2. Discuss the advantages and disadvantages of POCT.
3. State the regulations required for POCT and the qualifications required for health-care personnel to perform testing.
4. Explain the POCT quality control procedures for Clinical Laboratory Improvements Amendments (CLIA) compliance.
5. Describe the tests and instrumentation commonly used in POCT.

Key Terms

Calibration
Control
Critical value
Point-of-care testing
Proficiency testing
Quality control
Reagent
Shift
Trend
Turnaround time

Point-of-care testing (POCT), previously referred to as alternate site testing, near-patient testing, decentralized testing, bedside testing, or ancillary testing, is the performance of laboratory tests at the patient's bedside or nearby rather than in a central laboratory. POCT is particularly beneficial to patient care in the critical care or intensive care units, operating suites, emergency department, or neonatal intensive care units. Other POCT locations include satellite laboratories, physician offices, ambulatory clinics, ambulances or helicopters, long-term care facilities, workplace screenings, health fairs, dialysis centers, and home settings.

Factors that have motivated the practice of POCT include the increased acuteness of inpatient illnesses that require a faster *turnaround time* (TAT) of results and the decreased length of hospital stays that require the increased performance of procedures and care on an outpatient basis. TAT is defined as the time from when the health-care provider orders the test until the result is returned to the health-care provider. The shorter the TAT, the sooner the health-care provider can treat the patient. In critical care units or surgical suites, the TAT of stat tests is of the utmost importance in providing the best possible patient care.

POCT is well suited for the concepts of decentralization of laboratory testing and cross-training of personnel to perform certain tests at the patient's bedside. The immediate availability of test results provides convenience to both the patient and the health-care provider by decreasing the time required for diagnosis and treatment, resulting in faster patient recovery. This streamlined workflow provides more effective health-care provider-patient interaction because the clinical signs, symptoms, and test results can be evaluated immediately for patient treatment, reducing follow-up visits for patients. Quick and accurate test results enable the patient to be treated immediately, thereby improving patient outcomes.

The growing popularity and scope of POCT is a result of the rapidly evolving technology. Small, handheld, user-friendly instruments provide mobility, low maintenance, ease of use, cost effectiveness, decreased sample volume, decreased potential for sample handling and processing errors, compliance with the Clinical Laboratory Improvement Amendments of 1988 (CLIA '88), and most important, reliable test results when properly used. Most tests require only a drop of whole blood obtained by dermal puncture using a single lancet versus collecting a tube of blood using venipuncture equipment. This feature not only decreases the sample acquisition cost but also is an advantage for geriatric or pediatric patients in whom iatrogenic anemia is a concern. Another advantage of POCT is the decreased chance of preexamination errors that occur with sample labeling, transporting, and processing.

POCT technology benefits also have been realized in many traditional laboratory settings. Decreased sample volume, small analyzer size and portability, ease of use, and fast TAT have made POCT technology a replacement option for laboratory equipment in many traditional laboratories.

POCT also has several identified drawbacks. Because POCT is laboratory testing, it also is governed by all of the same regulations that apply to laboratory testing in a traditional laboratory. Accreditation requirements, charging and billing mechanisms, documentation of patient results, *quality control* (QC), testing and documentation, and inventory management are all processes that can be problematic. A large number of patient-care providers perform POCTs compared with a much smaller number of laboratory staff that would be performing the test in a traditional laboratory setting. The large number of operators can have a dilution effect on operator competency. This is particularly apparent when the volume of POCTs is low and the number of operators is high. The operators have fewer opportunities to maintain their skill level because the test is performed at a very low frequency.

There are many tests available from a variety of reputable manufacturers, and new POCT procedures and instruments are continuously being developed. Whole blood, plasma, urine, and direct swabs from an infected area are still the most common sample types, but saliva and other body fluids also are being used. Some newer technologies do not require a collection of a sample, such as the devices that perform transcutaneous bilirubin and noninvasive glucose testing. These technologies are capable of obtaining a laboratory result by placing the POCT device directly on the patient's skin without obtaining a sample from the patient. As technology has advanced, the scope of POCT and its role in providing quality patient care has rapidly expanded to bring a large test menu of laboratory tests to the patient's bedside. Table 15-1 lists commonly performed POCTs and their associated laboratory section.

The importance of proper instrument maintenance and *calibration*, QC, and documentation is the same for all instruments and procedures. Health-care

TABLE 15-1 ● Common Point-of-Care Testing Associated With Laboratory Departments	
LABORATORY DEPARTMENT	**TESTS**
Hematology	Hemoglobin, hematocrit, erythrocyte sedimentation rate (ESR)
Chemistry	Glucose, arterial blood gases (ABGs), bilirubin, lipid panels, blood urea nitrogen (BUN), electrolytes, creatinine, comprehensive metabolic profile, cardiac markers, liver function, human chorionic gonadotropin, hemoglobin A1c
Serology	Human immunodeficiency virus, mononucleosis, *Helicobactor pylori*
Urinalysis and body fluids	Reagent strip urinalysis, occult blood, gastroccult, body fluid pH
Urine toxicology (drugs of abuse)	Amphetamines, marijuana, cocaine, benzodiazepines, barbiturates, ethanol
Microbiology	Group A *Streptococcus*, influenza A/B, bacterial vaginosis, detection of biowarfare agents, respiratory synctial virus (RSV)
Coagulation	Prothrombin time (PT)/international normalized ratio (INR), activated partial thromboplastin time (APTT), activated clotting time (ACT)

professionals performing POCT must be trained to collect the sample correctly and understand the quality assessment criteria involved in performing laboratory tests. Although POCT is laboratory testing, the majority of POCT is performed by nonlaboratory personnel. Persons performing POCT are called operators and are usually primary patient providers. Operators include phlebotomists, nurses, physicians, respiratory therapists, radiographers, medical and nursing assistants, ambulance personnel, patient-care technicians, medical laboratory scientists, and patients. Medical laboratory scientists perform the least number of POCTs, but the laboratory is often responsible for administering the POCTs program. CLIA '88 regulates the qualifications for health-care personnel authorized to perform POCT.

REGULATION OF POCT

The CLIA '88 encompasses all laboratory testing and requires every testing site examining "specimens derived from the human body for the purpose of providing information for the diagnosis, prevention or treatment of disease, or impairment of or assessment of health" to be regulated. All testing sites are subject to the federal law CLIA '88 that defines the standards and guidelines for performing laboratory testing and must be licensed based on the test complexity model regardless of the number of tests performed or whether there is a charge for the test.

The Center for Medicare and Medicaid Services (CMS) administers CLIA '88 and requires CLIA certification for reimbursement of laboratory tests. CMS grants deemed status to accrediting organizations that have demonstrated equivalency with CLIA standards. These agencies include the Commission on Laboratory Assessment (COLA) that is popular with physician office laboratories and The Joint Commission (JC) and the College of American Pathologists (CAP) that primarily serve larger laboratories. Compliance with CLIA and accrediting organizations' regulatory standards is mandatory and is normally evaluated using a biannual inspection process. Failure to comply with the regulatory standards can lead to federal sanctions and loss of accreditation and the ability to legally perform all laboratory testing.

Under CLIA, all clinical laboratories, regardless of location, size, or type, must meet standards based on the complexity of the tests that they perform. Test complexity is determined by the testing characteristics such as stability of the reagent, preparation of the reagent, operational steps, calibration, and QC. Complexity also depends on the degree of knowledge, training, experience, troubleshooting, and interpretation required in the testing process. The complexity level of the highest complexity test performed determines the level of certification required. The Food and Drug Administration (FDA) has the responsibility for categorizing tests and classifying testing devices and systems. Laboratory testing is classified into four complexity categories: waived, moderate complexity, high complexity, and provider-performed microscopy procedures (PPM). Laboratories performing moderate or high complexity (nonwaived) testing must meet requirements for *proficiency testing,* patient test management, QC, quality assessment, and personnel. The major differences in regulatory requirements between moderate and high complexity testing are in the QC and personnel standards. POCTs may be waived, moderate, or even high complexity if performed under the oversight of a laboratory that is CLIA certified for nonwaived testing.

Waived Tests

Waived tests are defined as simple procedures that are cleared by the FDA for home use; employ methodologies that are easy to perform and the likelihood of erroneous results is negligible; or pose no reasonable risk of harm to the patient if the test is performed incorrectly. Waived tests are considered simple to perform and interpret, require no special training or educational background, and require only minimum QC. This category has been greatly expanded from the original eight tests that were listed as meeting these criteria in 1988 (Box 15-1) to more than 80 today. Table 15-2 lists the current CLIA waived tests. This list continues to grow as new test kits and instrumentation are developed. To perform waived testing, the organization must obtain a Certificate of Waiver from the CMS and follow manufacturers' directions for the testing process. Many waived tests, such as glucose monitoring and pregnancy tests, are available over the counter to all consumers.

 Technical Tip 15-1. Tests are continually being developed and added to the waived test category. For an up-to-date listing of waived tests, refer to www.cms.hhs.gov/clia.

BOX 15-1 Original CLIA '88–Waived Tests

Blood glucose
Reagent strip or tablet reagent urinalysis
Erythrocyte sedimentation rate (nonautomated)
Fecal occult blood
Hemoglobin by copper sulfate (nonautomated)
Ovulation tests
Spun hematocrit
Urine pregnancy tests

Moderate Complexity

Moderate complexity tests are more difficult to perform than are waived tests and require documentation of training in testing principles, instrument calibration, and QC. Moderate complexity testing requires that testing personnel have a minimum of a high school diploma or equivalent. Many laboratory tests in chemistry and hematology have been assigned to this category. Facilities performing moderate complexity tests are subject to proficiency testing and on-site inspections. In institutions with CAP, JC, and COLA accreditation, waived tests also must adhere to most of the moderate complexity test standards. In most hospitals and large institutions, the clinical laboratory administers the training, proficiency testing, and monitoring of QC. Persons performing POCT are required to demonstrate testing competency on a periodic basis.

High Complexity

High complexity tests require sophisticated instrumentation and a high degree of interpretation by the testing personnel. Personnel performing high complexity tests must have formal education with a degree in laboratory science. Most tests performed in microbiology, immunology, immunohematology, and cytology are in this category.

Provider-Performed Microscopy Procedures

The first CLIA '88 modification created a new certificate category for PPM. The new category included certain procedures that can be performed in conjunction with any waived test and includes clinical microscopy procedures only.

The tests within this new category can be performed only by physician's assistants, nurse practitioners, midwives, physicians, and dentists during a patient's examination. In addition, laboratories performing these tests must meet the moderate complexity requirements for proficiency testing, patient test management, QC, and QA as required by the accreditation agency. CLIA PPM tests are listed in Box 15-2.

QUALITY ASSESSMENT

Laboratories performing moderate or high complexity tests must be inspected every 2 years. Waived laboratories are not subject to routine inspection,

TABLE 15-2 ● **Current CLIA '88–Waived Tests**	
Adenovirus	Gastric pH
Aerobic/anaerobic organisms–vaginal	Glucose
Alanine aminotransferase (ALT)	Glycated hemoglobin, total
Albumin	Glycosylated hemoglobin (HgA1c)
Albumin, urinary	HCG, urine pregnancy test
Alcohol, saliva	HDL cholesterol
Alkaline phosphatase (ALP)	*Helicobacter pylori*
Amines	*Helicobacter pylori* antibodies
Amphetamines	Hematocrit
Amylase	Hemoglobin
Aspartate aminotransferase (AST)	Hemoglobin by copper sulfate, HemoCue
B-type natriuretic peptide (BNP)	HIV antibodies
Barbiturates	Infectious mononucleosis antibodies (mono)
Benzodiazepines	Influenza tests
Bilirubin, total	Ketones (blood and urine)
Bladder tumor–associated antigen	Lactic acid (lactate)
Blood lead	LDL cholesterol
Buprenorphine	Leukocyte esterase, urinary
Calcium, ionized	Lithium
Calcium, total	Luteinizing hormone (LH)
Cannabinoids (THC)	Lyme disease antibodies
Carbon dioxide, total (CO_2)	Methadone
Catalase, urine	Methamphetamines, amphetamine
Chloride	Methylenedioxymethamphetamine (MDMA)
Cholesterol	Microalbumin
Cocaine metabolites	Morphine
Collagen type I crosslink, N-telopeptides (NXT)	Nicotine and/or metabolites
Creatine kinase (CK)	Nitrite, urine
Creatinine	Opiates
Erythrocyte sedimentation rate (nonautomated)	Ovulation test (LH)
Estrone-3 glucuronide	Oxycodone
Ethanol (alcohol)	pH (blood and urine)
Fecal occult blood	Phencyclidine (PCP)
Fern test	Phosphorus
Follicle-stimulating hormone (FSH)	Platelet aggregation
Fructosamine	Potassium
Gamma-glutamyl transferase (GGT)	Propoxyphene
Gastric occult blood	Protein, total

Continued

TABLE 15-2 ● **Current CLIA '88–Waived Tests—cont'd**	
Prothrombin time (PT)	Triglyceride
Respiratory syncytial virus	Urea
Semen	Uric acid
Sodium	Urine dipstick (ascorbic acid, bilirubin, blood, chemistries, creatinine, glucose, ketone, leukocytes, nitrite, pH, protein, specific gravity, urobilinogen)
Spun hematocrit	
Streptococcus, group A	Urine HCG
Thyroid-stimulating hormone (TSH)	Vaginal pH
Trichomonas	Whole blood qualitative dipstick glucose
Tricyclic antidepressants	

BOX 15-2 CLIA '88 Provider-Performed Microscopy Tests

Fecal leukocyte examination
Fern test
Potassium hydroxide (KOH) preparation
Nasal smear for eosinophils
Pinworm examination
Postcoital direct, qualitative examinations of vaginal or cervical mucous
Qualitative semen analysis
Urine sediment examination
Wet mounts (vaginal, cervical, skin, or prostatic secretions)

although a certain number are inspected to ensure compliance or when a complaint has been filed. Inspections must be announced and are done within the first 2 years of certification. CAP performs an initial inspection for sites seeking CAP accreditation and every 2 years thereafter. When requested, the JC accepts CAP and COLA inspections and reinspects waived testing as part of hospital accreditation. CMS has state inspectors who inspect testing sites seeking only CLIA accreditation. CLIA inspection standards are the federal standards of CLIA '88 and are listed in the Federal Register. Requirements of each agency follow CLIA regulations, but other requirements may differ. Each testing site must decide on an accrediting agency and follow its standards. CLIA '88 regulations include patient test management assessment, QC

assessment, proficiency testing assessment, comparison of test results, relationship of patient information to patient test results, personnel assessment, communications, complaint investigation, QA review with staff, and QA records.

Patient Test Management

Patient test management includes methods of patient preparation, proper sample collection, sample identification, sample preservation, sample transportation, sample processing, and accurate result reporting. The testing site must have and follow written procedures for these methods so that specimen integrity and identification are maintained from the pretesting through the posttesting process.

Quality Control Assessment

QC must include records of the date, results, testing personnel, lot numbers, and expiration dates for reagents and controls. These must be retained for 2 years. It is recommended that records be reviewed daily, as well as monthly, in order to detect trends, shifts, unstable test systems, or operator difficulties.

Proficiency Testing Assessment

All laboratories performing moderate or high complexity testing must enroll in an approved proficiency testing program. This program involves three events per year, with five challenges per analyte in the survey material. All survey specimens are tested in the same manner as patient specimens. No communication with other laboratories is permitted.

Personnel Assessment

Personnel assessment includes education and training, continuing education, competency assessment, and performance appraisals. Each complexity level has its own requirements and is identified per CLIA requirements.

Each new employee must have documentation of training during orientation to the laboratory. This is a checklist of procedures and must include date and initials of the person doing the training and of the employee being trained.

CLIA mandates continuing education, although no minimum hours are given. A record of all applicable continuing education sessions should be maintained. The personnel file must include a certificate of the education level of each employee performing laboratory testing.

Competency Assessment

Competency assessment is required by CLIA regulations for all POCT personnel who perform moderate and high complexity testing at 6 months and 1 year after initial training. After the first year, competency must be assessed and validated annually. Most accrediting agencies also require annual competency assessment for staff performing waived tests. Methods for assessing competency include direct observation, review of QC records and review of proficiency testing records, blind testing of specimens with known values, and written assessments. Performance appraisals are done according to institution protocol and include standards of performance linked to the job description. The standards may include evaluation of organizational and communication skills and attitude.

Quality Assessment Records

The laboratory must maintain patient test records for 2 years, blood banking for 5 years, and pathology/cytology for 10 years. Other records that must be kept include QC, reagent logs, proficiency testing, competency assessment, education and training, equipment maintenance, service calls, documentation of problems, complaints, and communications, inspection files, and certification records.

QUALITY CONTROL

QC of testing procedures is part of a much larger system referred to as quality assurance (QA) the purpose of which is to provide overall quality patient care. QA includes written policies and documented actions that are used to evaluate the entire testing process from test ordering and sample collection through reporting and interpreting of results. QC procedures are performed to ensure that acceptable standards for accuracy and precision are being met during the process of specimen testing to provide reliable results. QC includes internal, external, and electronic QC, proficiency testing, calibration or calibration verification, and equipment maintenance. Performance and monitoring of QC are a major part of POCT, performed to verify that instrumentation is functioning properly and has been accurately calibrated, that *reagents* are stable and are reacting appropriately, and that the testing is being performed correctly (methodology and standards of performance). The person performing patient testing must be the person performing the QC. However, QC does not verify the integrity of the patient sample. Collection procedures discussed in previous chapters must be followed.

Specific QC information regarding the type of control specimen, preparation and handling, frequency of use, tolerance levels, and method of recording the QC results are included in the procedure for each test. QC is performed at scheduled times, such as at the beginning of each shift and before testing patient specimens, and it must always be performed if an instrument is dropped or if test results are questioned by the health-care provider. Laboratory guidelines depend on the accrediting agency and the manufacturer's recommendation. POCT procedures or instruments may include electronic *controls*, calibration verification, optical checks, procedural controls, and external manufactured controls.

External Controls

External controls are tested in the same manner as a patient specimen and are used to verify test systems that use urine or blood samples. The external commercial controls are manufactured specimens with known values, and they are available in several strengths, such as abnormal low, normal, and abnormal high ranges, or positive and negative depending on the test being performed. The concentration of controls should be at medically significant levels and should be as much like the human specimen as possible. At least two levels of assayed controls are used to evaluate daily performance of instruments. External controls for POCT methods are often required each time a new test kit is opened, or with each new lot and each new shipment of testing supplies.

Internal Controls

Internal controls are contained within the test system and are sometimes referred to as procedural controls. Internal controls are commonly used in test kit systems, which verify that the test kit and any added reagents performed as expected. Many waived tests have internal procedural controls that indicate that the test was performed correctly and that it was completed. Internal QC procedural controls are usually performed more frequently and are often performed with each test.

Electronic Controls

Electronic quality control (EQC) uses a mechanical or electrical specimen in place of a liquid QC specimen. This type of QC can be internal to the POCT device or an external component inserted into the POCT device. Although EQC can verify the functional ability of the POCT device, it does not verify the integrity of the testing supplies. EQC is usually performed on a timed schedule, which can be daily, or every few hours, depending on the manufacturer's recommendations and laboratory regulations. Many test systems use a combination of external and internal controls to verify the entire test system is working properly. Many POCT devices have a safety feature that locks the device to prevent any patient testing until the QC error is resolved.

 Technical Tip 15-2. Light, moisture, cleaning agents, or premature deterioration can affect point-of-care testing supplies. Frequent quality control testing verifies the integrity of the supplies and test system.

Documentation of QC

Documentation of QC testing is required. Some POCT devices can capture this information electronically, and other methods require manual documentation. When interpreting the QC result, it is imperative to verify that the controls performed as expected. Any time a QC result does not perform as expected (the results are not within the predetermined range), no further patient testing should be performed until the QC result error is corrected. The test procedure should provide guidance to resolve the error. Additional information can be obtained from the test manufacturer. Documentation of successful QC performance is required to confirm that the test system was able to produce valid test results on the same day that patient testing was performed.

Documentation of QC includes dating and initialing the material when it is first opened and recording the manufacturer's lot number and the expiration date each time a control is run and the test result obtained (Fig. 15-1). Controls are plotted on QC charts, usually Levy-Jennings charts, which indicate the mean and the control range. Results should fall within the range of two standard deviations (± 2 SD) 95 % of the time, and the values should be evenly distributed on either side of the mean, confirming precision and accuracy. Two consecutive values cannot fall outside of the two standard deviations, and no value should exceed three standard deviations. Controls should be plotted at the time of testing and in the order of measurement. Separate charts are required for each test and each level of control. Some POCT instruments have QC data management software that does this automatically (Fig. 15-2). These instruments can be programmed to lock out all patient testing if a control value falls outside the established control ranges and if QC has not been performed within the allotted time frame. Six sudden consecutive values on one side of the mean indicate a *shift* that may be caused by a malfunction of the instrument or a new lot number of reagents. A gradual increase or decrease for six consecutive values indicates a *trend* that may be caused by a gradual deterioration of reagents or deterioration of instrument performance. QC charts provide a visual display of statistical information that monitors shifts or trends in the testing procedure or instrument (Fig. 15-3).

Patient results must not be reported if QC is out of control. Patient results are reported with reference and interpretive ranges. There must be written procedures for handling abnormal control and patient results. Corrective action for abnormal control results or errors in reporting patient results must be taken and documented. Individuals performing the testing

SURESTEP WHOLE BLOOD GLUCOSE
PATIENT/QUALITY CONTROL LOG

Test Strip Lot # _____ Control Code: _____ Exp. Date: _____

Low Control Lot # _____ Low Control QC Range: _____ Exp. Date: _____

High Control Lot # _____ High Control QC Range: _____ Exp. Date: _____

DATE	PATIENT NAME (Or use patient label)	PATIENT ID	PATIENT RESULT	LOW CONTROL	HIGH CONTROL	TECH

Reviewed by: _____ Date: _____

FIGURE 15-1 SureStep whole blood glucose patient/quality control log. *(From Di Lorenzo, MS, and Strasinger, SK: Blood Collection: A Short Course, ed. 2. FA Davis, 2010, Philadelphia, with permission.)*

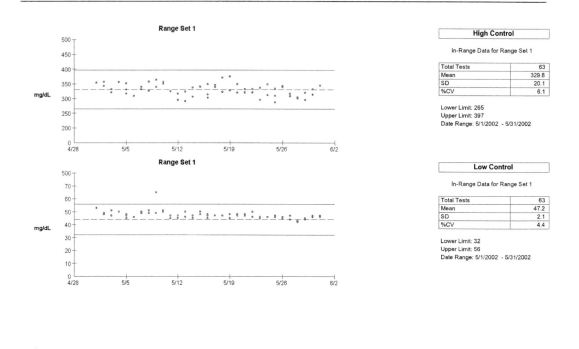

Location: NMH - Emergency Dept

Trend Graph Report

Time Report Generated: 14:38
Glucose Units: mg/dL
Test Strip Lot Number: 173416A004

High Control

In-Range Data for Range Set 1

Total Tests	63
Mean	329.8
SD	20.1
%CV	6.1

Lower Limit: 265
Upper Limit: 397
Date Range: 5/1/2002 - 5/31/2002

Low Control

In-Range Data for Range Set 1

Total Tests	63
Mean	47.2
SD	2.1
%CV	4.4

Lower Limit: 32
Upper Limit: 56
Date Range: 5/1/2002 - 5/31/2002

FIGURE 15-2 LifeScan DataLink data management system trend graph report. *(Courtesy of Lifescan, Milpitas, CA.)*

must be identified on the patient report. Various POCT instruments require that an operator use a unique personal identification number, which allows all QC testing to be identified and monitored. Instrument maintenance checks and function checks must be performed and documented. A designated supervisor reviews all patient results, QC, and instrument maintenance results.

 Technical Tip 15-3. Patient test results can never be reported if the quality control test results are not in range. The problem must be resolved and the test repeated.

COMMON POCT ERRORS

Each time a POCT is performed, there are multiple opportunites to make an error that could result in a negative patient outcome. Incorrect results influence the way the patient is treated or not treated and the sequence of ordering additional diagnostic tests based on those results. Table 15-3 lists the common errors associated with POCT.

Prevention of common POCT errors is good laboratory practice and include

- Patient identification—Identify the correct patient. Use the full name and a second identifier on all samples, requisitions, and reports.
- Proper sample collection—Ensure the correct sample type is collected, use correct collection technique, label all samples, and handle and transport samples according to procedure.
- Proper storage of testing supplies—Store reagents at the correct storage temperature and never use an expired test reagent or collection device.
- QC—Always perform and document QC as required and confirm that QC results are within the expected range before any patient testing is performed.

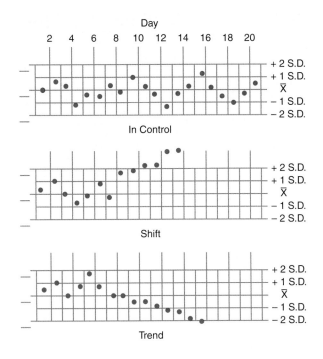

Day

FIGURE 15-3 **Levy-Jennings charts showing in-control results, trend, and shift.** *(From Strasinger, SK, and Di Lorenzo, MS: Urinalysis and Body Fluids, ed. 5. FA Davis, 2008, Philadelphia, with permission.)*

- Sample application and test performance—Always follow manufacturer's instrucions for applying the sample to the test device and strictly follow test-timing instructions.
- Result interpretation—Refer to the test procedure for correct interpretation of test results, confirmatory testing that may be required, and guidance for identification and communication of critical results.
- Documentation of results—Results must be recorded in the permanent medical record, legible, and easily retrieved.

PROCEDURES

Laboratory testing is performed in three phases: preexamination, examination, and postexamination (see Chapter 13). Procedures must be available that address all three phases of testing for each POCT. The preexamination phase encompasses the test ordering process, patient identification and patient preparation, sample collection and handling, reagent storage, and preparing materials, equipment, and the test area. The examination phase is

TABLE 15-3 • Common Errors Associated with Point-of-Care Tests	
TESTS	**ERRORS**
Hemoglobin	Failure to adequately fill the cuvette
	Bubbles in the cuvette
Glucose	Use of compromised or expired reagent strips
	Failure to adequately cleanse and dry the capillary puncture site
	Failure to adequately or correctly apply sample to testing area
	Failure to run controls and document as required
i-STAT profiles	Failure to identify the patient correctly in the meter
	Failure to observe cartridge warm-up time
	Failure to comply with room termperature expiration dates
	Returning room temperature cartridges to refrigerated storage
	Underfilled or overfilled cartridges
	Squeezing the cartridge when closing
	Moving the device while analyzing a specimen
	Failure to upload meter for timely data transfer

Continued

TABLE 15-3 ● **Common Errors Associated with Point-of-Care Tests—cont'd**	
TESTS	**ERRORS**
Urinalysis	Use of compromised or expired reagent strips
	Incorrect reaction timing
	Leaving reagent strips in the sample too long
Occult blood (guaiac slide methods)	Failure to allow the sample to dry on the testing area prior to adding reagent
	Patients not given precollection instructions
	Failure to use the correct sample type for the test
	Failure to apply the correct amount of specimen on the slide
	Failure to wait specified time after sample is applied to add the developer reagent
Toxicology profile	Use of incorrectly stored or expired kits
	Misinterpretation of patient and control results
Group A *Streptococcus*	Using cotton or calcium alginate collection swabs
	Use of compromised or expired reagent kits
	Failure to observe the internal control
	Incorrect collection or timing
Urine pregnancy test	Failure to test a first morning sample
	Addition of reagents in the wrong order
	Misinterpretation of test and control results
Immunoassay kits	Using reagents from different kits
	Failure to follow the step-by-step instructions
	Use of incorrectly stored or expired kits
	Misinterpretation of test and control results
	Failure to observe and document internal control results
Coagulation tests	Failure to adequately cleanse and dry the capillary puncture site
	Failure to follow manufacturer's instructions for sample collection
	Prematurely performing the capillary puncture before test strip/test cartridge is ready to accept the specimen
	Inadequate application of specimen
	Failure to identify the patient correctly in the meter
POC meters (analyzers with data management)	Failure to follow correct timing for application of sample to test strip/test cartridge
	Failure to follow correct timing for placing test strip/test cartridge in the meter
	Failure to upload meter for timely data transfer

when the actual test is performed and includes QC testing and result interpretation. The postexamination phase involves recording and reporting results, addressing critical values when indicated, following through for confirmatory testing, and disposing of biohazard waste.

It is important to note that the majority of all laboratory testing errors occur in the preexamination and postexamination phases of testing. Because the technology for most POCT is designed to be user-friendly, the potential of performing a test incorrectly and the direct impact of that error is often underestimated. Care must be taken at all stages of testing to ensure a quality result.

Preexamination Phase

Patient identification is the primary concern prior to performing laboratory tests. With POCT, many times no collection tube or sample cup is required to contain the specimen prior to performing the test. This eliminates the ability to verify positive patient identification. Many POCT devices enable the operator to enter the patient identification directly into the POCT device where the information is captured and stored electronically. Newer technology also has the ability to capture patient identification and operator identification using a bar-code scanner. Failure to identify the patient correctly in the POCT device can result in failure to document a test result that was needed to treat a patient or the results may be reported on the wrong patient.

 Technical Tip 15-4. Patient identification must be verified at the bedside and entered correctly in the point-of-care testing device.

Other preexamination factors that can affect patient outcomes include correct collection and proper storage of equipment and supplies. Many POCT supplies have very specific storage requirements. Many are sensitive to heat, light, and moisture. Others require refrigeration and warm-up to room temperature prior to use. The expiration date for some testing supplies changes when moved from refrigerated storage to room temperature, or whenever the primary container is opened. No testing supplies should be used past their expiration dates.

Examination Phase

The examination phase is the phase when the actual test is performed. For all POCT, it is imperative that manufacturers' instructions are followed. Application of the sample to the test device and test timing are common errors associated with the examination phase. For some tests, especially coagulation methods, the time between the actual collection of the sample and application to the POCT device is critical because coagulation starts immediately after the blood sample is removed from the patient. Test methods that utilize a color formation are especially sensitive to critical timing. A test that is read too early or too late can be misinterpreted due to the lack of color development, color over development, or degradation of the color that is to be measured. Although POCT devices are designed to be portable, many cannot be moved when analyzing a specimen, since movement may disrupt the flow of specimen through the device.

Test interpretation also is part of the examination phase. Many POCT devices, both automated and manual test kit methods, have built-in procedural QC mechanisms to monitor the examination phase of testing and alert the operator that a test is invalid or the device simply does not display a test result. Kit methods often include a "control" line that aids in correct interpretation of the test. The presence of the control line indicates that the test was performed correctly. If the control line does not appear, the test is invalid and the patient result cannot be interpreted or reported. The invalid tests may be caused by compromised integrity of the testing supplies or addition of test reagents in the wrong order.

POCT results can be qualitative, semiquantitative, or quantitative. Qualitative results are reported as positive or negative. A urine pregnancy test is an example of a qualitative test because the result is reported as either positive or negative. Semiquantitative results are reported in terms of reaction intensity (1+, 2+, 3+) that equates to a range of numeric values. Quantitative results are numeric results, such as a whole blood glucose result.

 Technical Tip 15-5. Careful attention to collection technique and specimen application to the test device is critical for point-of-care coagulation tests.

➤ *Technical Tip 15-6.* Incorrect patient results may be obtained if the exact test procedure is not followed.

➤ *Technical Tip 15-7.* Follow manufacturers' storage requirements for reagent strips. Testing strips may not be stored in an open container and exposed to light, moisture, or heat.

➤ *Technical Tip 15-8.* When working for a different organization, do not assume that you will be using the same procedure kits. Read the procedure manual for all kits and instruments before performing tests.

➤ *Technical Tip 15-9.* The Joint Commission mandates that point-of-care tests be described as a screening or definitive test.

Postexamination Phase

The postexamination phase of testing is the documentation of the results. Many POCT devices have the capability to capture results electronically and transmit those results to the permanent medical record.

Manual documentation of POCT results is not uncommon. When manual documentation is employed, duplicate transcription is often required to document the result in the patient's permanent medical record and on a laboratory log. The patient's name, identification number, date and time of result, testing operator, and test results are required documentation. Results are usually reported with normal patient reference ranges, although it also is common to include therapeutic ranges for most coagulation results (Fig 15-4). A written record of lot numbers and expiration dates for supplies also may be required, depending on the test complexity and accrediting organization (see Figure 15-1).

POCT operators must be familiar with the critical values for each test and the processes for notification of attending staff and/or initiating treatment adjustments. For some POCTs, a result may require confirmatory testing. The confirmatory testing process may include obtaining an additional order, getting patient consent, and/or collection of a new sample. The operator must properly dispose of all biohazard items.

PROCEDURE MANUALS AND PACKAGE INSERTS

CLIA requires that laboratories performing POCT follow manufacturer's guidelines; therefore, procedure manuals must contain the information provided by the manufacturer and the specific institution operational requirements (quality control and calibration procedures). Operators must read the entire package insert and procedure manual before performing the test. The information in the manual and package insert lists all of requirements for each stage of testing and includes:

- Sample collection and handling
- Safety precautions regarding biological, chemical, electrical, and mechanical hazards
- Instrument maintenance and calibration
- Reagent storage requirements
- Acceptable control ranges
- Specimen requirements
- Procedural steps
- Interpretation of results and normal values and sources of error
- Troubleshooting assistance

Areas in which POCT is performed are required to maintain a procedure manual that is readily available to all testing personnel. The procedure manual contains the information provided in the package inserts from the instrumentation, reagents, and controls for each procedure. It also contains site-specific information, such as the location of supplies, instructions for reporting and recording results, and the protocol to follow when critically low or high test results (*critical values*) are encountered. Training for personnel performing POCT includes reading both the package inserts and the procedure manual thoroughly and demonstrating an understanding of the information. It is important to understand that POCT procedures vary among manufacturers; therefore, package inserts and procedures in the procedure manual are not interchangeable.

This chapter provides a general overview of some of the commonly performed POCT procedures and does not include all of the material that would be found in the package inserts or a procedure manual.

LABORATORY REPORT FORM

Patient Name: _____   Test Date: _____

Patient ID: _____

Test	Results	Reference Ranges
Urinalysis (adult)	Clean Catch YES NO	
Specific gravity		1.001–1.030
pH		5–6
Leukocytes		Neg
Nitrate		Neg
Protein (mg/dL)	mg/dL	Neg
Glucose (mg/dL)	mg/dL	Neg
Ketone		Neg
Urobilinogen (mg/dL)	mg/dL	<1
Bilirubin		Neg
Blood (RBC/uL)	RBC/uL	Neg
Stool for Occult Blood	Internal Pos/Neg Controls: OK	Neg
Hemoglobin by HemoCue (g/dL)	g/dL	4 to 10 months 10.0–14.0 g/dL
		10 mo to 3 yrs 11.0–14.0 g/dL
		4 to 9 yrs 11.5–15.0 g/dL
		9 to 14 yrs 12.0–15.6 g/dL
		Adult Female 11.6–16.1 g/dL
		Adult Male 13.3–17.7 g/dL
Mono Test	Internal Pos/Neg Controls: OK	Neg
Rapid Strep A/Throat	Internal Pos/Neg Controls: OK	Neg
Glucose (Whole Blood)	mg/dL	70–99 mg/dL (fasting)
		If patient not fasting—
		Time of last food intake:
		Time of test: _____
Urine Pregnancy Test (hCG)	Internal Pos/Neg Controls: OK	Neg (LMP)
Vaginal Wet Prep/KOH		Neg
(PPMP, performed only by		
Nurse Practitioner)		
Comments:		

Person performing test (Initial): _____   Practitioner: _____

FIGURE 15-4 Laboratory report form with reference ranges. *(From Di Lorenzo, MS, and Strasinger, SK: Blood Collection: A Short Course, ed. 2. FA Davis, 2010, Philadelphia, with permission.)*

It also does not include all of the many currently available tests and instruments.

Blood Glucose

Measurement of blood glucose is performed as POCT primarily to monitor persons with diabetes mellitus to determine whether their diet and insulin dosage are maintaining an acceptable level of glucose in the body. It is a definitive test used to measure the concentration of glucose in blood. Normal values for blood glucose vary slightly among testing procedures and are higher when serum or plasma, instead of whole blood, is tested in the clinical laboratory. POCT must be performed on whole blood; however, most of the newer bedside glucose meters report a plasma equivalent result. It is important to know what type of result the glucose meter reports so that the glucose results are interpreted correctly. POCT glucose normal values are approximately 60 to 115 mg/dL in a fasting blood sugar sample. Levels below 60 mg/dL are termed hypoglycemic, and increased levels are termed hyperglycemic. The phlebotomist should be aware of the established critical value levels for blood glucose and notify the appropriate personnel immediately when they are encountered.

Another tool for monitoring glucose levels in a patient with diabetes is glycosylated hemoglobin. Glycosylated hemoglobin, HbA1c, is measured using a waived POCT analyzer that provides an average plasma glucose level over a 3- to 4-month time period. The test measures the glucose within a red blood cell and is valuable in monitoring the long-term effectiveness of blood glucose control.

Research has shown that maintaining a normal glucose level in nondiabetic hospitalized patients particularly in the intensive care areas results in decreased length of stay, costs, and mortality. This has led to a marked increase in POC glucose testing for inpatients.

Many varieties of blood glucose POCT instrumentation are available, and the specific manufacturer's instructions for each instrument must be followed. The methodology may be photometric (Lifescan SureStep) or electrochemical (Roche Comfort Curve) and use different reagents in the test strip. The SureStep (LifeScan, Inc., Milpitas, CA), Accucheck II (Boehringer Mannheim Diagnostics, Indianapolis, IN), and ONE TOUCH II (Life Scan, Inc., Milpitas, CA) employ dry reagent technology using a special reagent test strip (Fig. 15-5). A glucose oxidase reaction occurs between the blood and reagents in the test strip, resulting in the formation of a blue color. The intensity of the blue color formed correlates with the concentration of glucose in the sample.

The reagent test strips must be stored in tightly closed containers and protected from heat, and they should not be used if they appear discolored or are past their expiration date. Care must be taken not to contaminate the testing area by rubbing it against the patient's skin or touching the pad before collection. Each container of test strips has a code number. The analyzer code number must be set to match the code number of the reagent strip container.

Whole blood obtained by dermal puncture is preferred, but some instruments can use blood samples

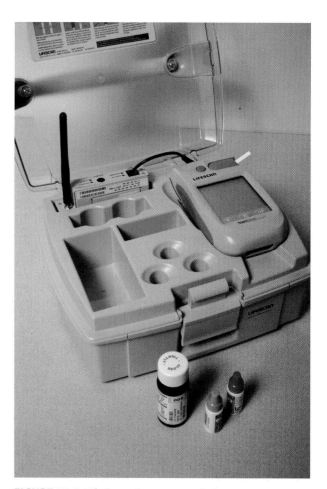

FIGURE 15-5 Life Scan glucose meter (Milpitas, CA).

collected in citrate, heparin, or ethylenediaminete-traacetic acid (EDTA) anticoagulant tubes. The appropriate area of the reagent strip is covered with a drop of blood and is inserted into the instrument. Applying too small a drop of blood to the test strip may cause falsely decreased values, and too much blood may falsely elevate results. The level of blood glucose is measured, and the results are displayed on a screen. Error codes appear if the specimen did not completely cover the test area.

▶ *Technical Tip 15-10.* If incorrect amounts of blood are applied to the test strip, use a new strip because the meter cannot accurately read glucose results when blood is reapplied to the original test strip.

▶ *Technical Tip 15-11.* Falsely low glucose values can result when the first drop of blood (contains tissue fluid) is not wiped away from the finger before applying the second drop to the glucose test strip.

🗒 *Preexamination Consideration 15-1.*
Glucose strips must not be allowed to sit in an open container on the phlebotomist's tray because the strips will absorb moisture and cannot absorb the correct amount of blood producing falsely low results.

The HemoCue Glucose 201 Analyzer (HemoCue, Inc., Mission Viejo, CA) analyzes arterial, venous, and capillary whole blood specimens. HemoCue technology uses dual wavelength photometry and specially designed cuvettes containing freeze-dried reagents instead of a test strip. Five microliters of blood is drawn into the disposable cuvette by capillary action, where it mixes with the freeze-dried reagents. The plasma equivalent result is displayed on completion of the reaction (Fig. 15-6).

The phlebotomist must know about possible sources of test error, understand and perform daily maintenance and QC of the instrument and the QC of the reagent strips, and document all actions taken. Some of the POCT glucose instruments have software capability to store data such as user identification number, patient identification number, calibration and QC results, and patient results for CLIA compliance.

Transcutaneous Bilirubin Testing

As discussed in Chapter 12, newborns are frequently tested to detect and monitor increased levels of bilirubin (hyperbilirubinemia). In addition to hemolytic disease of the newborn (HDN) and premature birth, a variety of other risk factors for hyperbilirubinemia exist. However, these factors may not be considered in healthy-appearing, nonjaundiced infants. Of particular concern is the failure to visually detect jaundice in infants with dark skin.

The JC has released a sentinel event alert (see Chapter 3) that addresses hyperbilirubinemia in the healthy newborn, recommending that risk assessment criteria be established. The JC suggests implementation of earlier neonatal bilirubin testing on patients determined to be at risk by noninvasive transcutaneous bilirubin (TcB) testing or capillary serum bilirubin testing.

Noninvasive TcB testing is ideally suited to provide increased monitoring of infants who do not appear jaundiced but who may have risk factors associated with hyperbilirubinemia. TcB testing is performed at the patient bedside, using a portable, hand-held Bilichek meter (Respironics, Inc., Murrysville, PA) (Fig. 15-7). The test is complete in less than 1 minute, which facilitates excellent TAT for newborn bilirubin testing. The noninvasive technology also eliminates most infection control issues associated with capillary punctures, including wound care, lancing devices, blood exposure, and biohazard disposal.

The Bilichek noninvasively directs white light into the skin of the newborn and measures the intensity of the specific wavelength that is returned. The Bilichek measures the intensity of more than 100 wavelengths of reflected light. The intensity of the reflected light is converted to absorbance units/optical density for analysis. Interfering components in the skin are subtracted from the known spectral properties of the normal skin by the instrument before displaying the bilirubin concentration. When the disposable tip is placed on the Bilicheck meter, the instrument initiates a self-test for integrity and an electronic check (Fig. 15-8). After a successful calibration, the protective covering and calibration material are removed from the tip. The unit is activated and the tip is pressed flat against the infant's forehead. The indicator light will change from amber to green when proper pressure is applied. On completion of five measurements, a tone sounds and the test results are displayed with the current time and date.

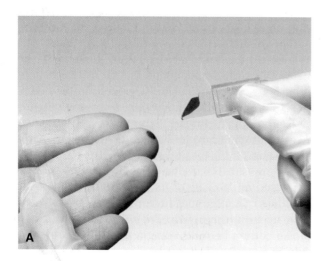

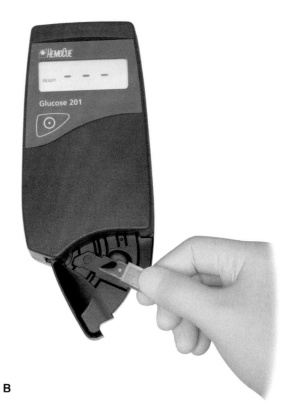

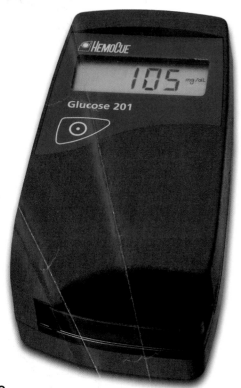

FIGURE 15-6 HemoCue Glucose 201 Analyzer and test procedure. A, Fill the cassette. B, Place the filled cassette into the instrument. C, Read the result. *(Courtesy of HemoCue, Inc., Mission Viejo, CA.)*

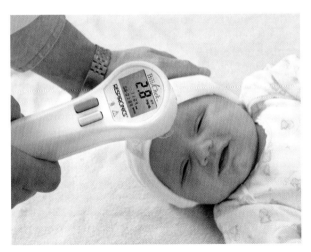

FIGURE 15-7 **Bilichek being performed on an infant.** *(Courtesy of Respironics, Inc., Murrysville, PA.)*

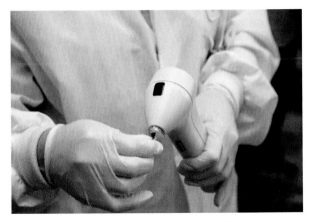

FIGURE 15-8 **Bilicheck meter electronic check.**

TcB testing is approved for use on newborns of 27 to 42 weeks' gestational age, 0 to 20 days postnatal age, and 950 to 4,995 g infant weight. The test is not affected by skin pigment and is appropriate for use on all races. Testing is not indicated for newborns who have received an exchange transfusion. A dermal puncture should be performed for closer monitoring of the bilirubin level.

 Technical Tip 15-12. Transcutaneous bilirubin measurements are performed only on the forehead of an infant. Avoid areas with bruising, birthmarks, hematomas, or excessive hair.

Hemoglobin

The primary function of the red blood cell (RBC) protein hemoglobin (Hgb) is to transport oxygen to all cells in the body. A decrease in the number of RBCs or the amount of Hgb in the cells (anemia) results in a decrease in the amount of oxygen reaching the cells. Normal values for Hgb vary with age and gender, with values for adult women ranging between 12 and 15 g/dL and for adult men between 14 and 17 g/dL. Measurement of Hgb is one of the most frequently performed screening tests in all health-care settings and also provides a means to monitor patients known to have anemia.

Varieties of POCT analyzers that measure Hgb include instruments that provide Hgb concentration as part of a larger test menu that may analyze glucose and electrolytes, as well as instruments designed only to measure Hgb. The HemoCue Hemoglobin System is designed to measure Hgb specifically (HemoCue, Inc., Mission Viejo, CA) (Fig. 15-9) using arterial, venous, or capillary whole blood samples. A fresh capillary or anticoagulated whole blood sample is placed into a microcuvette and inserted into the instrument. The Hgb measurement is determined photometrically using a dry reagent system. The reagents in the microcuvette lyse the RBCs to release hemoglobin, which is converted to azide methemoglobin by sodium nitrite and sodium azide to produce a color reaction. A dual-wavelength photometer reads the absorbance of the reaction and corrects the hemoglobin value for lipemia and leukocytosis.

The HemoCue hemoglobin analyzer is available with data management systems that can transfer

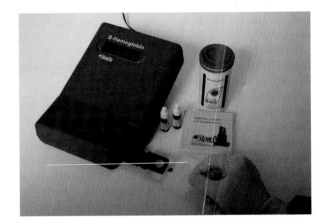

FIGURE 15-9 **HemoCue B Hemoglobin Analyzer, cassettes, and control.**

QC and patient data to a laboratory information system (LIS). Expanded analyzer functions include bar coding, linearity checks, proficiency testing, and more control levels for compliance with regulatory agencies. The HemoCue Hb 201+ Analyzer is the latest smaller version hemoglobin monitor from HemoCue.

 Technical Tip 15-13. Fill the cuvette with the blood in a continuous process without bubbles, making sure that the drop of blood is big enough to fill the cuvette completely.

Urinalysis

A routine urinalysis consists of a physical and chemical examination of urine and a microscopic examination when indicated. The microscopic portion of the urinalysis is not a part of POCT and should not be performed by phlebotomists.

Urine is a readily available and usually easy-to-collect sample that contains information about many of the body's major functions. It is important to obtain a patient history before testing urine, because ingestion of highly pigmented foods, medications, and vitamins can interfere with results. Information regarding collection and sample types can be found in Chapter 16. Urine should be tested within 2 hours of collection. Table 15-4 describes the most significant changes that may occur in a sample allowed to remain unpreserved at room temperature for longer than 2 hours.

Physical examination of urine describes the color and clarity of the sample. Abnormal colors and increased turbidity can be indications of pathological conditions. Normal urine color is yellow, and the intensity of the color is related to the concentration. A dilute urine is pale yellow, and a concentrated (first morning) urine is dark yellow. Common color descriptions of normal urine include pale yellow, light yellow, yellow, dark yellow, and amber and may vary among institutions. If there are no interfering substances, red or brown-black urine is abnormal and could indicate a disease process. Amber urine that produces yellow foam when shaken is also abnormal, if there are no interfering substances, and could indicate a disease process associated with liver disease.

Normal urine is usually clear; however, normal substances such as epithelial cells may increase the turbidity. Describing clarity also varies from one facility to another. Common terms related to appearance include clear, hazy, cloudy, and turbid. A cloudy or turbid appearance in a fresh sample may be cause for concern.

Routine chemical examination of urine is performed using plastic strips containing reagent-impregnated test pads that test for specific gravity,

TABLE 15-4 • **Changes in Unpreserved Urine**		
ANALYTE	**CHANGE**	**CAUSE**
Color	Modified/darkened	Oxidation or reduction of metabolites
Clarity	Decreased	Bacterial growth and precipitation of amorphous material
Odor	Increased	Bacterial multiplication or breakdown of urea to ammonia
pH	Increased	Breakdown of urea to ammonia by urease-producing bacteria/loss of CO_2
Glucose	Decreased	Glycolysis and bacterial use
Ketones	Decreased	Volatilization and bacterial metabolism
Bilirubin	Decreased	Exposure to light/photo-oxidation to biliverdin
Urobilinogen	Decreased	Oxidation to urobilin
Nitrite	Increased	Multiplication of nitrate-reducing bacteria
Red and white blood cells and casts	Decreased	Disintegration in dilute alkaline urine
Bacteria	Increased	Multiplication

pH, glucose, bilirubin, ketones, blood, protein, urobilinogen, nitrite, and leukocytes. A color-producing chemical reaction occurs when the reagent pads come in contact with urine. The color reaction can be read visually by comparing the strip against a color chart on the container (Fig. 15-10) or by inserting the strip into an automated instrument such as the Bayer Clinitek 50 Urine Chemistry Analyzer (Bayer Healthcare Diagnostics, Tarrytown, NY) that reads the strip and prints the results (Fig. 15-11).

Correct handling and storage of reagent strips is critical for obtaining accurate results. Strips are stored at room temperature in their original opaque bottles that contain a desiccant to protect them from exposure to excess light, moisture, and chemical contamination. Containers should be uncapped only long enough for a strip to be removed. When performing the test, strips should be briefly and completely dipped into the urine. They should not be left in the sample because reagents will wash out of the pads, causing false-negative results. Failure to read the reactions within the time frame specified by the manufacturer will also produce inaccurate results. Table 15-5 summarizes routine chemical testing of urine.

Preexamination Consideration 15-2.

Results of a routine urinalysis can be seriously affected if the urine is not tested within 2 hours of collection or preserved by refrigeration.

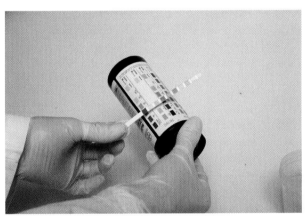

FIGURE 15-10 **Chemical examination of urine comparing reagent strip color reactions.**

Occult Blood

The purpose of occult (hidden) blood testing in stool (feces) is to detect gastrointestinal bleeding that is not visible to the naked eye. Detection of occult blood is a valuable aid in the early diagnosis of colorectal cancer and gastric ulcers. Most test kits for occult blood consist of a packet containing filter paper areas impregnated with guaiac reagent on which small amounts of feces are placed, positive and negative control areas, and a bottle of color-developing reagent (Fig. 15-12). The sample can be collected and tested at the patient setting, or the packets can be sent home with the patient to collect the sample and return the packet by mail. Hgb present in the stool sample reacts with hydrogen peroxide in the color-developing reagent to release oxygen, which then reacts with the guaiac reagent to produce a blue color (Fig. 15-13). Test kits are available from several manufacturers, and it is important not to combine materials from different kits. Samples should be collected following instructions provided by the test kit manufacturer. Contamination of the sample with urine or toilet water should be avoided.

Test kits for fecal occult blood must be sensitive enough to detect a very small amount of blood; therefore, they are highly subject to interference by diet and medications. A patient's diet should exclude red meat and certain vegetables that are sources of peroxidase and may cause false-positive results. Patients should be instructed to avoid the following items 72 hours before testing: red meat, turnips, radishes, melons, horseradish, alcohol, high doses of vitamin C, and excessive amounts of vitamin C–enriched foods. Aspirin and other nonsteroidal anti-inflammatory

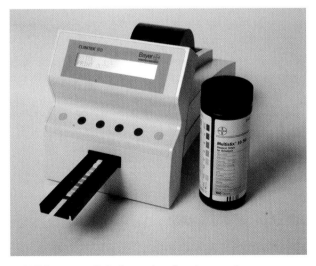

FIGURE 15-11 **Clinitek 50 urine chemistry analyzer.**

TABLE 15-5 ● **Summary of Chemical Testing by Reagent Strip**

TEST	PRINCIPLE	POSSIBLE REACTION INTERFERENCE		CORRELATIONS WITH OTHER TESTS
		FALSE-POSITIVE TESTS	**FALSE-NEGATIVE TESTS**	
pH	Double-indicator system	None	Run-over from the protein pad may lower	Nitrite Leukocytes Microscopic
Protein	Protein error of indicators	Highly alkaline urine, quaternary ammonium compounds (antiseptics), detergents, strip exposure to heat, light, moisture	High salt concentration	Blood Nitrite Leukocytes Microscopic
Glucose	Glucose oxidase, double sequential enzyme reaction	Peroxide, oxidizing detergents	Ascorbic acid, 5-hydrdoxyindoleacetic acid homogentisic acid, aspirin, levodopa, ketones, high specific gravity with low pH, strip exposure to heat, light, moisture, and chemicals	Ketones
Ketones	Sodium nitroprusside reaction	Levodopa, phthalein dyes, phenylketones	Strip exposure to heat, light, moisture, and chemicals	Glucose
Blood	Pseudoperoxidase activity of hemoglobin	Oxidizing agents, vegetable and bacterial peroxi-dases, cleaning agents (bleach)	Ascorbic acid, nitrite, protein, pH below 5.0, high specific gravity, captopril	Protein Microscopic
Bilirubin	Diazo reaction	Iodine Pigmented urine Indican	Ascorbic acid, nitrite	Urobilinogen
Urobilinogen	Ehrlich's reaction	Ehrlich-reactive compounds (Multistix), medication color	Nitrite, formalin	Bilirubin
Nitrite	Greiss's reaction	Pigmented urine on automated readers	Ascorbic acid High specific gravity	Protein Leukocytes Microscopic

TABLE 15-5 ● **Summary of Chemical Testing by Reagent Strip—cont'd**			
		POSSIBLE REACTION INTERFERENCE	
TEST	**PRINCIPLE**	**FALSE-POSITIVE TESTS**	**FALSE-NEGATIVE TESTS**	**CORRELATIONS WITH OTHER TESTS**
Leukocytes	Granulocytic esterase reactions	Oxidizing detergents	Glucose, protein, high specific gravity, oxalic acid, gentamycin, tetracycline, cephalexin, cephalothin	Protein Nitrite Microscopic
Specific gravity	pK change of polyelectrolyte	Protein	Alkaline urine	None

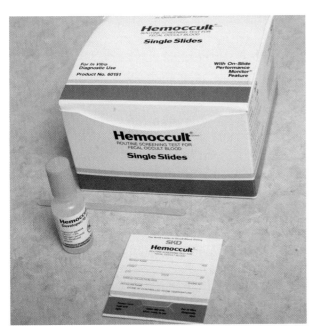

FIGURE 15-12 Hemoccult fecal occult blood test kit.

drugs that may cause gastrointestinal irritation should be avoided 7 days before testing.

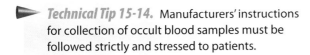

Technical Tip 15-14. Manufacturers' instructions for collection of occult blood samples must be followed strictly and stressed to patients.

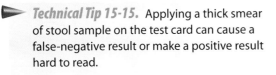

Technical Tip 15-15. Applying a thick smear of stool sample on the test card can cause a false-negative result or make a positive result hard to read.

Preexamination Consideration 15-3.

Stool samples must be allowed to soak into the Hemoccult card for 3 to 5 minutes before adding the developer to avoid missing a positive result. Hemoglobin must be completely absorbed onto the test card before a positive result can occur.

Pregnancy Testing

Pregnancy testing is based on the detection of human chorionic gonadotropin (HCG) hormone in urine or serum. HCG is produced by cells of the placenta and, depending on the sensitivity of the test kit, can be detected approximately 10 days after conception. False-negative results are obtained if not enough HCG has been produced to be detected at the time of testing. It is also important to perform urine pregnancy testing on a first-morning sample to achieve maximum concentration. Cloudy urine samples should be centrifuged or allowed to settle before testing to avoid interference with the test reaction.

No special instrumentation is required for pregnancy testing, and a variety of commercial test kits are available. Most pregnancy testing kits use monoclonal antibodies that react with different regions of the HCG molecule. Antibodies to HCG molecules are impregnated on a permeable membrane, and urine is added. If HCG is present in the urine, the antibodies will bind it on the membrane. The placement of the antibody on the membrane determines the shape of the color reaction, such as a plus or minus sign, line, or circle. Internal procedural controls are also included on the test kit membranes.

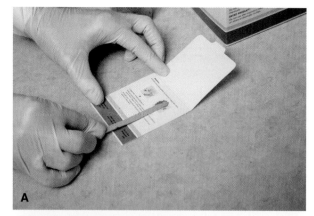

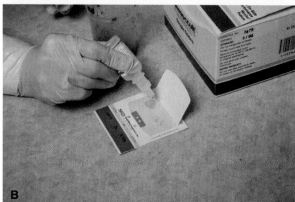

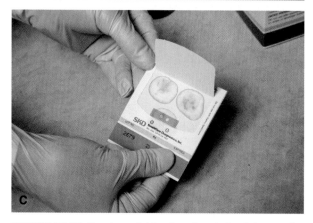

FIGURE 15-13   Fecal occult blood testing. A, Applying stool sample to test slide. B, Adding color developer to specimen on test card. C, Reading test and controls.

Reagents, timing, and methodology vary with each manufacturer's kit, and the directions must be followed exactly. Never mix components from different kits (Fig. 15-14).

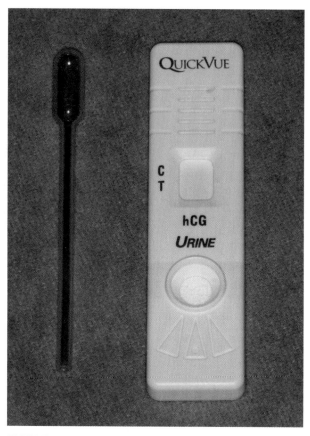

FIGURE 15-14   Pregnancy test kit.

 Technical Tip 15-16. Package inserts indicate the sensitivity of the human chorionic gonadotropin assay and list interfering substances.

Strep Tests

Symptoms of a sore throat are an indication to test for group A *Streptococcus* (strep throat). Although only a small percentage of children and adults with sore throat symptoms have positive results for group A *Streptococcus*, complications of untreated positive infections are serious; therefore, all symptomatic patients are usually tested.

Detection of group A streptococci using a rapid test kit can be accomplished in a matter of minutes as opposed to the 1 or 2 days required when using conventional culture methods. Rapid tests work well when a high number of bacteria are collected on the throat swab. Fewer numbers of bacteria reduce the accuracy of the rapid tests, and it is common policy to perform a throat culture on patients with negative results on rapid tests. Therefore, it may be necessary to collect two throat swabs: one for the rapid test, and one to hold for possible culture. Samples should be collected from the throat using a swab that does not have a cotton or calcium alginate tip and does not have a wooden shaft. When swabbing the throat, the procedures discussed in Chapter 16 should be followed.

Group A *Streptococcus* tests employ various methodologies and different reagents. An example of a waived test kit is the QuickVue In-Line One-Step Strep A test (Quidel, San Diego, CA) that uses a lateral flow immunoassay in which the antigen extraction takes place in the test cassette. The swab is placed in the cassette. The extraction solution is mixed and added to the test cassette. Bacterial antigens are extracted from the swab within the testing device using a mild acid solution. The extracted solution flows onto a test strip by capillary action and flows through a label pad consisting of anti-group A *Streptococcus* antibodies. If the extracted solution contains group A *Streptococcus* antigen, the antigen will bind to the antibody on the test label and will then bind additional color-producing anti-group A *Streptococcus* antibody on the membrane. Results are read at 5 minutes, and the test result pattern is compared with the interpretation chart. The test line indicates a positive or negative patient result, and the control line indicates that the reagents were mixed and added properly, that the proper volume of fluid entered the test cassette, and that capillary flow occurred (Fig. 15-15).

Influenza A and B

Influenza is a contagious viral infection of the respiratory tract caused by influenza viruses A and B. Type A viruses are the most prevalent and are most often associated with serious epidemics. Detection of Type A virus can also be used as a screening test for the H1N1 influenza virus. Type B produces a milder illness. Waived POCT test kits provide a quick diagnosis within 10 minutes; however, negative results may need to be confirmed by cell culture.

The influenza antigens may be detected directly from a nasal swab, nasopharyngeal swab, nasal aspirate, and nasal wash samples collected from the patient (see Chapter 16). The patient sample is placed in an extraction reagent tube where the virus particles in the

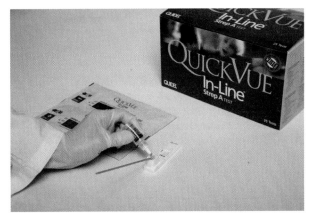

FIGURE 15-15 QuickVue In-Line Strep A test kit. Test cassette, swab, and extraction reagent.

sample are disrupted to expose the internal viral nucleoproteins. A test strip containing specific monoclonal antibodies is then placed into the extracted specimen. If influenza antigens are present in the extracted specimen, they will react with the monoclonal antibodies on the test strip. The test line indicates a positive or negative result accompanied by a control line indicating that the reagents were performing correctly.

Whole Blood Immunoassay Kits

In addition to the kits for pregnancy and group A *Streptococcus* testing, a large variety of CLIA waived kits are available for detection of abnormal whole blood components. Complete kits include reaction cassettes or cards, color developer, positive and negative controls, and detailed instructions. Depending on the test methodology, the color developer and controls may be impregnated into the reaction cassettes or cards, or added by the person performing the test. The previously described group A *Streptococcus* test is an example of a kit in which the controls are included in the test cassette.

To avoid using the wrong reagents, it is important that all components of a kit be stored in their designated box. Kits contain enough reagents to perform a specified number of tests, and reagents from a different kit should not be used. Many kits require refrigeration and must be allowed to warm to room temperature before use. All kits contain a package insert that provides information concerning the stability, sensitivity, and storage of reagents; sample collection guidelines; sources of error; and detailed step-by-step instructions. It is essential that all instructions be followed strictly.

All immunoassay kits use the same basic principle—that is, the appearance of a color reaction when antigens and antibodies combine. The color, size, and shape of the reaction will vary among kits and manufacturers. In addition, some procedures are designed to detect antibodies in the patient's blood and others are designed to detect antigens in blood and body substances. Antibodies are produced by the body when a foreign substance (antigen) enters the body. Detection of antibodies is often used to diagnose bacterial and viral infections caused by microorganisms that are difficult to culture or obtain on a swab. Antigen testing is used to identify substances produced by the body in specific conditions or bacteria that can be obtained on a swab. The previously discussed pregnancy and group A *Streptococcus* tests are examples of antigen testing by immunoassay. Reagent antibodies known to be specific for HCG or group A *Streptococcus* antigens are used to detect their presence (Fig. 15-16).

 Technical Tip 15-17. When working for a different organization, do not assume that you will be using the same immunoassay procedures. Read the procedure manual.

Three frequently used immunoassays detect the antibodies present in infectious mononucleosis (IM) and gastrointestinal disorders caused by *Helicobacter pylori* and the antigen troponin T present in a myocardial infarction (MI). Several different manufacturers produce kits for the detection of these substances. The actual kit used is a matter of laboratory preference.

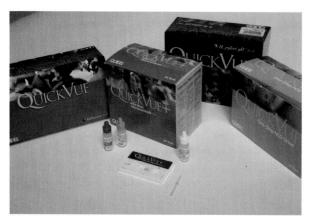

FIGURE 15-16 **Various waived test kits.**

IM is an acute, self-limiting infection caused by the Epstein-Barr virus. Symptoms include fatigue, swollen lymph glands, sore throat, and enlargement of the liver. The diagnosis can be confirmed by detection of unique heterophile antibodies formed in response to the infection. The manufacturer's instructions must be followed closely to ensure that only the heterophile antibodies specific for IM are detected.

Helicobacter pylori is the causative agent of several gastrointestinal disorders, of which the most common are duodenal and gastric ulcers. The rapid detection of antibodies specific for *H. pylori* in the blood of a patient with symptoms of gastrointestinal pain alerts the health-care provider to prescribe antibiotics. Early treatment prevents the bacteria from causing additional damage to the gastrointestinal tract.

Early diagnosis of an MI can be critical to patient survival. Troponin T is a protein specific to heart muscle and is only released into the blood after an MI. It can be detected within 4 hours of damage to the heart and remains elevated for 14 days. Troponin T is one of the earliest markers present in MI, and the ability to detect it by rapid immunoassay is a valuable diagnostic aid. The test is well suited for use in outpatient settings and the emergency department.

Blood Coagulation Testing

Several POCT instruments are available to monitor blood coagulation therapy and clotting deficiencies in patients. The anticoagulant heparin is administered intravenously to patients to prevent the formation of clots after certain surgeries and clinical procedures that can initiate the clotting process such as cardiac catheterization, hemodialysis, and coronary angioplasty. Heparin is a fast-acting anticoagulant that must be monitored closely because too much heparin can produce internal hemorrhaging and too little heparin may lead to clot formation. An oral anticoagulant, Coumadin, is frequently given to outpatients at risk for clot formation. The prothrombin time (PT) test is used to monitor the anticoagulant, Coumadin, used for patients with deep vein thrombosis, heart valve replacement, atrial fibrillation, and other conditions according to clinical guidelines. The international normalized ratio (INR) is a calculation used to standardize the results from the PT between testing devices. The activated partial thromboplastin time (APTT) test is used to monitor heparin therapy. The activated clotting time (ACT) also monitors heparin therapy.

Depending on the manufacturer, POCT instruments for coagulation testing are capable of providing a combination of PT (INR), APTT, and ACT results or only PT (INR) results. The type of instrument chosen depends on the needs of the POCT site. As mentioned previously, surgical areas must be able to monitor heparin therapy, and therefore an instrument that performs an APTT or ACT is required. In contrast, outpatient sites are monitoring Coumadin therapy and need only to perform a PT (INR).

> ▶ *Technical Tip 15-18.* The international normalized ratio (INR) standardizes prothrombin time results between different reagent manufacturers. The INR should be reported for patients taking Coumadin for at least 2 weeks.

The ProTime 3 Microcoagulation System (International Technidyne Corporation, Edison, NJ.) is a system for PT testing consisting of the ProTime instrument, a three-channel reagent cuvette with built-in QC, and the Tenderlett Plus LV sample collection system. It is a CLIA waived test that performs PTs from finger-stick whole blood and displays the results as the PT result in seconds and the more standardized INR. ProTime runs two levels of QC with each patient's sample (Fig. 15-17).

The CoaguChek system (Roche Diagnostics, Indianapolis, IN) performs a PT using a drop of fingerstick whole blood applied to a test strip containing dried thromboplastin reagent and tiny iron particles. The specimen, dried reagent, and iron particles move through alternating magnetic fields that cause the iron particles to move. The endpoint is reached when a clot forms and stops the iron particles from moving. The analyzer displays the INR result (Fig. 15-18).

The HEMOCHRON Jr. Signature Whole Blood Microcoagulation System (International Technidyne Corporation, Edison, NJ) is a POCT instrument that performs ACT, APTT, and PT tests using one drop of whole blood per test. Specific cuvettes containing dried reagents for each test are placed into the instrument, blood is added, and the timing begins. The timing stops when a clot is detected and the result is displayed. The instrument has data management capabilities to identify, store, and print both patient and QC results (Fig. 15-19).

> ▶ *Technical Tip 15-19.* Point-of-care testing coagulation tests often specify that the first drop of blood obtained by dermal puncture be used for testing.

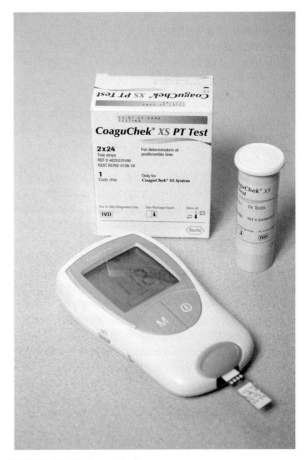

FIGURE 15-18 CoaguChek system.

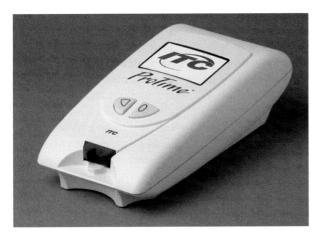

FIGURE 15-17 ProTime 3 Microcoagulation System. *(Courtesy of International Technidyne Corporation, Edison, NJ.)*

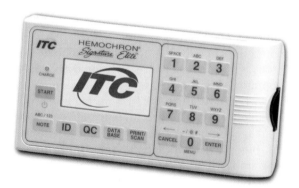

FIGURE 15-19 HEMOCHRON Jr. Signature Whole Blood Microcoagulation System. *(Courtesy of International Technidyne Corporation, Edison, NJ.)*

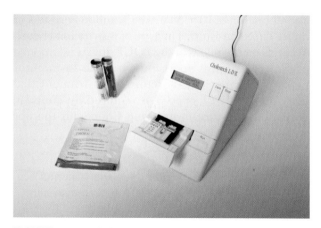

FIGURE 15-20 Cholestech LDX with optics cassette and capillary tubes.

Cholesterol

Cholesterol is a lipid manufactured by the body for use in cell membranes and as a precursor to steroid hormones. It is found in high concentrations in animal fats; therefore, additional cholesterol enters the body through ingestion. When excessive amounts of cholesterol are ingested or produced by the body, the increased cholesterol circulating in the blood adheres to the walls of the blood vessels, resulting in blockage of blood flow and subsequent coronary artery disease.

Normal values for cholesterol vary with age. The ideal value is less than 200 mg/dL. Studies show that lowering cholesterol to acceptable levels reduces the risk of developing coronary heart disease. The studies also suggest that increases in high-density lipoprotein (HDL) reduce coronary heart disease risk. The National Institutes of Health (NIH) has recommended aggressive efforts to identify and treat those at risk for coronary heart disease. Several POCT instruments are available that can perform cardiac risk profiles from a single drop of whole blood.

The Cholestech LDX (Cholestech Corporation, Hayward, CA) analyzer measures total cholesterol, HDL cholesterol, and triglycerides using a cassette containing dry reagents capable of performing an enzymatic reaction when blood is added to the cassette (Fig. 15-20). Estimated low-density lipoprotein (LDL) cholesterol, very–low-density lipoprotein (VLDL) cholesterol, and a total cholesterol/high-density lipoprotein (TC/HDL) ratio are calculated using the measured values. Each cassette has a magnetic stripe containing calibration information; therefore, no operator calibration is required. The analyzer is designed to go into a locking mode if QC testing is not within acceptable limits. The

operator must then contact a technical service representative at Cholestech, Inc.

 Technical Tip 15-20. Hold the cassette by the short sides only. Do not touch the black bar or the brown magnetic stripe.

Arterial Blood Gas and Chemistry Analyzers

Arterial blood gases (ABGs), electrolyte testing, and cardiac markers are used for the stat analysis of a critical patient population because delayed results would significantly affect patient care. ABGs include the pH, the partial pressure of carbon dioxide (Pco_2), and the partial pressure of oxygen (Po_2) in the blood. Electrolytes commonly measured are sodium (Na^+), potassium (K^+), chloride (Cl^-), bicarbonate ion (HCO_3^-), and ionized calcium (iCa^{++}). Cardiac markers include troponin I, B-type natriuretic peptide (BNP), and CK-MB. POCT for electrolytes uses small instruments located in emergency departments, operating suites, and intensive care and critical care units.

ABGs are obtained to determine if the patient is well oxygenated and to determine the acid-base status of the patient. Electrolytes maintain osmotic pressure, proper pH, regulation of heart and other muscles, and oxidation-reduction potential and participate as catalysts for enzymes. Disturbance of K^+ homeostasis causes muscle weakness and affects heart rate. Sodium maintains normal distribution of water through osmotic pressure. Ionized calcium is the active form of calcium and is useful in evaluation of renal function and endocrine disorders during cardiac surgery and in neonatology. Cardiac markers indicate heart function and myocardial damage.

Chemistry Analyzers

Various analyzers are available for waived POC chemistry testing. Instruments are portable, self-contained, and most include quality control and data management programs. Cartridges or reagent disks for the instruments contain the reagents and methodologies for performing one test or are designed to perform a specific panel of tests. They are equipped to perform a variety of chemical profiles ranging from single organ profiles to basic and comprehensive metabolic profiles. This chapter describes only a few of the available instruments.

The IRMA TruPoint Blood Analysis System (ITC, Edison, NJ) measures analytes using a single-use cartridge containing reagents and electrodes for the determination of each analyte or group of analytes. Cartridges are automatically calibrated when inserted into the instrument. A small sample of blood is injected into the system's sensor cartridge and a test is performed in 2 minutes. Results are displayed on a screen and a hard copy can be printed (Fig. 15-21).

The hand-held i-STAT Portable Clinical Analyzer (Abbott, Princeton, NJ) uses test cartridges. Separate cartridges are available for the different batteries of tests. Only a few drops of blood are inserted into the cartridge, which is placed into the analyzer and the result is available within 2 minutes (Fig. 15-22). The Nova STAT Profile Analyzer (Nova Biomedical, Waltham, MA) uses optical and electrode technology

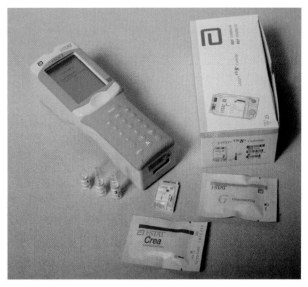

FIGURE 15-22 **i-STAT Portable Clinical Analyzer.**

and provides an automated QC system for POCT with controls that are analyzed automatically on a preset schedule or on demand. Out-of-range results can be followed by an optional system shutdown. A single snap-in reagent pack contains all required blood gas and chemistry reagents, plus a self-sealing waste container. The 10-test menu requires 100 μL of whole blood, and a blood gas panel requires 40 μL of arterial blood (Fig. 15-23).

The Piccolo Xpress point-of-care chemistry analyzer brings comprehensive CLIA waived diagnostics to physician offices. In three easy steps, the

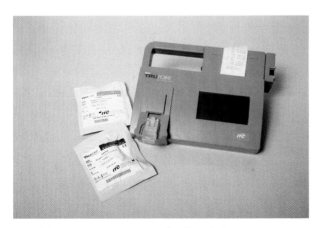

FIGURE 15-21 **IRMA TruPoint Blood Analysis System.**

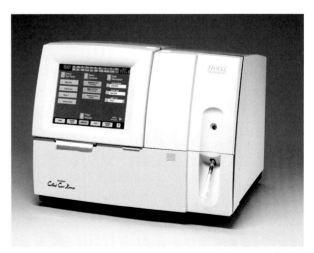

FIGURE 15-23 **Nova STAT Profile Analyzer.** *(Courtesy of Nova Biomedical, Waltham, MA.)*

Piccolo delivers laboratory-accurate chemistry re-sults in minutes, using a unique menu of 14 single-use reagent panels. With the Piccolo, doctors can make better-informed treatment decisions, reduce time spent reviewing labs, and increase profitability (Fig. 15-24).

 Technical Tip 15-21. Tests included in chemistry panels can be found in Chapter 2, Table 2-4.

FUTURE APPLICATIONS

The evolving technological advances have allowed POCT to expand to all areas of laboratory analysis with techniques for noninvasive sample collection and the use of nonblood samples, including saliva and nasal swabs, for analysis. POC device technology will continue to develop portable, stand-alone devices with diverse test menus. Data management and con-nectivity to the patient electronic medical record will become the standard of care. New therapies also will force the evolution of new tests and test methods.

The advancements in technology coupled with im-proved instrument connectivity and wireless interfac-ing capabilities will continue to facilitate the rapid expansion of POCT to provide clinically relevant in-formation accurately and rapidly.

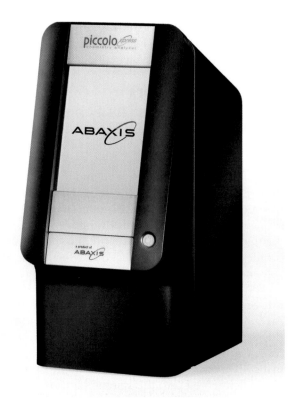

FIGURE 15-24 **Piccolo Xpress POCT chemistry analyzer.** *(Courtesy of Abaxis, Union City, CA.)*

Key Points

✦ POCT is laboratory testing at or near the patient bedside often by nonlaboratory personnel. Tests can be waived, moderate, or high complexity classification. The qualifications of personnel eligible to perform the tests in each classification are regulated by the federal law CLIA '88. Locations include
  - ✦ Specialized areas of the hospital
  - ✦ Home health care
  - ✦ Physician's offices
  - ✦ Health fairs
✦ Advantages of POCT include
  - ✦ Decreased TAT
  - ✦ Decreased sample volume
  - ✦ Elimination of sample transport
  - ✦ Ease of use
  - ✦ Mobility
  - ✦ Increased interpersonal interaction between patient and health-care personnel
✦ Drawbacks of POCT include
  - ✦ Large number of operators causing diluted competency
  - ✦ Capturing documentation of QC and patient results
  - ✦ Charging and billing mechanisms
✦ POC sample types are usually whole blood but also can include anticoagulated samples, direct swabs from infected areas, saliva, and noninvasive transcutaneous, transdermal methods.
✦ The three phases of laboratory testing are preexamination, examination, and postexamination. Procedures must address all three stages of laboratory testing.
✦ QC ensures the reliability of the test system and must comply to regulatory requirements.
  - ✦ External controls are commercial controls that are tested like a patient specimen to verify that the test system is working properly and the operator is performing the test correctly.
  - ✦ Internal controls are procedural controls and are contained within the system to ensure that the test kit and reagents are performing as expected.
  - ✦ Electronic controls use a mechanical or electrical calibrator in place of a QC specimen.
✦ Two levels of QC are required each day a test is performed and the results must be in the expected range before patient test results are reported.
✦ Various test kits, test methodologies, and POC analyzers are available for the many POC tests. The phlebotomist must read the package insert and the procedure manual for each procedure before performing the test. Reagents from various kits must not be interchanged.

BIBLIOGRAPHY

CDC and CLIA information. http://wwwn.cdc.gov/clia/default.aspx.

CLIA Home Page and CLIA Regulations. http://www.cms.hhs.gov/CLIA/

Di Lorenzo, MS, and Strasinger, SK: Blood Collection: A Short Course, ed. 2. FA Davis, 2010, Philadelphia.

FDA Test Complexity. http://www.accessdata.fda.gov/scripts/cdrh/cfdocs/cfCLIA/search.cfm.

Good Laboratory Practices for Waived Testing Sites (Centers for Disease Control and Prevention). http://www.cdc.gov/dls/bestpractices/

Rubaltille, FF, Gourley, GR, Loskamp, N, Modi, N, Roth-Kleiner, M, Sender, A, and Vert, P: Transcutaneous Bilirubin Measurement: A Multicenter Evaluation of a New Device. *Pediatrics* 2001;107(6):1264–1271.

Strasinger, SK, and Di Lorenzo, MS: Urinalysis and Body Fluids, ed. 5. FA Davis, 2008, Philadelphia.

Wager, EA, Yasin, B, and Yuan, S: Point-of-Care Testing: Twenty Years' Experience. *Lab Medicine* 2008;39(9) 560–563.

Study Questions

1. Preexamination errors in POCT include all of the following **EXCEPT:**
   a. improper storage of test materials
   b. failure to check reagent expiration dates
   c. performing the test too near the patient
   d. performing the test on the wrong patient

2. Acceptable QC can ensure all of the following **EXCEPT:**
   a. correct patient identification
   b. integrity of testing materials
   c. correct performance of the test
   d. correct functioning of the testing device

3. Procedural controls that verify that the test kit and added reagents are performing correctly are called:
   a. electronic controls
   b. external controls
   c. internal controls
   d. proficiency testing

4. When performing POCT, the operator must be sure to document results of:
   a. patient tests
   b. quality control
   c. electronic controls
   d. all of the above

5. The most common POCT test performed at home and in the hospital is a:
   a. glucose
   b. bilirubin
   c. strep test
   d. urinalysis

6. A waived test performed on the HemoCue analyzer that will indicate whether a patient may have an anemia is:
   a. glucose
   b. hemoglobin
   c. bilirubin
   d. Monotest

7. The recommended sample for urine pregnancy testing is a:
   a. random sample
   b. first morning sample
   c. midstream clean-catch sample
   d. timed sample

8. The test used to monitor Coumadin therapy is:
   a. APTT
   b. ACT
   c. PT (INR)
   d. bleeding time

9. Errors most commonly associated with incorrect PT(INR) results include all of the following **EXCEPT:**
   a. failure to adequately cleanse and dry the capillary puncture site
   b. prematurely performing the capillary puncture before test strip/cartridge is ready to accept the sample
   c. using the first drop of dermal puncture blood
   d. inadequate application of specimen

10. A POCT analyzer that can perform metabolic chemistry panels is:
    a. Bilichek
    b. Glucometer
    c. Cholestech LDX
    d. I-STAT

Clinical Situations

1 A phlebotomist performs daily bedside glucose tests on an inpatient using a POCT glucose meter. Daily results for the patient were:

Day 1: 100 mg/dL
Day 2: 105 mg/dL
Day 3: 98 mg/dL
Today the phlebotomist gets a result of 48 mg/dL. The patient states no change in diet or routine in the past 24 hours.
a. What should the phlebotomist do?
b. What three things could be a cause of an incorrect glucose value?

2 A phlebotomist performed the daily morning QC on the glucose meter. The results were:
Abnormal low = 50 mg/dL
Abnormal high = 200 mg/dL
The range for the abnormal low is 33 to 57 mg/dL; the abnormal high range is 278 to 418 mg/dL.

a. Can the phlebotomist report patient results?
b. What actions are required by the phlebotomist?
c. What is a possible cause of any discrepancy?

3 An outpatient urine sample was delivered to the clinic at 8:00 a.m. and placed on the counter in the laboratory. The phlebotomist finished the blood collections at 11:30 a.m. and then performed the urinalysis on this sample. The results were:

COLOR: Yellow	PROTEIN: Negative	BILIRUBIN: Negative
CLARITY: Cloudy*	GLUCOSE: Negative	UROBILINOGEN: Normal
SP. GRAVITY: 1.020	KETONES: Negative	NITRITE: Positive*
pH: 9.0*	BLOOD: Negative	LEUKOCYTE: Negative

* Significant results
a. What could be a possible cause for the abnormal results?
b. What should have been done with this specimen?

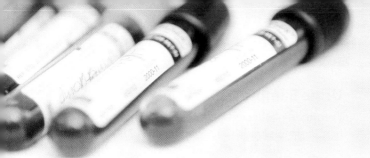

CHAPTER 16

Additional Duties of the Phlebotomist

Learning Objectives

Upon completion of this chapter, the reader will be able to:

1. Provide patients with instructions and containers for the collection of random, first morning, midstream clean-catch, and 24-hour urine samples.
2. Provide patients with instructions and containers for the collection of random and timed fecal samples.
3. Provide patients with instructions and containers for the collection of semen samples.
4. Correctly collect a throat culture.
5. Correctly obtain a nasopharyngeal sample.
6. Briefly describe the purpose of and the collection procedure for sweat electrolytes, including the precautions to protect sample integrity.
7. Describe the purpose of and the collection procedure for bone marrow samples.
8. Discuss the major components and concerns of the blood donor selection process.
9. Compare and contrast the blood donor collection process and the routine venipuncture.
10. Describe the purpose of and the tests performed on various nonblood samples.
11. Discuss the responsibilities of a phlebotomist when accessioning samples into the laboratory and shipping samples from the laboratory.
12. Describe the safety precautions associated with sample processing.
13. State four rules for safe operation of a centrifuge.
14. State three routine phlebotomy duties that can involve a phlebotomist in the use of a laboratory information management system.

Key Terms

Aliquot
Apheresis
Autologous donation
Iontophoresis
Pilocarpine
Pneumatic tube system
Sweat electrolytes
Therapeutic phlebotomy

Although collection of quality blood samples is the primary duty of phlebotomists, they are frequently assigned other responsibilities related to sample collection and handling of nonblood samples. These additional duties may include:

1. Providing instructions and materials to patients for the collection of urine, fecal, and semen samples
2. Collecting throat cultures and nasopharyngeal swabs
3. Performing sweat electrolyte collections
4. Assisting the physician with bone marrow aspirations
5. Interviewing blood donors
6. Performing donor blood collections and therapeutic phlebotomies
7. Transporting and receiving nonblood samples
8. Preparing specimens for delivery to laboratory sections or shipment to reference laboratories
9. Transporting samples from off-site collection areas
10. Using the laboratory computer system to enter and retrieve patient and specimen information

The extent to which phlebotomists are assigned these duties varies greatly among laboratories, as do the protocols for performing them. This chapter is intended to provide phlebotomists with basic information associated with these additional functions.

PATIENT INSTRUCTION

The phlebotomy department is usually located in or near the laboratory patient and sample reception area. Therefore, phlebotomists often provide instructions to patients and may receive calls from the health-care provider's office personnel requesting instructions. Instructions may be given verbally, using guidelines stated in the laboratory procedure manual, or may be handed to the patient in written form. The phlebotomist should be prepared to answer questions regarding the instructions. Depending on the test requested, patients may be collecting the sample while at the laboratory or collecting the sample at home and returning it to the laboratory. The facilities for sample collection should be at a location convenient to the laboratory.

 Technical Tip 16-1. Always confirm with the patients that they have understood the instructions.

Urine Sample Collection

Frequently collected urine samples include random, first morning, midstream clean-catch, 24-hour (timed) samples, catheterized, and suprapubic aspirations. Phlebotomists should explain to patients that the composition of urine changes quickly and samples should be delivered promptly to the laboratory or refrigerated. Types of urine samples are summarized in Table 16-1.

Random Specimen

Random samples are collected by patients while at the laboratory and are used primarily for routine urinalysis. Patients should be provided with a disposable urine container and directed to the bathroom facility.

First Morning Sample

A first morning sample is the specimen of choice for urinalysis because it is more concentrated. It may be used to confirm results obtained from random specimens. Patients are provided with a container and instructed to collect the sample immediately after arising and to return it to the laboratory within 2 hours or refrigerate the sample.

Midstream Clean Catch

Midstream clean-catch samples are used for urine cultures. Patients are provided with sterile containers

TABLE 16-1 • Types of Urine Specimens and Their Purposes

TYPE OF SPECIMEN	PURPOSE
Random	Routine screening
First morning	Routine screening
	Pregnancy tests
	Orthostatic protein
Fasting	Diabetic screening/ monitoring
24-hour (or timed)	Quantitative chemical tests
Catheterized	Bacterial culture
Midstream clean-catch	Routine screening
	Bacterial culture
Suprapubic aspiration	Bladder urine for bacterial culture
	Cytology

and antiseptic materials for cleansing the genitalia. Mild antiseptic towelettes are recommended. The procedures for collecting a clean-catch sample vary slightly between men and women and are described in Procedures 16-1 and 16-2. Midstream clean-catch samples are collected at the laboratory and delivered immediately to the microbiology section.

PROCEDURE 16-1 ✦ Midstream Clean-Catch Urine Collection for Women

EQUIPMENT:

Requisition form

Sterile urine container with label

Sterile antiseptic towelettes

Written instructions for cleansing and voiding

PROCEDURE:

Step 1. Wash hands.

Step 2. Remove the lid from the container without touching the inside of the container or lid.

Step 3. Separate the skin folds (labia).

Step 4. Cleanse from front to back on either side of the urinary opening with an antiseptic towelette, using a clean one for each side.

Step 5. Hold the skin folds apart and begin to void into the toilet.

Step 6. Bring the urine container into the stream of urine and collect an adequate amount of urine. Do not touch the inside of the container or allow the container to touch the genital area.

Step 7. Finish voiding into the toilet.

Step 8. Cover the sample with the lid. Touch only the outside of the lid and container.

Step 9. Label the container with the name and time of collection and place in the specified area or hand to the phlebotomist for labeling.

PROCEDURE 16-2 ✦ Midstream Clean-Catch Urine Collection for Men

EQUIPMENT:

Requisition form

Sterile urine container with label

Sterile antiseptic towelettes

Written instructions for cleansing and voiding

PROCEDURE:

Step 1. Wash hands.

Step 2. Remove the lid from the sterile container without touching the inside of the container or lid.

Step 3. Cleanse the tip of the penis with an antiseptic towelette and let dry. Retract the foreskin if uncircumcised.

Step 4. Void into the toilet. Hold back foreskin if necessary.

Step 5. Bring the sterile urine container into the stream of urine and collect an adequate amount of urine. Do not touch the inside of the container or allow the container to touch the genital area.

Step 6. Finish voiding into the toilet.

Step 7. Cover the sample with the lid. Touch only the outside of the lid and container.

Step 8. Label the container with the name and time of collection and place in the specified area or hand to the phlebotomist for labeling.

> **Technical Tip 16-2.** Posting instructions for collection of midstream clean-catch samples on bathroom walls is very helpful to patients.

Preexamination Consideration 16-1.

If a routine urinalysis is also requested, the culture should be performed first to prevent contamination of the sample.

24-Hour (or Timed) Sample

A carefully timed (usually 24 hours) sample is required for quantitative measurement of urine constituents. Patients are provided with large plastic containers that may contain a preservative. Phlebotomists should check the procedure manual or with a laboratory supervisor to be sure the appropriate preservative is supplied. Patients should be cautioned to avoid contact with the preservative in the container because some preservatives are caustic. For accurate results, it is critical that the patient understand that all urine produced during the collection period be placed in the container. Patients who indicate they have not been able to collect a complete sample should obtain a new sample. To obtain an accurate timed sample, it is necessary for the patient to begin and end the collection period with an empty bladder. Addition of urine produced before the start of the collection time or failure to include urine produced at the end of the collection period will affect the accuracy of the analysis. Sample labels must provide correct patient identification, the time of sample collection, the type of preservative used, and applicable precautions. Procedure 16-3 describes the 24-hour urine collection. Examples of urine sample containers and supplies are shown in Figure 16-1.

PROCEDURE 16-3 ✦ 24-Hour (Timed) Urine Sample Collection Procedure

EQUIPMENT:

> Requisition form
> 24-hour urine sample container with lid
> Label
> Container with ice, if required
> Preservative, if required

PROCEDURE:

Step 1. Provide patient with written instructions and explain the collection procedure.

Step 2. Issue the proper collection container and preservative.

Step 3. Day 1: 7 a.m. Patient voids and discards specimen.

Step 4. Patient writes the exact time on the sample label and places the label on the container.

Step 5. Patient collects all urine for the next 24 hours.

Step 6. Refrigerate the sample after adding each urine collection.

Step 7. Patient should collect urine sample before bowel movement to avoid fecal contamination.

Step 8. Continue to drink normal amounts of fluid throughout the collection time.

Step 9. Day 2: 7 a.m. Patient voids and adds this urine to the previously collected urine.

Step 10. Sample is transported to the laboratory in an insulated bag or portable cooler.

Step 11. Upon arrival in the laboratory, the entire 24-hour sample is thoroughly mixed, and the volume is accurately measure and recorded.

Step 12. An aliquot is saved for testing and additional or repeat testing. The remaining urine is discarded.

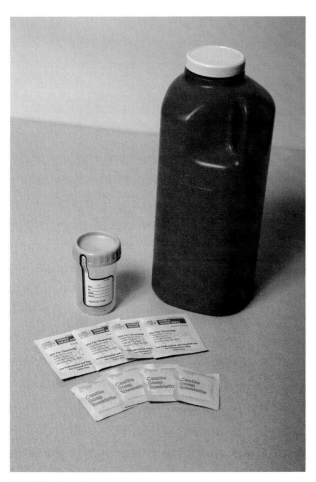

FIGURE 16-1 **Containers for urine samples.**

Preexamination Consideration 16-2.
Failure to collect a complete timed sample causes falsely decreased results.

Catheterized Sample

This sample is collected under sterile conditions by passing a sterile hollow tube through the urethra into the bladder. The most commonly requested test on a catheterized sample is a bacterial culture. This type of sample is collected on a patient unable to void, babies, or bedridden patients.

Suprapubic Sample

A suprapubic sample is collected by external introduction of a needle through the abdomen into the bladder. Suprapubic aspiration is used when a sample must be completely free of extraneous contamination, particularly in infants or children. The sample can be used for bacterial cultures and cytological examination.

 Technical Tip 16-3. Catheterized and suprapubic samples are collected by personnel in the nursing units and delivered to the laboratory. Be sure to maintain their sterility and deliver them to the appropriate laboratory section.

Urine Drug Sample Collection

Phlebotomists may be involved in the urine drug sample collection from both outpatients and in-house health-care workers. Sample collection is the most vulnerable part of a drug-testing program. For urine samples to withstand legal scrutiny, it is necessary to prove that no tampering (e.g., adulteration, substitution, or dilution) took place. Acceptable identification of the person requires picture identification, and as discussed in Chapter 11, the chain of custody (COC) must be carefully documented.

Urine sample collection may be "witnessed" or "unwitnessed." The decision to obtain a witnessed collection is indicated when it is suspected that the donor may alter or substitute the sample, or it is the policy of the client ordering the test. If a witnessed sample collection is ordered, a same-gender collector will observe the collection of 30 to 45 mL of urine. Witnessed and unwitnessed collections should be immediately handed to the collector.

The urine temperature must be taken within 4 minutes from the time of collection to confirm the sample has not been adulterated. The temperature should read within the range of 32.5°C to 37.7°C. If the sample temperature is not within range, the sample temperature should be recorded and the supervisor or employer contacted immediately. Urine temperatures outside of the recommended range may indicate sample contamination. Recollection of a second sample as soon as possible is necessary. The urine color is inspected to identify any signs of contaminants. A urine pH of greater than 9.0 suggests adulteration of the urine sample and requires that the sample be recollected if clinically necessary. A specific gravity of less than 1.005 could indicate dilution of the urine sample and would require recollection of the sample. The sample is labeled, packaged, and transported following laboratory-specific instructions. A typical urine drug sample collection procedure is described in Procedure 16-4.

PROCEDURE 16-4 ✦ **Urine Drug Sample Collection Procedure**

EQUIPMENT:

Requisition form
Gloves
Bluing agent (dye)
Sample container
Label
Chain of custody (COC) form
Temperature strip

PROCEDURE:

Step 1. The collector washes hands and wears gloves.

Step 2. The collector adds bluing agent (dye) to the toilet water reservoir to prevent an adulterated sample.

Step 3. The collector eliminates any source of water other than toilet by taping the toilet lid and faucet handles.

Step 4. The donor provides photo identification or positive identification from employer representative.

Step 5. The collector completes step 1 of the COC form and has the donor sign the form.

Step 6. The donor leaves his or her coat, briefcase, or purse outside the collection area to avoid the possibility of concealed substances contaminating the urine.

Step 7. The donor washes his or her hands and receives a sample cup.

Step 8. The collector remains in the restroom but outside the stall, listening for unauthorized water use, unless a witnessed collection is requested.

Step 9. The donor hands sample cup to the collector.

Step 10. The collector checks the urine for abnormal color and for the required amount (30 to 45 mL).

Step 11. The collector checks that the temperature strip on the sample cup reads between 32.5°C and 37.7°C. The collector records the in-range temperature on the COC form (COC step 2). If the sample temperature is out of range or the sample is suspected to have been diluted or adulterated, a new sample must be collected and a supervisor notified.

Step 12. The sample must remain in the sight of the donor and collector at all times.

Step 13. With the donor watching, the collector peels off the sample identification strips from the COC form (COC step 3) and puts them on the capped bottle, covering both sides of the cap.

Step 14. The donor initials the sample bottle seals.

Step 15. The date and time are written on the seals.

Step 16. The donor completes step 4 on the COC form.

Step 17. The collector completes step 5 on the COC form.

Step 18. Each time the sample is handled, transferred, or placed in storage, every individual must be identified and the date and purpose of the change recorded.

Step 19. The collector follows laboratory-specific instructions for packaging the sample bottles and laboratory copies of the COC form.

Step 20. The collector distributes the COC copies to appropriate personnel.

Fecal Sample Collection

The laboratory provides patients with several types of containers for collection of fecal (stool) samples (Fig. 16-2). Detailed instructions and appropriate containers should be provided.

Random samples used for cultures, ova and parasites (O&P), microscopic examination for cells, fats and fibers, and detection of blood are collected in cardboard containers with wax-coated interiors or plastic containers with wide openings and screw-capped tops similar to those used for urine samples. Containers with preservatives may be required for certain microbiology tests, including ova and parasites, and can be kept at room temperature. Kits containing

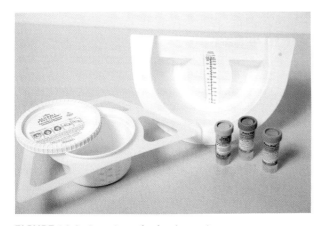

FIGURE 16-2 Containers for fecal samples.

reagent-impregnated filter paper are provided to screen for the presence of occult (hidden) blood (see Chapter 15). Phlebotomists should check the procedure manual before distributing containers for fecal samples.

For quantitative testing, such as for fecal fats and urobilinogen, timed samples are required. Large paint can–style or plastic hat–style containers are used for collection of 72-hour samples for fecal fats. It may be necessary to collect the specimen in a large container, such as a bedpan or disposable container, and then transfer it to the laboratory container. Patients should be instructed to collect the sample in a clean container and return the sample to the laboratory as soon as possible and to avoid contaminating the sample with urine or toilet water, which may contain chemical disinfectants. Samples must be refrigerated during the collection time.

Containers that contain preservatives for O&P must not be used to collect samples for other tests. For purposes of safety, the outside of the container must not be contaminated.

Semen Sample Collection

Semen samples are collected and tested to evaluate fertility and postvasectomy procedures. Patients presenting requisitions for semen analysis should be instructed to abstain from sexual activity for 3 days and not longer than 5 days before collecting the sample. Ideally, the sample should then be collected at the laboratory in a warm sterile container. Samples for fertility studies must not be collected in a condom because condoms frequently contain spermicidal agents.

If the sample is collected at home, it must be kept warm and delivered to the laboratory within 1 hour. When accepting a semen sample, it is essential that the phlebotomist record the time of sample collection, and the sample receipt, on the requisition form because certain parameters of the semen analysis are based on specimen life span. Sample should be kept at 37°C.

Written instructions should be available for patients required to collect semen samples.

COLLECTION OF THROAT CULTURES

The duties of the phlebotomist may include collection of throat culture samples from outpatients, often children. They are performed primarily for the detection of a streptococcal infection, "strep throat." Samples may be collected for the purpose of performing a culture or a rapid immunological Group A Strep test (see Chapter 15). A throat culture is collected using a collection kit that contains a sterile swab in a transport medium collection tube (Fig. 16-3). The procedure for collecting a throat culture sample is shown in Procedure 16-5.

▶ *Technical Tip 16-4.* The purpose of the transport media in a culture swab kit is to keep the bacteria to be cultured alive during transport to the microbiology laboratory.

▶ *Technical Tip 16-5.* Swabs for rapid streptococcal tests do not require transport media.

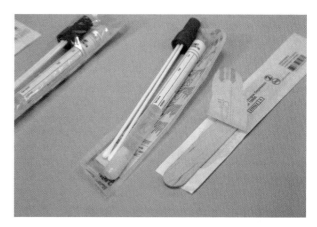

FIGURE 16-3 Throat swab and transport tube collection kit.

PROCEDURE 16-5 ✦ **Collection of a Throat Culture Sample**

EQUIPMENT:

Requisition form
Tongue depressor
Collection swab in a sterile tube containing transport media
Flashlight

PROCEDURE:

Step 1. Wash hands and put on gloves.

Step 2. Have the patient tilt the head back and open the mouth wide.

Step 3. Remove the cap with its attached swab from the tube using sterile technique.

Step 4. If necessary, use a flashlight to illuminate the back of the throat.

Step 5. Gently depress the tongue with the tongue depressor. Ask the patient to say, "Ah."

Step 6. Being careful not to touch the cheeks, tongue, or lips; swab the area in the back of the throat, including the tonsils, and any inflamed or ulcerated areas.

Step 7. Return the swab to the sterile transport tube.

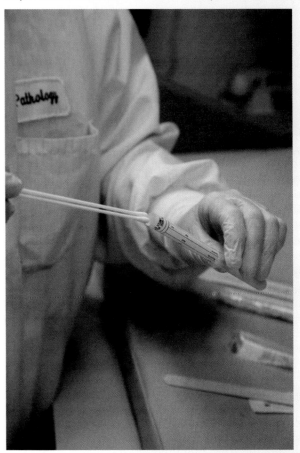

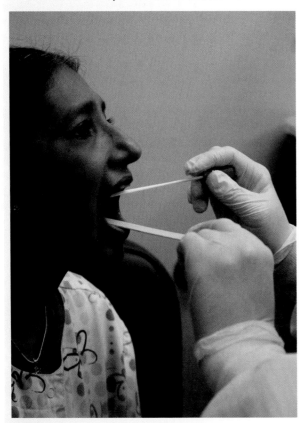

PROCEDURE 16-5 ✦ **Collection of a Throat Culture Sample** (Continued)

Step 8. Close the cap.

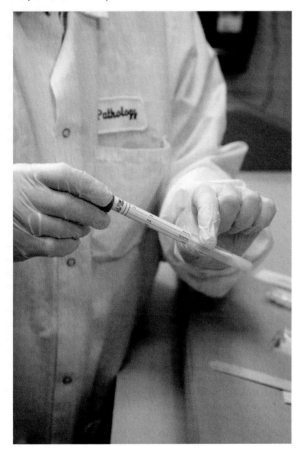

Step 9. Crush the ampule of transport medium (if necessary), making sure the released medium is in contact with the swab.

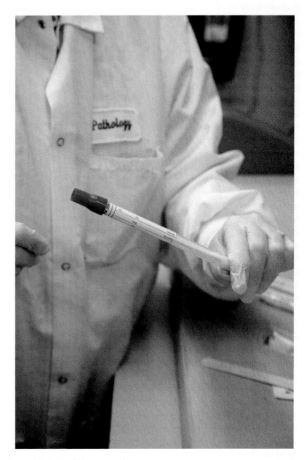

Step 10. Label the sample.

Step 11. Remove gloves and wash hands.

Step 12. Deliver the sample immediately to the microbiology laboratory.

COLLECTION OF SWEAT ELECTROLYTES

Measurement of the *sweat electrolytes,* sodium and chloride, is performed to confirm the diagnosis of cystic fibrosis, a genetic disorder of the mucous-secreting glands. Because cystic fibrosis involves multiple organs, many clinical symptoms can lead the physician to suspect its presence. Symptoms usually appear early in life; therefore, sweat electrolytes are frequently collected from infants. Although genetic methods are now predominately used to determine cystic fibrosis, sweat electrolytes remain an important diagnostic tool. Chloride levels in sweat that are two to five times the normal value indicate the presence of cystic fibrosis.

Sample collection is time consuming and must be performed under very controlled conditions to ensure that the small amount of sample collected is not altered by contamination or evaporation.

Patients are induced to sweat using a technique called pilocarpine *iontophoresis. Pilocarpine,* a sweat-inducing chemical, is applied to an area of the forearm or leg that has been previously cleansed with deionized water. The pilocarpine is then iontophoresed into the skin by the application of a mild electrical current provided by a device designed for pilocarpine iontophoresis. After iontophoresis, the area exposed to the pilocarpine is again thoroughly cleansed with deionized water and dried.

▶ *Technical Tip 16-6.* Be sure to use deionized water to cleanse the sweat collection area.

Several methods are available for collection of sweat for electrolyte analysis, including the use of preweighed gauze, filter paper pads, or coil collectors. The collection apparatus is placed on the stimulated area, covered securely with plastic if the collection material is gauze or filter paper, and allowed to remain for a specified length of time, usually 30 minutes. Regardless of the collection method used, it is essential that:

1. The collection apparatus is handled only with sterile forceps or powder-free gloves and not contaminated by use of the fingers.
2. The collection apparatus is tightly sealed during the collection period to prevent evaporation of the collected sweat.
3. The collected sweat is tightly sealed during transportation to the laboratory to prevent evaporation.

Phlebotomists may be required to perform sweat electrolyte collections or to assist personnel from the chemistry section with the collection. If the collection of sweat electrolytes is one of the phlebotomist's duties, the phlebotomist is usually required to notify the chemistry section when a collection is requested and to obtain collection materials (which may have to be preweighed) from the department.

COLLECTION OF NASOPHARYNGEAL (NP) SAMPLES

NP secretions are collected to detect acute respiratory diseases caused by respiratory syncytial virus (RSV) from infants and small children using rapid membrane enzyme immunoassay tests. NP secretions can also detect influenza A and B and the organisms that cause pertussis, diphtheria, meningitis, and pneumonia. The procedures for collecting NP swabs and NP wash samples from the nasal cavity are described in Procedures 16-6 and 16-7, respectively.

PROCEDURE 16-6 ✦ Collection of Nasopharyngeal Swab

EQUIPMENT:

Requisition form
Sterile mini-tip Dacron polyester or rayon-tipped swab
Transport medium (saline)
Ice slurry

PROCEDURE:

Step 1. Identify patient.

Step 2. Wash hands and put on gloves.

Step 3. Gently insert a mini-tip culture swab through the nose into the nasopharynx.

Step 4. Gently rotate the swab and carefully remove.

Step 5. Place swab sample in 0.75 to 3 µL of transport medium (saline).

Step 6. Mix the swab and transport medium vigorously.

Step 7. Express excess liquid from the swab.

Step 8. Dispose of the swab in the appropriate biohazard container.

Step 9. Label the sample.

Step 10. Place the sample/transport medium in a slurry of ice.

Step 11. Deliver the sample to the laboratory immediately after collection.

PROCEDURE 16-7 ✦ Collection of Nasopharyngeal Wash

EQUIPMENT:

Requisition form
Prepackaged sterile 0.9% sodium chloride solution
Sterile ear syringe
Sterile mini-tip Dacron polyester or rayon-tipped swab
Transport medium (saline)
Ice slurry

PROCEDURE:

Step 1. Identify the patient.

Step 2. Wash hands and put on gloves.

Step 3. Lay the child down and have another person hold the child's head firmly.

Step 4. Swab the inside of each naris with a sterile cotton-tipped swab to remove any extraneous mucus and to disturb the epithelial cells where the virus is harbored.

Step 5. Using a prepackaged sterile 0.9% sodium chloride solution, squeeze the vial and inject half of the solution (1.5 mL) into each naris.

Step 6. Using a sterile ear syringe, immediately suction the solution back.

Step 7. Inject the sample into the RSV transport medium.

Step 8. Repeat the procedure for the other naris using the same transport medium.

Step 9. Label the transport medium.

Step 10. Place the sample in a slurry of ice.

Step 11. Transport the sample to the laboratory immediately after collection.

BONE MARROW COLLECTION

In some facilities, phlebotomists assist the physician, usually an oncologist or radiologist, with bone marrow aspiration procedures. Bone marrow is the site of blood cell production. A bone marrow aspiration and biopsy is performed to diagnose various blood diseases. Bone marrow samples are collected by inserting a Jamshidi needle into the center of the iliac crest or sternum and aspirating liquid bone marrow and a bone core biopsy for evaluation. The bone marrow collection procedure is described in Procedure 16-8.

PROCEDURE 16-8   ✦   **Bone Marrow Collection**

EQUIPMENT:

Requisition form
Consent form
Ethylenediaminetetraacetic acid (EDTA) tubes, sodium heparin tubes
Glass slides
Transfer devices
10% formalin jars
"Isolator" tubes for culture studies
Petri dish
Sterile 4 × 4 gauzes
Wooden applicator sticks
Jamshidi aspiration needle
Sharps container
5 mL syringe
12 mL syringe
1% lidocaine ampules
Identification labels

PROCEDURE:

Step 1. Obtain the requisition form

Step 2. Confirm that the patient has signed the consent form.

Step 3. Identify the patient.

Step 4. Wash hands and put on gloves.

Step 5. Set up prep table/counter space to process the bone marrow aspirate/biopsy.

Step 6. Assist the physician during the procedure.

Step 7. The physician inserts the Jamshidi needle into the iliac crest after anesthetizing the area with lidocaine. The phlebotomist hands the physician a large syringe that is attached to the needle to aspirate the liquid bone marrow.

Step 8. A bone core biopsy is then collected. The core biopsy is placed on a sterile 4 × 4 gauze. Three to four touch prep slides are made by gently touching the specimen onto the slide three times to make imprints of the specimen. The biopsy is then placed in a 10% formalin container.

Step 9. Dispense three to four drops of the liquid marrow to run down the center of a slide that is angled down and sitting in a Petri dish for spicule collection and preparation of thin prep slides.

Step 10. As the drops of marrow run down the slide, pick up spicules of marrow and spread onto a spreader slide. Gently pull the spreader slide across another glass slide resulting in a thin smear of the marrow. Six to eight thin prep slides are made.

Step 11. Transfer 1 to 2 mL of the liquid bone marrow in the syringe into the EDTA and sodium heparin tubes. Mix tubes by inversion.

Step 12. Allow the remaining liquid marrow to clot in the syringe. When a clot has formed, place the clotted marrow into another 10% formalin container and label appropriately.

Step 13. Label all slides with patient's name and date, using pencil on the frosted end of the slide. Use patient identification labels for tubes and formalin containers. Include date, time, initials, and bone marrow site on the tubes.

Step 14. Deliver specimens to the histology department for processing and examination.

Step 15. Slides are delivered to the hematology department for staining and examination under the microscope.

BLOOD DONOR COLLECTION

Phlebotomists may be assigned to work in the blood donor collection station as a part of their routine duties, or they may obtain employment in an independent blood collection center. In the blood collection center, units of blood are collected to provide the blood bank with a supply of blood and blood components for transfusions. A unit of blood consists of 405 to 495 mL of blood mixed with 63 mL of anticoagulant and preservative, citrate-phosphate-dextrose (CPD) or CPDA (when adenine is added). After collection, a unit of blood can be separated by centrifugation into its individual components, including red blood cells, white blood cells, platelets, plasma, and plasma proteins. Experienced phlebotomists are needed to perform donor unit collections, assess and screen donors, and operate specialized equipment. Blood donor collections are performed following guidelines established by the American Association of Blood Banks (AABB) and the Food and Drug Administration (FDA) for donor selection and unit collection and processing. The responsibilities of the phlebotomist include the following:

- Donor interview and screening
- Donor identification
- Donor informed consent
- Venipuncture
- Product collection
- Postdonation care
- Complication management

Donor Selection

Persons volunteering to donate blood must be interviewed and tested to ensure that the donation will not be physically harmful to them, as well as to determine that their blood is unlikely to cause an adverse condition in the recipient. In addition to testing each donor unit for ABO blood group and Rh blood type, donor units are always tested with all available tests for bloodborne pathogens (Box 16-1); however, exclusion of donors with possible exposure to these pathogens provides additional protection for the recipient.

 Technical Tip 16-7. The phlebotomist must conduct a thorough interview and screening procedure to ensure the safety of both the donor and recipient.

Donor Registration and Identification

Donor registration requires identification (including name, address, telephone number, date of birth, social security number, and sex) and date of last donation (at least 8 weeks is required between whole blood donations). This information is needed in case the donor must be contacted in the future. Donors must also sign a consent form permitting the laboratory to draw the blood and test it for bloodborne pathogens.

 Technical Tip 16-8. Always follow specific facility's identification protocol for donor identification.

BOX 16-1 Infectious Diseases Tested for on Each Unit of Donor Blood

Chagas disease *(Trypanosoma cruzi)*
HIV 1 and 2
Hepatitis B (HBV)
Hepatitis C (HCV)
Syphillis
West Nile virus (WNV)
Human T-cell lymphotropic virus (HTLV)

Physical Examination

Eligibility requirements for blood donors include:

- Appear to be in good health
- No evidence of skin infections, rashes, or track marks
- 17 years old, or in some states 16 years old with parental consent
- Weigh at least 110 pounds
- Temperature of 99.5°F or lower
- Blood pressure no higher than 180/100 mm Hg
- Pulse rate between 50 and 100
- Hemoglobin level of 12.5 g/dL or higher or a hematocrit of 38% or higher

 Technical Tip 16-9. The risk of contamination of blood products is increased in units of blood collected from a patient with an obvious skin rash or infection.

Medical History Interview

Donors are asked an extensive list of questions regarding their previous medical history that includes:

- Past and current medications and antibiotics
- Injected drug use, exposure to infectious diseases
- History of infectious disease, venereal disease
- Social habits, particularly related to bloodborne pathogen exposure

Information can be checked with a donor referral registry to determine if a donor has been previously disqualified. Phlebotomists performing this interview must be certain that all questions are fully understood by the donor and that the donor understands the importance of a truthful answer to the future health of the recipient. The phlebotomist must explain risks of the procedure and the screening tests that will be performed on the donor blood. It is also required that all donors be given a private opportunity to indicate that after the unit is collected, it should not be used for transfusion. There are two boxes on the donor consent form, one giving permission to use the blood for transfusion and one denying permission to use the blood. A donor who for social reasons wants to donate blood but who knows the blood should not be used can check the "do not transfuse" box. The form is sealed until the unit is being processed. Another method is to provide the donor with two barcode labels (Use or Do Not Use), and the donor attaches the appropriate label to the collected unit. The unit is then scanned for acceptability during processing.

 Technical Tip 16-10. Be very careful to put donors at ease during the interview process and to conduct the interview in a private area.

Donor Collection

Units of blood are collected into sterile, closed systems consisting of one or more plastic bags connected to tubing and a sterile needle. Large-gauge needles (15 to 16 regular gauge or 17 gauge thin-walled) are used for collection of donor units, both to prevent hemolysis and to facilitate collection of the large amount of blood. Thin-walled needles provide a larger bore without increasing the diameter of the needle, so that there is less discomfort for the donor. The plastic bags fill by gravity and must be located below the collection site. They are frequently placed in an automatic mixing device that is also designed to stop when the unit reaches a weight that is consistent with the appropriate volume of blood. Hemostats may be applied to the tubing to start and stop the flow of blood into the bag.

A large vein, usually located in the antecubital area, is necessary to accommodate the large needle and supply the required amount of blood. A tourniquet or blood pressure cuff is used to facilitate vein selection. Aseptic site preparation is essential to prevent introduction of microorganisms into the unit of blood. Cleansing is a two-step process, beginning with a soap or detergent scrub and followed by application of more concentrated iodine or chlorhexidine that is allowed to dry for 30 seconds.

 Technical Tip 16-11. Failure to practice aseptic technique can result in the contamination of the unit of blood with skin microorganisms or the transmission of infectious disease to several recipients from a unit of whole blood that has been divided into its various components.

Technical Tip 16-12. Normal skin flora is the major source of blood product contamination.

Venipuncture is performed in the usual manner, and when blood appears in the tubing, the needle is securely taped to the donor's arm. Donors are encouraged to open and close their fists during the collection to speed the flow of blood. In contrast to routine venipuncture, hemoconcentration is acceptable in donor blood. After removal of the needle, donors are instructed to elevate the arm and apply firm pressure to the puncture site. The phlebotomist completes any required procedures such as transferring blood from the tubing into tubes for testing and discards the needle. Labels corresponding to those on the unit collection bag must be attached to all additional tubes.

After confirming that bleeding has stopped, the phlebotomist should place a sterile gauze and bandage over the site and instruct the donor to keep the bandage on for 4 hours. Donors should not be left alone during the collection period and should be carefully observed for dizziness or nausea during and after the collection. They are usually offered fruit juice and a snack before they leave the donor blood collection station.

Additional Donor Collection

A specialized area of blood donation is *apheresis.* Apheresis is performed to collect a specific blood component such as double red cells, platelets, or plasma. Under sterile conditions, donor blood is anticoagulated and sent directly to a specialized separation instrument (centrifuge). The desired component is removed, and the remainder of the blood is returned to the donor. Apheresis donors are able to donate more frequently than whole blood donors. Donors frequently have blood components that can be necessary for specific patients or can be of value for the manufacture of certain blood bank reagents. Phlebotomists must receive additional training to perform apheresis procedures.

Autologous Donation

Patients scheduled for elective surgery may choose to donate units of their own blood to be transfused back to them during their surgery if blood is needed. This is referred to as an *autologous donation* and has become a common procedure because of the concern about transmission of bloodborne pathogens. Patients may donate as often as every 72 hours, providing they have their health-care provider's approval and a hemoglobin level of at least 11.0 g/dL. The autologous units are specifically designated for autologous donor.

Therapeutic Phlebotomy

Phlebotomists may also perform a procedure called a *therapeutic phlebotomy*. In this procedure, a unit of blood is collected from patients with conditions causing overproduction of red blood cells (polycythemia) or iron (hemochromatosis). Patients requiring therapeutic phlebotomy are not as healthy as routine blood donors and should be carefully monitored during the collection period. Frequently, therapeutic phlebotomy is performed in a designated area of the laboratory or in a hospital unit and not in the donor blood collection station.

Because of the requirements of additional personnel, equipment, documentation of compliance with the regulations imposed by the AABB and the FDA and the legal responsibilities, not all hospitals have donor collection stations. However, most hospitals do perform therapeutic phlebotomy.

RECEIVING AND TRANSPORTING SAMPLES

Phlebotomists encounter a variety of samples other than those they personally collect. When collecting blood in the hospital units, they are often asked to transport nonblood samples back to the laboratory. Many inpatient and outpatient samples are delivered to the central processing area, and phlebotomists must be knowledgeable about any special handling requirements, the laboratory sections that analyze the samples, and the laboratory policy for accepting samples. A procedure manual detailing specimen requirements should be present in the central processing area.

In addition to urine, fecal, and semen samples, common samples received in the laboratory that are not collected by phlebotomists include cerebrospinal, synovial, pleural, pericardial, peritoneal (ascitic), and amniotic fluids and sputum, hair, saliva, and tissue samples. It is extremely important that phlebotomists recognize that these samples are collected using procedures that are more invasive than phlebotomy. Patients are subjected to more discomfort and possible complications. Therefore, samples should be transported in the appropriate biohazard bags or containers and delivered to the laboratory department with high priority.

Preexamination Consideration 16-4.
Many nonblood samples such as cerebrospinal fluid must be analyzed immediately to prevent loss of glucose and cellular elements.

Technical Tip 16-13. Always consult the procedure manual whenever you are unsure of a sample handling procedure.

Technical Tip 16-14. Samples that are collected by invasive procedures must be transported by hand and not delivered to the laboratory via the pneumatic tube system.

When delivering samples to laboratory sections, phlebotomists should be sure to alert the technical personnel about the sample. If samples are delivered to sections where no personnel are present, as may be the case on evening and night shifts, the phlebotomist must be aware of sample preservation requirements. This information should be available in the procedure manual or may be posted in the section; it varies with the type of sample and the section to which it is delivered. For example, cerebrospinal fluid (CSF) samples are refrigerated in hematology and left at room temperature in microbiology.

Samples accepted by phlebotomists, either on the units or in the laboratory, must be accompanied by a requisition form containing appropriate information and must have a label containing information that correlates with the requisition form. Labels should be attached to the actual collection container and not the lid to avoid a sample mix-up when lids are removed from containers. Samples must be transported in biohazard bags.

Preexamination Consideration 16-5.

Failure to follow temperature and exposure-to-light requirements during sample transport may alter certain analytes.

In some hospitals, samples are transported to the laboratory through a *pneumatic tube system.* Delivery of samples through a pneumatic tube system is a very efficient method because both personnel time and delivery time are saved. Samples must be properly cushioned to prevent breakage or red blood cell (RBC) hemolysis and enclosed in leak-proof material. Gloves should be worn when removing samples from the sample container (Fig. 16-4).

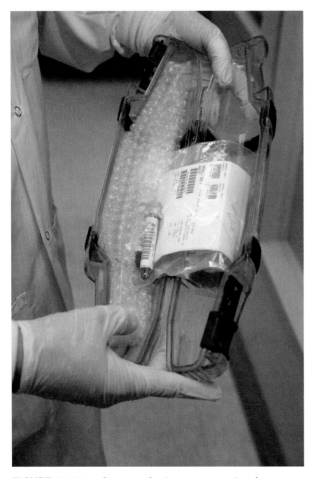

FIGURE 16-4 Loading samples into a pneumatic tube system.

NONBLOOD SAMPLES

Cerebrospinal Fluid

CSF surrounds the brain and spinal cord to supply nutrients to the nervous tissue, remove metabolic wastes, and produce a barrier to cushion the brain and spinal cord against trauma. CSF is routinely collected by lumbar puncture between the third, fourth, or fifth lumbar vertebrae. Normal CSF appears clear and colorless. Cerebrospinal fluid is collected to diagnose meningitis, subdural hemorrhage, and other neurological disorders.

Samples are collected in sterile tubes usually numbered 1 through 3, representing the order in which the sample was collected:

- Tube No. 1 is designated for chemistry.
- Tube No. 2 is designated for microbiology.
- Tube No. 3 is designated for hematology.

An alternate procedure is to collect four tubes numbered one through four. When this is done, Tubes No. 1 and 4 are sent to hematology, Tube No. 2 to chemistry, and Tube No. 3 to microbiology. The RBC counts in Tubes 1 and 4 are compared to determine possible contamination of Tube No. 1.

With both procedures it is important that tubes be delivered in this order because tube No. 1 is always more likely to contain cells or microorganisms obtained during the punctures and not actually present in the CSF.

CSF samples should be handled with extreme care, and delivered to the laboratory immediately, and tests are performed on a stat basis.

Synovial Fluid

Synovial fluid, often referred to as "joint fluid" is a viscous liquid found in the cavities of the movable or synovial joints that lubricates and reduces friction between bones during joint movement. Normal synovial fluid appears colorless to pale yellow. Synovial fluid is increased in inflammatory diseases, arthritis, and gout. Samples are collected by needle aspiration and collected into tubes based on the required tests: a sterile heparinized tube for Gram stain and culture and sensitivity, a heparin or EDTA tube for cell counts and crystal identification, a sodium fluoride tube for glucose analysis, and a non-anticoagulated tubes for other tests.

Serous Fluid

Serous fluid is located between the parietal membrane and visceral membrane of the pleural, pericardial, and peritoneal cavities and provides lubrication to prevent the friction between the two membranes as a result of movement of the enclosed organs. In congential heart failure, hypoproteinemia, inflammation and infection, or lymphatic obstruction, the amounts of fluid become increased. Fluids for laboratory examination are collected by needle aspiration from the respective body cavities as follows:

- Pleural fluid: obtained from between the pleural cavity membranes surrounding the lungs
- Pericardial fluid: obtained from between the pericardial cavity membranes surrounding the heart
- Peritoneal fluid: obtained from between the membranes surrounding the abdominal cavity

Samples are collected into EDTA evacuated tubes for cell counts and differential, sterile heparinized evacuated tubes for microbiology and cytology, and heparinized tubes for chemistry. The type of fluid should be noted on the sample label.

 Technical Tip 16-15. Samples such as synovial (joint), pleural (chest), pericardial (heart), and peritoneal (abdominal) fluids are frequently collected in evacuated tubes corresponding to those used for similar tests performed on blood.

Amniotic Fluid

Amniotic fluid collected from the fetal sac may be tested for the presence of bilirubin, to monitor hemolytic disease of the newborn and lipids, to determine fetal lung maturity. In addition, it may be examined by the cytogenetics section for the presence of abnormal chromosomes. Samples for bilirubin analysis must be protected from light in the same manner as blood samples, and samples for cytogenetic analysis should be delivered immediately for processing to preserve the limited number of cells present. Handling and processing of amniotic fluid varies with the tests requested. Refer to the laboratory procedure manual.

Gastric Fluid

Gastric fluid is tested to determine stomach acid production. Samples are obtained by inserting a gastric tube through the mouth or nose into the stomach. An initial sample is collected and a gastric stimulant, such as histamine, is injected. Subsequent samples are collected at timed intervals. Samples are collected into sterile containers and labeled properly including the time of each collection. The phlebotomist may collect blood samples for gastrin levels concurrently.

Sputum

Sputum is mucus or phlegm collected from the trachea, bronchi, and lungs and is tested for active tuberculosis (TB) and pneumonia. Sputum is obtained by deep coughing to bring the sputum up from the lungs and then expelled into a sterile container. The largest amount of sputum is collected in a first morning sample. Samples should be collected from patients who have abstained from eating, drinking, or smoking. Before collecting the sample, the patient is asked to rinse his or her mouth with water (do not swallow) to minimize contamination with saliva. Samples are immediately delivered to the laboratory and kept at room temperature before processing.

 Technical Tip 16-16. Extreme caution must be followed when collecting and transporting sputum samples that are potentially infectious for active tuberculosis. Instruct the patient to cough away from people and to avoid contaminating the outside of the container.

Buccal Swabs

Cells for DNA analysis may be obtained from a buccal (cheek) swab. The sample is collected by rubbing the inner lining of the cheek for 20 seconds with a sterile Dacron-tipped cotton swab. In the laboratory, the cells collected on the swab are extracted for DNA testing. Often, these samples are collected for legal purposes such as paternity testing; therefore, follow strict COC protocol.

Saliva

Saliva samples can be used to test for HIV antibodies, hormone levels, and drug and alcohol abuse. Advantages of testing saliva are that the detection of drugs and alcohol can be made immediately and the tests are difficult to adulterate. Saliva is a less invasive technique for HIV testing. Several techniques and point-of-care kits are available for collecting and testing saliva.

Hair

Hair samples can detect chronic use of drugs, alcohol, heavy metals, poisons, and toxins. Hair sample testing is becoming more prominent because of the ease of collection and the sample cannot be easily adulterated. Hair samples also may be used for DNA paternity testing.

Breath

The presence of *Helicobacter pylori*, a bacteria that damages the lining of the stomach and causes peptic ulcers, can be detected by the C-urea breath test. The test measures the amount of CO_2 in the patient's breath. A baseline breath sample is collected by breathing into a balloon-like collection device. The patient then ingests urea labeled with a nonradioactive carbon isotope. A second breath sample is then collected. Urease produced by *H. pylori* degrades the urea and produces carbon dioxide, which is absorbed into the bloodstream and exhaled. The carbon dioxide level in the two samples is compared. Increased amounts of carbon in the postingestion sample indicate the presence of *H. pylori* in the stomach.

A hydrogen breath test can be used to diagnose lactose intolerance, overgrowth of bacteria in the small bowel, and the rapid passage of food through the small intestine. Prior to testing, the patient must have fasted for 12 hours. A baseline breath sample is collected by having the patient exhale into a balloon-type collecting device and the amount of hydrogen is measured. The patient ingests a prescribed amount of lactose and breath samples are collected and analyzed for hydrogen every 15 minutes for 3 and up to 5 hours. Increased hydrogen levels indicate a problem with the digestion or absorption of lactose resulting in increased lactose in the intestinal tract, perhaps indicating lactose intolerance.

Breath samples also are used in the detection of alcohol use. Various breath-testing devices are available and are often used by law enforcement.

Tissue Samples

Tissue samples are routinely received in a preservative solution and are processed by the histology section. Samples that are not preserved must be immediately delivered to the histology section. Samples with a large quantity of fluid designated for cytology may also be received.

SAMPLE PROCESSING, ACCESSIONING, AND SHIPPING

In some laboratories, particularly in large hospitals, phlebotomists may be involved in centrifuging, *aliquoting*, and assigning accession numbers or bar codes to specimens before their delivery to the laboratory sections. They may also process and package specimens sent to reference laboratories.

Standard precautions must be strictly followed when processing all samples. In accordance with Occupational Safety and Health Administration (OSHA) regulations, protective apparel must include gloves, fluid-resistant laboratory coats that are completely closed, and goggles or chin-length face shields with protective sides. Samples must never be centrifuged in uncapped tubes.

Sample Processing

Sample processing involving centrifugation and aliquoting is primarily associated with laboratory tests performed on plasma and serum. An instrument, called a centrifuge, spins blood tubes at a high relative centrifugal force to separate serum or plasma from the blood cells. Plasma is obtained by centrifugation of anticoagulated blood, and serum is similarly obtained from clotted blood (Fig. 16-5). To prevent contamination of plasma and serum by cellular constituents, it is recommended that samples be separated within

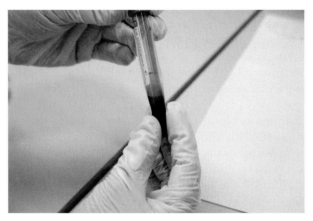

FIGURE 16-5 A centrifuged gel serum tube.

2 hours. Anticoagulated samples can be centrifuged immediately after collection, and the plasma removed. Samples collected without anticoagulant must be fully clotted before centrifugation. Clotting time can vary from 5 minutes, when clot activators are present, to an hour, for samples from patients receiving anticoagulant therapy or when samples have been chilled.

Preexamination Consideration 16-6.

By 2 hours after blood collection significant changes in some analytes, such as decreased glucose, increased potassium, and increased lactate dehydrogenase, are seen in blood that has not been centrifuged.

Preexamination Consideration 16-7.

Fibrin strands in a sample that has not completely clotted can interfere with chemistry analyzers and lead to erroneous results.

Preexamination Consideration 16-8.

Loosening clots from the side of the tube (rimming) before centrifugation is not recommended because it may cause hemolysis.

Technical Tip 16-17. Blood samples should be stored in an upright position while clotting.

Preexamination Consideration 16-9.

Blood tubes must remain closed before, during, and after centrifugation to avoid contamination with dust or glove powder, accidental spills, formation of aerosols, and evaporation of the specimen. Specimen pH increases when the cap is removed and may cause erroneous pH, ionized calcium, and acid phosphatase results.

Centrifugation

In the accessioning area, there are a number of types of centrifuges available, including table models, floor models, and refrigerated models. The relative centrifugal force (RCF) of a centrifuge is expressed as gravity (*g*) and is determined by the radius of the rotor head and the speed of rotation (revolutions per minute [rpm]). Most laboratory samples are centrifuged at 850 to 1000 g for 10 minutes.

Preexamination Consideration 16-10.

Refer to the manufacturer's literature for sample speeds and times of centrifugation for various analytes.

Preexamination Consideration 16-11.

Chilled samples received in the laboratory should be centrifuged in a temperature-controlled centrifuge.

Rules for Centrifugation of Samples

Improper use of the centrifuge can be dangerous, and the following rules of operation must be observed:

1. Tubes placed in the cups of the rotor head must be equally balanced. This is accomplished by placing tubes of equal size and volume directly across from each other. Failure to follow this practice will cause the centrifuge to vibrate and possibly break the tubes. A final check for balancing should be made just before closing the centrifuge lid (Fig. 16-6).
2. A centrifuge should never be operated until the top has been firmly fastened down, and the top should never be opened until the rotor head

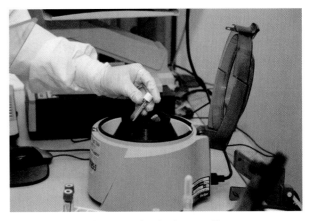

FIGURE 16-6 **Balancing tubes in the centrifuge.**

has come to a complete stop. Should a tube break during centrifugation, pieces of glass and biohazardous aerosols will be sprayed from a centrifuge that is not covered.

3. Do not walk away from a centrifuge until it has reached its designated rotational speed and no evidence of excessive vibration is observed.
4. When a tube breaks in the centrifuge, immediately stop the centrifuge and unplug it before opening the cover. Don puncture-resistant gloves before beginning the cleanup. The cup containing the broken glass must be completely emptied into a puncture-resistant container and disinfected. The inside of the centrifuge must also be cleaned of broken glass and disinfected. Deposit any cleaning materials that may contain broken glass into a puncture-resistant container.
5. Samples should not be recentrifuged. This can cause hemolysis and erroneous tests results. When the serum or plasma has been removed from the tube, the volume ratio of plasma to red blood cells has been altered. Substances from the cellular leakage or exchange, caused by the blood clotting, will then be centrifuged into the serum or plasma and alter test results.

Preexamination Consideration 16–12.
Potassium levels will be falsely increased in recentrifuged samples.

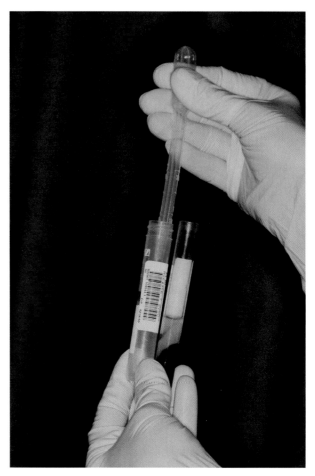
FIGURE 16-7 Using a disposable pipette to transfer a specimen to an aliquot tube.

Sample Aliquoting

Separation of serum and plasma from the cellular elements and sample aliquoting require careful attention to detail so that specimens are placed in properly labeled tubes. An aliquot is a portion of the sample that is placed in a separate tube. Care must also be taken to prevent the formation of aerosols when stoppers are removed from evacuated tubes. As discussed in Chapter 8, stoppers should be covered with gauze and twisted rather than "popped" off. Specimens must never be poured from one tube to another, because this will produce aerosols. Disposable pipettes should be used to transfer the specimen from one tube to another (Fig. 16-7). A Plexiglas shield should be used when aliquoting specimens (Fig. 16-8).

A variety of transfer systems is available. All systems are designed to prevent the formation of aerosols

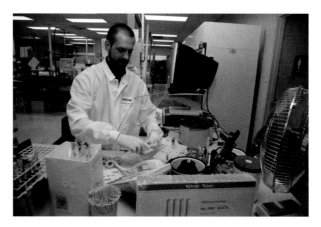
FIGURE 16-8 Sample processing using a plexiglass shield.

and to provide minimum contact with the sample by laboratory personnel. Some automated instruments are equipped to sample directly from the sealed tube.

Specimen Storage

Based on the tests requested, separated serum or plasma may remain at room temperature for 8 hours. If testing has not been completed in 8 hours, the specimen should be refrigerated (2°C to 8°C). If testing is not complete in 48 hours, the serum or plasma should be frozen at or below −20°C. Refer to the procedure manual for specific analyte instructions.

Technical Tip 16-18. Serum can be stored on the gel in gel separator tubes for up to 48 hours at 4°C. Confirm the gel barrier integrity.

Preexamination Consideration 16-13.

Samples collected for electrolytes must not be stored at 2°C to 8°C before centrifugation and testing.

Preexamination Consideration 16-14.

Specimens can only be thawed once. Repeated freezing and thawing of the specimen can destroy substances for testing.

Specimen Shipping

Samples collected from home health care or nursing home patients and samples being transported between laboratories must be appropriately packaged for transport. The United States Department of Transportation regulates the interstate shipping of infectious substances and diagnostic samples and stipulates strict guidelines for packaging and labeling. Many of these requirements can apply to local sample transport.

Samples for local transport should be placed in securely closed, leak-proof primary containers (tubes and screw-top containers). The primary containers are enclosed in a secondary leak-proof container with sufficient absorbent material present to separate the samples and absorb the contents of the

primary containers in case of leakage or breakage. Containers should be labeled as biohazardous. Samples can be kept cool by transporting them in Styrofoam containers using plastic refrigerant packs. Refrigerant packs should not be placed directly on or against sample containers. Samples that must remain frozen are packaged in carbon dioxide permeable containers with dry ice.

When preparing samples for transport to reference laboratories, information provided by the reference laboratory regarding sample stability, type of sample, and volume required must be consulted. Many laboratories contract with a particular reference laboratory that may pick up samples on a daily basis or provide specific packaging materials. Personnel preparing samples for shipping must be sure all samples are properly labeled. Appropriate requisition forms must accompany the specimens. They should be protected from accidental sample contamination.

Samples requiring refrigeration can be shipped in Styrofoam containers with refrigerant packs of ice enclosed in a leak-proof bag. Samples that must remain frozen are packaged in containers with dry ice. Figure 16-9 is an example of packaging and labeling of Category B infectious substances.

USE OF THE LABORATORY COMPUTER

Computers are an essential part of the laboratory. Phlebotomists are in frequent contact with the laboratory computer through the generation of requisitions and sample labels, registration of outpatients, the logging in of samples personally collected or received from other locations, and identification of patients using barcode systems. They should understand the basic components of computer systems, be able to enter and retrieve data, be willing to learn new applications as the laboratory computer system expands, and realize that computers are intended to increase the efficiency and accuracy of patient care.

Most people have some experience using micro- or personal computers in school, in the workplace, or at home. The differences between these computers and laboratory computers are primarily the amount of information that can be processed, the speed of processing, and the ability to transfer information to other computers. Therefore, the actual computer operated by a phlebotomist appears to be no different

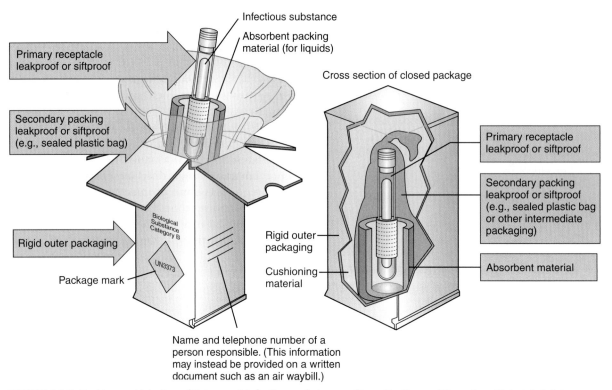

FIGURE 16-9 Packing and labeling of Category B infectious substances. *(From Pipeline and Hazardous Materials Safety Administration, US Department of Transportation.)*

than a familiar school or home model, although it may be connected to a higher-powered mainframe computer for transfer and storage of data. Phlebotomists may use hand-held computers or personal digital assistants (PDAs) for patient identification, test requests, and label printing at the patient's bedside. Point-of-care patient test results from portable hand-held instruments are directly transmitted to patient's charts. Data can be transferred among the laboratory sections or other hospital departments and by computer telephone cable, fiber optics, and wireless radiowave connections to outside agencies such as health-care providers' offices. In many laboratories, employees are assigned computer mailboxes through which they can receive intralaboratory communications, that is, notification of meetings, telephone messages, and procedural changes.

Laboratory Information Systems (LISs)

Many application programs for laboratory use are currently available, and the decision to use a particular program is determined by the requirements of the

laboratory. LISs may be used only by the laboratory or may be integrated into a hospital-wide computer system. Companies that provide LISs work closely with the laboratory staff to adapt the system to correspond with particular laboratory operations. LIS clinical applications include the following:

- Generate laboratory orders
- Print labels for sample collection
- Monitor sample status in the laboratory
- Interface with laboratory analyzers for direct reporting of results and autoverification
- Archive past patient results
- Provide billing of laboratory services
- Provide a mode for result viewing
- Monitor quality control and compliance

Phlebotomists first encounter an LIS through the receipt of computer-generated requisitions and sample labels (Fig. 16-10). They must learn to recognize the information provided, to be sure that it corresponds with the required information discussed in Chapter 9, and to compare this information with the

FIGURE 16-10 Computer requisition with barcode and tube labels.

information on the sample labels. Many computer-generated requisitions also provide the phlebotomist with the number and type of tubes to be collected.

 Technical Tip 16-19. Samples can be tracked through the preprocessing, testing, and eventual storage of the specimen.

Password

Phlebotomists required to input or retrieve data with the computer are assigned a password that allows them to use the computer. The purpose of the password is to provide computer security so that patient data is available only to authorized personnel. Phlebotomists should understand that any computer transaction performed when their password has been used to enter the computer can be traced back to them; therefore, the password should not be given to other persons. New government regulations to protect the privacy of patient health-care records (discussed in Chapter 3) have increased the importance of password protection.

Data Entry

Data are frequently entered or retrieved with computers with the help of codes, which can be numeric (1 = retrieve information) or memory-aiding abbreviations

(mnemonics), such as typing "RI" to retrieve information. The method varies with the system in use. Another method of data entry is the use of barcodes, from which information can be scanned into the computer by a specially designed light source (this method has been used in retail stores for many years) (Fig. 16-11). The black and white stripes of varying width on a barcode correspond to letters and numbers, and are grouped together to represent patient names, identification numbers, and laboratory tests. As discussed earlier, use of barcode systems decreases the possibility of laboratory error caused by clerical mistakes.

Reimbursement Codes

New reimbursement requirements for Medicare and other third-party payers require documentation of the medical necessity of laboratory and other medical procedures. This documentation requires the use of standardized codes by both the health-care provider and the department performing the tests or procedures. Patient conditions or symptoms are classified using the International Classification of Disease, 9th edition (ICD-9), which will continue to be updated. Health-care providers ordering tests primarily on outpatients must provide the ICD-9 code on the request.

Laboratory tests are also coded using Current Procedure Terminology (CPT) codes. For reimbursement purposes, the CPT code (laboratory test) should be consistent with the medical necessity of the ICD-9 code (patient diagnosis). Depending on the institution, phlebotomists may need to enter CPT codes into the computer, particularly when drawing from outpatients.

FIGURE 16-11 Barcode label printer.

Additional Computer Duties

Additional computer duties for phlebotomists may include generation and retrieval of collection lists and schedules, posting of patient charges, computing monthly phlebotomy workloads, and retrieving information for personnel in health-care providers' offices. Figure 16-12 illustrates a typical LIS workflow chart. Because of the variety of laboratory information systems available, the major learning requirement of a technically trained phlebotomist (or other laboratory worker) when entering a new job is usually the operation of the computer system. This can only increase as laboratories expand their computer applications (Fig. 16-13).

 Technical Tip 16-20. All information in the laboratory information system is traceable back to each person who has handled the sample and has significantly reduced errors in identification and documentation.

Test ordered by authorized person
↓
Test request entered into the computer
↓
Accession number assigned
↓
Requisition with labels printed
↓
Specimen collected
↓
Specimen delivered to laboratory
↓
Barcode label scanned
↓
Time of collection and receipt of specimen verified
↓
Test request uploaded to instrument
↓
Status of specimen available for review
↓
Specimen tested
↓
Results verified
↓
Results transmitted to patient chart
↓
Test charges sent to billing department

FIGURE 16-12 Laboratory information system workflow chart.

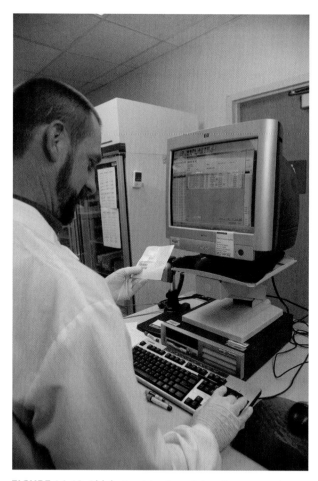

FIGURE 16-13 Phlebotomist using a laboratory computer.

Key Points

✦ Phlebotomists provide instructions and containers to patients for the collection of urine samples for random, first morning, midstream clean-catch, 24-hour (timed), and drug screening. Catheterized or suprapubic urine samples may be delivered to the laboratory.

✦ Phlebotomists provide instructions and containers to patients for the collection of random (used for cultures, ova and parasites, microscopic examination for cells, fats and fibers, and blood) and timed fecal samples (used for fecal fats and urobilinogen).

✦ Semen samples are collected for fertility studies and the effectiveness of a vasectomy. The phlebotomist provides specific instructions to the patient for the collection and transport of the sample to the laboratory. The phlebotomist must record the time of sample collection and delivery on the requisition form.

✦ Throat cultures and nasopharyngeal swabs and wash are collected to diagnose the cause of an acute respiratory infection. Proper collection technique is essential to a quality sample.

✦ Sweat electrolytes are collected for the diagnosis of cystic fibrosis. The sample is collected after pilocarpine iontophoresis is performed to induce sweat. Collection precautions must be taken to prevent contamination or evaporation of the sample.

✦ Phlebotomists may assist the physician in bone marrow aspiration procedures to diagnose blood disorders.

✦ A unit of whole blood collected from a donor is divided into the various components: red blood cells, white blood cells, platelets, plasma, and plasma proteins. The responsibilities of the phlebotomist include donor interview and screening, donor identification, donor informed consent, venipuncture, product collection, postdonation care, and complication management.

✦ Phlebotomists may transport or accept nonblood samples in the laboratory. Samples include CSF, synovial fluid, serous fluid, amniotic fluid, gastric fluid, sputum, saliva, buccal swabs, hair, breath samples, and tissue samples. Refer to the facilities procedure manual for specific collection and processing instructions for each type of sample.

✦ Standard precautions must be strictly adhered to when processing samples and include wearing personal protective equipment (PPE) that includes gloves, fluid-resistant laboratory coats, goggles or face masks, opening sample containers under a Plexiglass shield, transferring aliquot specimens with a disposable pipette, and not pouring from one tube to another.

✦ Plasma and serum must be removed from the cells within 2 hours. Specimens for electrolyte testing should not be chilled.

✦ Rules for centrifuge safety include:
  ✦ Balance tubes equally in the rotor head
  ✦ Always close the centrifuge cover
  ✦ Observe for excessive vibration
  ✦ Immediately stop and unplug the centrifuge when a tube has broken and wear puncture-resistant gloves when cleaning the broken pieces and disinfecting the centrifuge
  ✦ Do not recentrifuge samples

✦ Phlebotomists use a computer LIS to generate requisitions and sample labels, register outpatients, log-in samples personally collected or received from other locations, assign CPT codes, generate and retrieve collection lists and schedules, post patient charges, compute monthly phlebotomy workloads, and retrieve information for personnel in health-care providers' offices.

BIBLIOGRAPHY

American Association of Blood Banks. http://www.aabb.org/Content/Programs_and_Services/Government_Regulatory_Issues/donoreligibility.htm.

CLSI. Body Fluid Analysis for Cellular Composition: Approved Guideline, Clinical and Laboratory Standards Institute, document H56,Vol 26. CLSI, 2006, Wayne, PA.

CLSI. Procedures for the Handling and Processing of Blood Specimens for Common Laboratory Tests; Approved Guideline, ed. 4. CLSI, document H18-A4. CLSI, 2010, Wayne, PA.

Strasinger, SK, and Di Lorenzo, MS: Urinalysis and Body Fluids, ed. 5. FA Davis, 2008, Philadelphia.

Study Questions

1. If a urine sample for routine urinalysis cannot be delivered to the laboratory within 2 hours, how should the sample be stored?
   a. freeze the sample
   b. reject the sample and ask the patient to collect a new one
   c. refrigerate the sample
   d. add a boric acid preservative

2. What urine test would require a patient to collect a midstream clean-catch sample?
   a. culture and sensitivity
   b. pregnancy test
   c. 24-hour protein
   d. drug test

3. Which of the following tests would require a patient to collect a 72-hour fecal sample?
   a. fecal ova and parasites
   b. fecal occult blood
   c. fecal fat analysis
   d. fecal culture and sensitivity

4. All of the following are instructions that a patient must follow in the collection of a semen sample **EXCEPT:**
   a. abstain from sexual activity for 3 days but not longer than 5 days
   b. collect in a condom
   c. place in a warm sterile container
   d. record the time of collection

5. Areas that should be avoided when collecting a throat culture include all of the following **EXCEPT:**
   a. tonsils
   b. cheeks
   c. tongue
   d. lips

6. What type of sample is collected by inserting a flexible mini-tip culture swab through the nose?
   a. gastric
   b. NP
   c. serous fluid
   d. buccal

7. Sweat electrolytes are collected to confirm the diagnosis of:
   a. peptic ulcers
   b. RSV
   c. lactose intolerance
   d. cystic fibrosis

8. Which of the following would disqualify a person in the blood donor selection process?
   a. weight: 220 pounds
   b. hemoglobin: 11.0 g/dL
   c. blood pressure: 160/90 mm Hg
   d. temperature: 98°F

9. CSF samples labeled No. 1, No. 2, and No. 3 are delivered to the laboratory. What section should tube No. 3 be delivered to?
   a. hematology
   b. chemistry
   c. microbiology
   d. serology

10. Bone marrow is collected from the:
    a. femur
    b. lumbar vertebrae
    c. radius
    d. iliac crest

11. Sputum samples are collected to diagnosis:
    a. tuberculosis
    b. endocarditis
    c. strep throat
    d. cystic fibrosis

12. Pleural fluid is collected from the:
    a. heart
    b. lymph node
    c. joint
    d. chest

13. What special handling requirement is necessary for amniotic fluid that is to be tested for hemolytic disease of the newborn?
    a. protected from light
    b. placed in an ice slurry
    c. placed in a warm sterile container
    d. transported via the pneumatic tube system

Study Questions—cont'd

14. Serum or plasma must be separated from cells within:
  a. 30 minutes from collection
  b. 45 minutes from collection
  c. 60 minutes from collection
  d. 120 minutes from collection

15. The phlebotomist would use the LIS to perform all of the following **EXCEPT:**
  a. generate a requisition
  b. print sample labels
  c. check patient results
  d. collect from correct patient

Clinical Situations

1 A patient delivering a 24-hour urine sample to the laboratory mentions that he or she did not save a small amount of urine voided while visiting a neighbor.

  a. What should the patient be told?
  b. How would this affect the test result?

2 A supervisor counsels a phlebotomist because two computer entry errors on the previous day were traced back to the phlebotomist. The phlebotomist states that he or she did not use the computer that day.

  a. How could this have occurred?
  b. How could it be avoided?

3 A phlebotomist delivers Tube No. 1 of a CSF sample to the hematology department and Tube No. 3 to the chemistry department.

  a. Will the hematology result be affected? Explain your answer.
  b. Will the chemistry result be affected? Explain your answer.

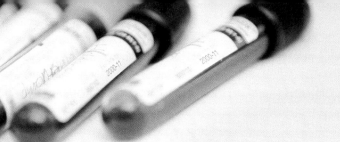
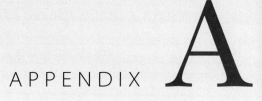

Laboratory Tests and the Required Type of Anticoagulants and Volume of Blood

TEST	COLLECTION TUBE	COMMENTS	DEPT.	CLINICAL CORRELATION
Acid phosphatase	Serum gel barrier tube	Freeze serum	C	Prostate cancer
Adrenocorticotropic hormone (ACTH)	Lavender, siliconized glass or plastic	Freeze plasma	C	Adrenal and pituitary gland function
Alanine aminotransferase (ALT)	Plasma or serum gel barrier tube		C	Liver disorders
Albumin	Serum gel barrier tube		C	Malnutrition or liver disorders
Aldosterone	Red		C	Adrenal function
Alkaline phosphatase (ALP)	Serum or plasma gel barrier tube		C	Bone disorders
Ammonia (NH_3)	Lavender	Send on ice slurry	C	Hepatic encephalopathy
Amylase	Serum or plasma gel barrier tube		C	Pancreatitis
Antibiotic assay (amikacin, gentamicin, theophylline, tobramycin, vancomycin)	Red; clear non-gel Microtainer	No gel barrier tubes	C	Broad-spectrum antibiotics
Antibody ID/screen	Lavender or pink	Blood bank ID	BB	Blood transfusion
Antidiuretic hormone (ADH)	Lavender	Freeze plasma	C	Pituitary function
Anti-hepatitis B surface antigen	Serum gel barrier tube; red		S	Immunity to hepatitis B

Continued

TEST	COLLECTION TUBE	COMMENTS	DEPT.	CLINICAL CORRELATION
Anti-hepatitis C virus	Serum gel barrier tube; red		S	Viral hepatitis
Anti-HIV	Red		S	Human immuno-deficiency virus
Antinuclear antibody (ANA)	Serum gel barrier tube; red		S	Systemic lupus erythematosus/ autoimmune disorders
Antistreptolysin O (ASO) titer	Red; serum gel barrier tube		S	Rheumatic fever
Antithrombin III	Light blue		CO	Coagulation disorders
Apo-A, Apo-B lipoprotein	Serum gel barrier tube		C	Cardiac risk
Aspartate aminotransferase (AST)	Plasma or serum gel barrier tube		C	Liver disorders, cardiac muscle damage
Beta human chorionic gonadotropin (Beta HCG)	Plasma or serum gel barrier tube		C	Pregnancy, testicular cancer
Blood culture	Blood culture bottles, yellow SPS tubes	Aseptic technique	M	Septicemia
Blood group and type (ABO and Rh)	Lavender or pink	Blood bank ID	BB	ABO group and Rh factor
Blood urea nitrogen (BUN)	Plasma or serum gel barrier tube		C	Kidney disorders
Bilirubin, total and direct (Bili)	Plasma or serum gel barrier tube; amber or green Microtainer	Protect from light	C	Liver disorders and hemolytic disorders
Brain natriuretic peptide (BNP)	Lavender; white plasma preparation tube, serum gel barrier tube	Stable for 4 hours	C	Congestive heart failure
Calcium	Plasma or serum gel barrier tube		C	Bone disorders
C-reactive protein (CRP)	Serum gel barrier tube		C	Inflammatory disorders
Chemistry panels (renal, hepatic, comprehensive, metabolic)	Plasma or serum gel barrier tube		C	Evaluates various organ systems

TEST	COLLECTION TUBE	COMMENTS	DEPT.	CLINICAL CORRELATION
Cholesterol	Plasma or serum gel barrier tube		C	Coronary artery disease
Creatine kinase (CK)	Plasma or serum gel barrier tube		C	Myocardial infarction, muscle damage
Creatine kinase isoenzymes (CK-MB, CK-MM, CK-BB)	Plasma or serum gel barrier tube		C	Myocardial infarction, muscle damage, brain damage
Cold agglutinins	Serum gel barrier tube	Must be kept at 37°C	S	Atypical pneumonia
Complement levels	Serum gel barrier tube		C	Immune system function/ autoimmune disorders
Complete blood count (CBC)	Lavender		H	Anemia, infection, leukemia, or bleeding disorders
Cortisol	Serum gel barrier tube; red	Serum only Timed specimen	C	Adrenal cortex function
Creatinine (Creat)	Plasma or serum gel barrier tube		C	Kidney disorders
Crossmatch	Lavender; pink	Blood bank ID remains on 72 hours	BB	Blood compatibility
Digoxin	Plasma or serum gel barrier tube; red		C	Heart stimulant
D-Dimer (DDI)	Light blue	Tube must be full (stable for 4 hours)	CO	DIC and thrombotic disorders
Direct anti-human globulin test (DAT) or direct Coombs	Lavender		BB	Anemia or hemolytic disease of the newborn
Disseminated intravascular coagulation panel (DIC)	Light blue		CO	Coagulation/fibrinolytic systems
Electrolytes (lytes)	Plasma or serum gel barrier tube		C	Fluid and acid-base balance
Ethanol/alcohol (ETOH)	Gray; red; plasma gel barrier tube	Do not open tube until testing; may require chain of custody	C	Intoxication
Fibrin degradation products (FDP)	Special light blue tube with thrombin	Tube will only fill to 2 mL and should clot immediately	CO	Disseminated intravascular coagulation

Continued

TEST	COLLECTION TUBE	COMMENTS	DEPT.	CLINICAL CORRELATION
Fibrinogen	Light blue	Tube must be full	C	Coagulation disorders
Fluorescent antinuclear antibody (FANA)	Serum gel barrier tube; red		S	Systemic lupus erythematosus/ autoimmune disorders
Fluorescent treponemal antibody-absorbed (FTA-ABS)	Serum gel barrier tube; red		S	Syphilis
Folate	Serum gel barrier tube		C	Anemia
Gastrin	Serum gel barrier tube		C	Gastric malignancy
Glucose (FBS)	Plasma or serum gel barrier tube; red; gray		C	Hypoglycemia or diabetes mellitus
Hemoglobin electrophoresis	Lavender		C	Hemoglobin abnormalities
Hemoglobin/ hematocrit (H&H); Hgb/Hct	Lavender		H	Anemia
Hepatitis panels	Serum gel barrier tube; red		C	
Human chorionic gonadotropin (Beta HCG)	Plasma or serum gel barrier tube		C	Pregnancy, testicular tumor
Immunoglobulin levels	Red; plasma or serum gel barrier tube		C	Immune system function
Insulin	Serum gel barrier tube		C	Glucose metabolism and pancreatic function
Ionized calcium (iCA^{2+})	Serum gel barrier tube; red; arterial blood gas syringe	Tube must be full; may use arterial blood gas syringe	C	Follow-up test for abnormal total calcium results
Iron	Plasma or serum gel barrier tube		C	Anemia
Lactate dehydrogenase (LD)	Plasma or serum gel barrier tube		C	Myocardial infarction
Lactate (lactic acid) (Lact)	Plasma gel barrier tube; arterial blood gas syringe	Send in ice; analyze in 15 minutes Draw without tourniquet	C	Muscle disorders
Lead (Pb)	Royal blue EDTA; tan EDTA; lavender Microtainer		C	Neurological function

TEST	COLLECTION TUBE	COMMENTS	DEPT.	CLINICAL CORRELATION
Lipase	Plasma or serum gel barrier tube; red		C	Pancreatitis
Lipoproteins (high-density lipoprotein [HDL], low-density lipoprotein [LDL], very-low density lipoprotein [VLDL])	Plasma or serum gel barrier tube		C	Coronary risk
Lithium (Li)	Serum gel barrier tube; red	Draw 12 hours post dose	C	Antidepressant drug monitoring
Magnesium	Plasma or serum gel barrier tube		C	Musculoskeletal disorders
MI panel (myoglobin, creatine kinase isoenzyme, troponin) (Myo, CK-MB, T)	Plasma gel barrier tube; white plasma preparation tube	Stable 4 hours; EDTA plasma from a lavender top tube or a white PPT	C	Myocardial infarction
Mononucleosis screen (Mono test)	Serum gel barrier tube; red		S	Infectious mononucleosis
pH	Green; non gel	Send on ice slurry	C	Acid-base balance
Parathyroid hormone (PTH)	Lavender		C	Parathyroid function
Partial thromboplastin time (PTT); activated partial thromboplastin time (APTT)	Light blue	Full tube; nonheparinized samples are stable at RT up to 4 hours; heparinized samples must be centrifuged within 1 hour and are stable up to 4 hours	CO	Heparin therapy and coagulation disorders
Phosphorus	Plasma or serum gel barrier tube		C	Endocrine and bone disorders
Platelet (Plt)	Lavender		H	Bleeding disorders
Potassium	Plasma or serum gel barrier tube; red		C	Muscle function, heart contraction/cardiac output
Prostate-specific antigen (PSA)	Serum gel barrier tube		C	Prostatic cancer
Prostatic acid phosphatase (PAP)	Serum gel barrier tube		C	Prostatic cancer
Protein electrophoresis	Serum gel barrier tube; red		C	Multiple myeloma/abnormal proteins

Continued

TEST	COLLECTION TUBE	COMMENTS	DEPT.	CLINICAL CORRELATION
Prothrombin time (PT)	Light blue	Full tube; stable at RT up to 24 hours	CO	Coumadin therapy and coagulation disorders
Quant proteins (C3, C4, IgG, IgA, IgM), haptoglobin	Plasma or serum gel barrier tube; red		S	Immunoglobulin disorders, hemolytic anemia
Reticulocyte count (Retic)	Lavender		H	Bone marrow function
Rheumatoid arthritis (RA)	Serum gel barrier tube; red		S	Rheumatoid arthritis
Rubella titer	Serum gel barrier tube; red		S	Immunity to German measles
Sedimentation rate (ESR)	Lavender		H	Inflammatory disorders
Sickle cell screening	Lavender		H	Sickle cell anemia
T-cell count	Lavender		S	Immune function/HIV monitoring
Testosterone	Serum gel barrier tube		C	Testicular function
Therapeutic drugs (digoxin, theo-phylline [theo], phenobarbital, phenytoin [Pheny], carbamazepine [Carb], valproic acid [val ac])	Red; clear non-gel Microtainer	No gel barrier; centrifuge and separate within 1 hour	C	Monitor medications for seizures, bipolar disorders, epilepsy, asthma
Thyroid-stimulating hormone/Free T4 (TSH/T4)	Plasma or serum gel barrier tube		C	Thyroid conditions
Total protein (TP)	Serum gel barrier tube		C	Kidney and liver disorders
Triglycerides	Plasma or serum gel barrier tube		C	Coronary heart disease
Troponin I and T	Serum gel barrier tube; lavender; white plasma preparation tube		C	Myocardial function
Type and screen	Lavender/pink	Blood bank ID	BB	Blood transfusion
Uric acid	Plasma or serum gel barrier tube		C	Kidney disorders, gout
Venereal Disease Research Laboratory (VDRL)	Serum gel barrier tube; red		S	Syphilis

TEST	COLLECTION TUBE	COMMENTS	DEPT.	CLINICAL CORRELATION
Viral load	Lavender; white plasma preparation tube; serum gel barrier tube	Freeze plasma immediately	S	HIV monitoring
Vitamin B_{12}	Plasma or serum gel barrier tube; red	Protect from light	C	Anemia
Vitamin D	Serum gel barrier tube		C	Calcium absorption
Western blot	Red		S	Human immunodeficiency virus
White blood cell count (WBC)	Lavender		H	Infection or leukemia

Lab department codes: BB = blood bank; C = chemistry; CO = coagulation; H = hematology; M = microbiology; S = serology. ID = identification; RT = room temperature sodioum polyanethol sulfonate.
*Follow evacuated tubes manufacturer's instructions when using gel barrier tubes for serology tests.

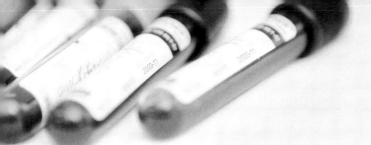
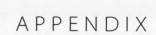

Answers to Study Questions

CHAPTER 1

1. a
2. a
3. c
4. c
5. d
6. d
7. a
8. d
9. b
10. b
11. d
12. b

CHAPTER 2

1. b
2. a
3. b
4. c
5. a
6. c
7. c
8. d
9. b
10. a
11. b
12. d

CHAPTER 3

1. d
2. b
3. d
4. a
5. c
6. a
7. a
8. b
9. d
10. a
11. d
12. c

CHAPTER 4

1. a
2. c
3. d
4. c
5. a
6. c
7. d
8. a
9. b
10. d
11. b
12. a
13. d
14. b
15. c

CHAPTER 5

1. b
2. a
3. d
4. b
5. b
6. d
7. c
8. a
9. b
10. d

CHAPTER 6

1. c, e, d, a, b
2. c
3. a
4. a
5. b
6. d
7. a
8. b
9. b
10. b
11. d
12. a
13. c
14. d, e, a, c, b

CHAPTER 7

1. c
2. a
3. d
4. d
5. a
6. d
7. d
8. d
9. d
10. c, d, b, e, a
11. c, d, a, a, b, c
12. c, c, d, b, d, a

CHAPTER 8

1. d
2. d
3. a
4. b
5. d
6. a
7. a
8. d
9. c
10. d

CHAPTER 9

1. d
2. d
3. a
4. c
5. a
6. b
7. a
8. d
9. b
10. c

CHAPTER 10

1. d
2. d
3. b
4. 5, 1, 2, 4, 3
5. d
6. a
7. d
8. c
9. b
10. b
11. b
12. c
13. c
14. d
15. d

CHAPTER 11

1. c
2. c
3. c
4. b
5. c
6. b
7. a
8. b
9. d
10. c
11. d
12. c

CHAPTER 12

1. c
2. d
3. a
4. b
5. c
6. a
7. b
8. d
9. a
10. c
11. d

CHAPTER 13

1. c
2. d
3. d
4. c
5. c
6. d
7. b
8. c
9. a
10. c
11. c
12. b

CHAPTER 14

1. c
2. b
3. a
4. d
5. b
6. d
7. c
8. a
9. c
10. d

CHAPTER 15

1. c
2. a
3. c
4. d
5. a
6. b
7. b
8. c
9. c
10. d

CHAPTER 16

1. c
2. a
3. c
4. b
5. a
6. b
7. d
8. b
9. a
10. d
11. a
12. d
13. a
14. d
15. d

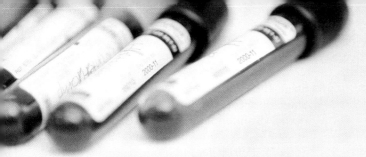

Answers to Clinical Situations

CHAPTER 1

1. a. Phlebotomists may be transferred to other areas such as the emergency department, outpatient services, and off-site collection areas in physician office buildings.
   b. Phlebotomists may be trained to perform basic patient-care tasks, point-of-care testing, and clerical duties.
   c. To increase efficiency and cost effectiveness by eliminating the need for health-care personnel to travel from a central testing area to the patient's room and then back to the testing area.
   d. Nurses, respiratory therapists, radiology technologists, and other patient-care personnel
2. a. The person answering the phone did not ask the patient if this was an emergency before putting the patient on hold.
   b. The person answering the phone did not repeat the request back to the caller or did not tell the phlebotomist what the actual request was.
   c. The phlebotomist was not observing the patient confidentiality rules.
   d. The instructions were not understood by the patient. Written instructions should have been given in the patient's native language.

CHAPTER 2

1. a. Enroll in an accredited 2-year associate degree medical laboratory technician program.
   b. Transfer the associate degree credits to an accredited 4-year baccalaureate program in clinical laboratory science.

   c. This person would have additional qualifications to become a department supervisor.
   d. Courses in administration or business that could apply to a Master's degree.
2. a. Acceptable—Urine specimens that cannot be tested within 1 or 2 hours should be preserved by refrigeration.
   b. Not acceptable—Cytologists, not histology technicians, examine Pap smears.
   c. Not acceptable—The gel interferes with the antigen-antibody reaction.
   d. Acceptable—If the specimen was a clean-catch specimen collected in a sterile container.
   e. Acceptable—It is a CLIA-waived test.
   f. Not acceptable—It must go to hematology.

CHAPTER 3

1. a. Yes, it is a breach of confidentiality (invasion of privacy).
   b. No, the results can only be released to the patient's health-care provider.
   c. Only with the patient's written consent.
2. a. Assault
   b. Negligence
   c. Slander
   d. Invasion of privacy

CHAPTER 4

1. a. Nosocomial
   b. The phlebotomist (gloves)
   c. The patients
   d. Direct contact

2. a. <u>PT</u> Only necessary equipment is brought into the room.
   b. <u>P</u> Sterile gloves are worn.
   c. <u>T</u> PPE is removed and disposed of inside the room.
   d. <u>PT</u> Duplicate tubes are taken into the room.
   e. <u>T</u> Specimens may require double bagging.
   f. <u>P</u> Equipment taken into the room is taken out of the room.
3. a. Proper training on the use of the safety device should have occurred before use.
   b. Immediately wash the site and report the incident to a supervisor so that a confidential medical examination can be started.
   c. Baseline blood tests for HBV, HCV, and HIV.
   d. When the source patient tests positive for HIV or HBV, within 24 hours.

CHAPTER 5

1. a. Immediately
   b. To rule out heart disease
   c. Not enough blood was drawn to perform the test
   d. Cardiovascular
   e. Phleb: vein; tom: cut; ist: specialist
2. a. Complete blood count; emergency department; lower right quadrant; fever of unknown origin; nothing taken by mouth
   b. An inflammation of the appendix
   c. Increased white blood cells with increased neutrophils

CHAPTER 6

1. a. Skeletal; b. Reproductive; c. Urinary; d. Lymphatic
2. a. Digestive; b. Reproductive; c. Respiratory; d. Digestive

CHAPTER 7

1. a. anti-B
   b. Groups A and O
   c. Groups A and AB
2. 1. Pulse; 2. Blood pressure

3. Stage 1: Bleeding time, platelet count
   Stage 2: Prothrombin time (PT), activated partial thromboplastin time (APTT)
   Stage 3: Thrombin time, fibrinogen level
   Stage 4: Fibrin degradation products (FDP), D-dimer test

CHAPTER 8

1. a. Theophylline level
   b. Red stopper tube
   c. It contains serum separator gel to prevent cellular contamination.
   d. The instrument methodology required plasma and not serum.
2. a. The tube was underfilled because a discard tube was not used to prime the winged blood collection tubing.
   b. The specimen was hemolyzed during the blood transfer process.
   c. The lavender stopper tubes are past their expiration date.
3. a. No, because EDTA interferes with factor V and the thrombin-fibrinogen reaction.
   b. No, because the sodium fluoride in the gray stopper tube will interfere with some enzyme analyses.
   c. The pink or lavender stopper tube.

CHAPTER 9

1. a. Improper patient identification.
   Tourniquet was not released while assembling the equipment and cleansing the site.
   Labeling the tube before blood collection.
   Blowing on the site to dry the alcohol.
   b. 1. The wrong patient may have been drawn or the wrong labeled tube used that could cause treatment errors based on the lab results.
      2. Hemoconcentration might cause the high molecular weight analytes to have erroneous results because the tourniquet was on too long.
      3. Microbes could be introduced into the site because the phlebotomist contaminated the site by blowing on it.

2. a. The phlebotomist should have been given the requisition and the labels.
   b. The secretary assumed all cancer patients were the same. The phlebotomist should have asked for the requisition to compare with the labels and the patient's identity.
   c. The patient's treatment was delayed and required the patient to return for another venipuncture.
   d. Poor customer service—patient anxiety and dissatisfaction
3. a. PT and glucose
   b. Potassium
   c. Cells must be separated from plasma and serum within 2 hours.

CHAPTER 10

1. a. On which side did you have the mastectomy?
   b. Lymphedema, infection
   c. Increased blood level of lymphocytes
   d. Contamination of specimen with waste products contained in the lymph fluid
2. a. The specimen contained small clots.
   b. The phlebotomist was busy with the patient and did not mix the specimen.
   c. Yes. Use one hand to mix the specimen as soon as the patient's head was lowered.
3. a. Try another light blue stopper tube and if unsuccessful request another phlebotomist to collect the specimen.
   b. Slowly advance the needle into the vein if the needle is only partially in the lumen of the vein.
   c. Pull back on a needle that may have gone through the vein.

CHAPTER 11

1. a. When was the last time the patient had anything to eat or drink?
   b. Cholesterol, triglycerides
   c. The patient should have been instructed to come to the lab early in the morning after a 12-hour fast.

2. a. Yes. The concentration of microorganisms fluctuates and is highest before the patient's temperature spikes.
   b. When the blood is collected using a winged blood collection set, the anaerobic bottle is inoculated second so that air does not enter the bottle.
   c. Improper site cleansing when the first set was drawn
   d. False-negative culture
3. a. A hematoma is forming because of the decreased collagen and elasticity in aging veins.
   b. Immediately remove the tourniquet and needle and put pressure on the site.
   c. Use a 23-gauge needle with a winged blood collection set attached to a syringe.

CHAPTER 12

1. a. The alcohol should be allowed to dry and the first drop of blood wiped away.
   b. Scraping the skin will cause hemolysis.
   c. Yes—Blood from a second puncture should be placed in a separate container to avoid microclots and hemolysis.
2. a. Yes—The red top Microtainers could have been collected first.
   b. The platelets will adhere to the puncture site producing a falsely low platelet count if the lavender Microtainer is not collected first.
   c. Excessive squeezing of the heel or scraping the Microtainer against the heel.
3. a. Specimen was exposed to light.
   b. Collect in an amber tube or cover tube with aluminum foil and notify chemistry technologists.
   c. Bilirubin is very sensitive to light and deteriorates quickly.

CHAPTER 13

1. a. Reason: Personnel from that unit are not ordering routine requests causing them to be ordered stat.
   Corrective action: Consult with the nursing supervisor to monitor the time between physician's orders and requisition generation.

b. Reason: Phlebotomists are not obtaining the right specimen or adequate volume of specimen, failing to completely read the requisition form, or missing requisitions printed in the laboratory prior to sweeps.

Corrective action: Provide additional training for phlebotomists that are not collecting specimens efficiently.

c. Reason: Specimens are hemolyzed.

Corrective action: Observe technique and provide continuing education to the staff illustrating ways to avoid hemolyzed specimens.

d. Reason: The phlebotomist has too many requests for blood draws at the same time.

Corrective action: Schedule additional phlebotomists for that time, rearrange scheduling patterns.

2. a. Monitoring of refrigerator or freezer temperatures
   b. Centrifuge calibration
3. Document the time of the call and the name of the person receiving the results.

CHAPTER 14

1. a. Collect the specimen 20 to 30 minutes after the patient has refrained from exercise and been reconnected to the bedside oxygen system to ensure the patient will be in a steady state.
   b. Indicate on the requisition the amount of oxygen the patient is receiving and the type of ventilation device in use.
2. a. The color of the blood
   b. Yes—The specimen may be venous rather than arterial blood.
   c. The P_{O_2} would be falsely decreased and the P_{CO_2} would be falsely in increased.
3. a. The color of the blood
   b. Brachial artery
   c. The phlebotomist should apply pressure for at least 5 minutes
   d. A hematoma

CHAPTER 15

1. a. Rerun the quality control—Repeat the fingerstick and repeat the glucose test.
   b. Insufficient specimen applied to testing strip
   Defective testing strip
   Instrument not correctly calibrated
2. a. No
   b. Rerun the QC.
   Test a new abnormal high control.
   c. Outdated reagent test strips
   Discolored reagent test strips
   Contaminated strips
   Test strips and analyzer code number don't match.
   Control is outdated or contaminated.
3. a. Bacteria in the specimen have multiplied.
   b. It should have been refrigerated.

CHAPTER 16

1. a. The patient must obtain a new specimen.
   b. Quantitative test results would be erroneously low.
2. a. Someone else used the phlebotomist's password to enter the computer.
   b. Passwords should not be given to other people.
3. a. Yes—The cell count could be higher due to contamination from cells entering the needle as it passes through the body to the spinal canal.
   b. No, the small amount of cells in the needle would not interfere with the chemistry results.

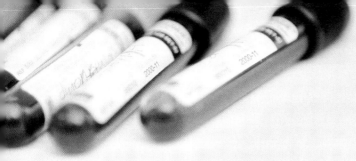

Abbreviations

AABB	American Association of Blood Banks
Ab	Antibody
ABGs	Arterial blood gases
ABO	Blood group
ACD	Acid citrate dextrose
ACT	Activated clotting time
ACTH	Adrenocorticotropic hormone
ADA	American Diabetes Association
ADH	Antidiuretic hormone
AFB	Acid-fast bacteria
Ag	Antigen
AHA	American Hospital Association
AIDS	Acquired immunodeficiency syndrome
ALP	Alkaline phosphatase
ALS	Amyotrophic lateral sclerosis
ALT	Alanine aminotransferase
AMT	American Medical Technologists
ANA	Antinuclear antibody
ANS	Autonomic nervous system
APTT (PTT)	Activated partial thromboplastin time
ARD	Antimicrobial removal device
ASAP	As soon as possible
ASCLS	American Society for Clinical Laboratory Science
ASCP	American Society for Clinical Pathology
ASO	Antistreptolysin O
ASPT	American Society of Phlebotomy Technicians
AST	Aspartate aminotransferase
AV	Atrioventricular
BaE	Barium enema
BB	Blood bank
bid	Twice a day
BNP	Brain natriuretic peptide
BP	Blood pressure
BSI	Body substance isolation
BT	Bleeding time
BUN	Blood urea nitrogen
Bx	Biopsy
C & S	Culture and sensitivity
Ca	Calcium

CAP	College of American Pathologists
CAT/CT scan	Computerized axial tomography
CBC	Complete blood count
CBGs	Capillary blood gases
CCU	Cardiac care unit
CDC	Centers for Disease Control and Prevention
CE	Continuing Education
CEA	Carcinoembryonic antigen
CEO	Chief Executive Officer
CEU	Continuing education unit
CFO	Chief Financial Officer
CHF	Congestive heart failure
CK	Creatine kinase
CK-BB, MB, MM	Creatine kinase isoenzymes
Cl	Chloride
CLSI	Clinical and Laboratory Standards Institute
cm	Centimeter
CMS	Centers for Medicare and Medicaid Services
CMV	Cytomegalovirus
CNA	Certified Nursing Assistant
CNS	Central nervous system
CO_2	Carbon dioxide
COC	Chain of custody
COLA	Commission on Laboratory Assessment
COPD	Chronic obstructive pulmonary disease
CPR	Cardiopulmonary resuscitation
CPT	Certified Phlebotomy Technician
CPT	Current Procedural Terminology
CQI	Continuous quality improvement
CRP	C-reactive protein
CSF	Cerebrospinal fluid
CT	Cytologist
ctO_2	Oxygen content
CTS	Carpal tunnel syndrome
CVA	Cerebrovascular accident
CVAD	Central venous access device
CVS	Chorionic villus sampling
Cx	Cervix
DAT	Direct antihuman globulin test
DI	Diabetes insipidus
DIC	Disseminated intravascular coagulation
Diff	Differential
DM	Diabetes mellitus
DNR	Do not resuscitate
DOA	Dead on arrival
DOB	Date of birth
DRG	Diagnosis-related group
Dx	Diagnosis
ECG/EKG	Electrocardiogram
ED	Emergency department
EDTA	Ethylenediaminetetra-acetic acid

EEG	Electroencephalogram
EIA	Enzyme immunoassay
EMG	Electromyogram
EMLA	Eutectic mixture of local anesthetics
EQC	Electronic quality control
ESR	Erythrocyte sedimentation rate
ETS	Evacuated tube system
FANA	Fluorescent antinuclear antibody
FDA	Food and Drug Administration
FDP	Fibrin degradation product
FIO_2	Fraction of inspired oxygen
FMS	Fibromyalgia syndrome
FSH	Follicle-stimulating hormone
FTA-ABS	Fluorescent treponemal antibody—absorbed
FUO	Fever of unknown origin
Fx	Fracture
g	Gravitational force
g, gm	Gram
GGT	Gamma glutamyl transferase
GH	Growth hormone
GI	Gastrointestinal
GTT	Glucose tolerance test
HAI	Health-care acquired infection
HBIG	Hepatitis B immune globulin
HB_sAg	Hepatitis B surface antigen
HBV	Hepatitis B virus
HCG	Human chorionic gonadotropin
HCl	Hydrochloric acid
HCO_3	Bicarbonate
Hct	Hematocrit
HCV	Hepatitis C virus
HDL	High-density lipoprotein
HDN	Hemolytic disease of the newborn
Hgb	Hemoglobin
HICPAC	Hospital Infection Control Practices Advisory Committee
HIPAA	Health Insurance Portability and Accountability Act of 1996
HIV	Human immunodeficiency virus
HLA	Human leukocyte antigen
HMO	Health maintenance organization
HT	Histology technician
HTL	Histology technologist
Hx	History
ICD-9	International Classification of Disease, 9th Edition
ICU	Intensive care unit
Ig	Immunoglobulin
IM	Intramuscular
IM	Infectious mononucleosis
INR	International normalized ratio
IOM	Institute of Medicine
IRDS	Infant respiratory distress syndrome
ISO	International Standardization Organization

IV	Intravenous
IVP	Intravenous pyelogram
JC	Joint Commission
K	Potassium
K_2EDTA	Dipotassium ethylenediaminetetra-acetic acid
K_3EDTA	Tripotassium ethylenediaminetetra-acetic acid
kg	Kilogram
KOH	Potassium hydroxide
L & D	Labor and delivery
LD	Lactic dehydrogenase
LDL	Low-density lipoprotein
LH	Luteinizing hormone
Li	Lithium
LIS	Laboratory information system
LLQ	Left lower quadrant
L/M	Liters per minute
LP	Lumbar puncture
LPN	Licensed Practical Nurse
LUQ	Left upper quadrant
Lytes	Electrolytes
MCH	Mean corpuscular hemoglobin
MCHC	Mean corpuscular hemoglobin concentration
MCV	Mean corpuscular volume
MD	Muscular dystrophy
mg	Milligram
Mg	Magnesium
MI	Myocardial infarction
mL	Milliliter
MLS	Medical Laboratory Scientist
MLT	Medical Laboratory Technician
mm	Millimeter
mm Hg	Millimeters of mercury
MRI	Magnetic resonance imaging
MS	Multiple sclerosis
MSDS	Material Safety Data Sheet
MSH	Melanocyte-stimulating hormone
Na	Sodium
NB	Newborn
NFPA	National Fire Protection Association
NHA	National Healthcareers Association
NIH	National Institutes of Health
NIOSH	National Institute of Occupational Safety and Health
NP	Nasopharyngeal
NPA	National Phlebotomy Association
NPO	Nothing by mouth
O & P	Ova and parasites
O_2	Oxygen
O_2Sat	Oxygen saturation
OGTT	Oral glucose tolerance test
OP	Outpatient
OR	Operating room

OSHA	Occupational Safety and Health Administration
OT	Occupational therapy
P	Phosphorus
Pap	Papanicolaou stain for cervical cancer
PAP	Prostatic acid phosphatase
PBT	Phlebotomy Technician
P_{CO_2}	Partial pressure of carbon dioxide
PEP	Postexposure prophylaxis
PET scan	Positron emission tomography
PF3	Platelet factor 3
PFT	Pulmonary function test
pH	Negative log of the hydrogen ion concentration (less than 7 is acid and above 7 is alkaline)
PICC	Peripherally inserted central catheter
PID	Pelvic inflammatory disease
PKU	Phenylketonuria
Plt	Platelet
PMS	Premenstrual syndrome
PNS	Peripheral nervous system
P_{O_2}	Partial pressure of oxygen
POCT	Point-of-care testing
POL	Physician office laboratory
post-op	After surgery
pp	Postprandial
PPD	Purified protein derivative
PPE	Personal protective equipment
PPMP	Provider-performed microscopy procedures
PPT	Plasma preparation tube
pre-op	Before surgery
PRL	Prolactin
PRN	Allowable as needed
PSA	Prostate-specific antigen
PST	Plasma separator tube
PT	Physical therapy
PT	Prothrombin time
PTH	Parathyroid hormone
q	Every
QA	Quality assessment
QC	Quality control
qh	Every hour
qid	Four times a day
QMS	Quality management system
QNS	Quantity nonsufficient
QSE	Quality system essential
RA	Rheumatoid arthritis
RBC	Red blood cell
RCF	Relative centrifugal force
RDS	Respiratory distress syndrome
RDW	Red cell distribution width
Retic	Reticulocyte
RF	Rheumatoid factor

RFID	Radio frequency identification
Rh	The D (Rhesus) antigen on red blood cells
RIA	Radioimmunoassay
RLQ	Right lower quadrant
RN	Registered Nurse
R/O	Rule out
rpm	Revolutions per minute
RPR	Rapid plasma reagin
RPT	Registered Phlebotomy Technician
RSV	Respiratory syncytial virus
RUQ	Right upper quadrant
Rx	Prescription/treatment
SA	Sinoatrial
SG	Specific gravity
SLE	Systemic lupus erythematosus
SOB	Shortness of breath
SP	Standard precautions
SPS	Sodium polyanethol sulfonate
SST	Serum separator tube
stat	Immediately
STD	Sexually transmitted disease
T & C	Type and crossmatch
T_3	Triiodothyronine
T_4	Thyroxine
TAT	Turn-around time
TB	Tuberculosis
TC	Throat culture
TC/HDL	Total cholesterol/high-density lipoprotein
TcB	Transcutaneous bilirubin
TDM	Therapeutic drug monitoring
TIBC	Total iron binding capacity
TP	Total protein
tPA	Tissue plasminogen activator
TPN	Total parenteral nutrition (IV feeding)
TPR	Temperature, pulse, respiration
TQM	Total quality management
TSH	Thyroid-stimulating hormone
TSS	Toxic shock syndrome
TT	Thrombin time
Tx	Treatment
UA	Routine urinalysis
μL	Microliter
URI	Upper respiratory infection
UTI	Urinary tract infection
UV	Ultraviolet
VDRL	Venereal Disease Research Laboratory
VLDL	Very low density lipoprotein
WBC	White blood cell
WHO	World Health Organization
ZDV	Zidovudine

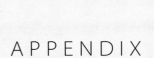

English-Spanish Phrases for Phlebotomy

ENGLISH PHRASE	SPANISH PHRASE	SPANISH PRONUNCIATION
Hello	*Hola*	(O-lah)
Good morning	*Buenos días*	(Bway-nos DEE-as)
Good afternoon	*Buenas tardes*	(Bway-nas TAR-des)
Good evening	*Buenas noches*	(Bway-nas NO-ches)
Mr.	*Señor*	(say-NYOR)
Mrs.	*Señora*	(say-NYO-rah)
Miss	*Señorita*	(say-nyo-REE-tah)
Please	*Por favor*	(por fah-VOR)
Thank you	*Gracias*	(GRAH-see-as)
You're welcome	*De nada*	(de NA-da)
Okay	*Muy bien*	(MU-e-byan)
My name is…	*Me llamo …* *or* *mi nombre es…*	(may-YAH-mo…) or (mee NOHM-bray es…)
I am from the laboratory.	*Soy del laboratorio.* *or* *Trabajo en el laboratorio.*	(soy dal lah-bo-rah-TOH-ree-o.) or (tra-BA-ho en el lah-bo-rah-TOH-ree-o.)
Your doctor has ordered some tests.	*Su médico [or doctor] ha ordenado unos análisises de laboratorio.*	(Soo MEH-dee-co ah or-de-NAH-doe OON-os ah-NAH-lee-sees de lah-bo-rah-TOH-ree-o)
I have to take some blood for testing.	*Tengo que sacarle sangre para un análisis.*	(TENG-go keh sah-CAR-leh SANG-gray PAH-rah oon ah-NAH-lee-sees.)
Please have a seat here.	*Por favor siéntese aqui.*	(por fa-VOR see-EN-tay-say a-KEY.)
What is your name?	*¿Cómo se llama usted?* *or* *¿Cuál es su nombre?*	(CO-mo say YA-ma oo-STED?) or (KWAL es soo nom-BRAY?)

Continued

May I see your identification bracelet?	*¿Puedo ver su brazalete de identificación?*	(PWAY-do vair soo bra-sa-LE-teh day ee-den-tih-fee-cah-see-ON?)
Have you had anything to eat or drink in the last 12 hours?	*¿Ha comido o bebido algo en las últimas doce horas?*	(ah co-MEE-doh oh beh-BEE-doh AL-go en las UL-tee-mas DOH-say OR-as?)
I am going to put a tourniquet on your arm.	*Le voy a poner un torniquete en el brazo.*	(lay boy ah po-NAIR un tor-ne-KAY-tay an el BRAH-so.)
Straighten your arm.	*Enderezca el brazo.*	(en-day-RAYZ-kah el BRAH-so.)
Please make a fist.	*Por favor haga un puño.*	(Por fa-VOR AH-ga oon POON-yo.)
You are going to feel a small prick.	*Usted va a sentir un pequeño pinchazo.*	(oo-STED vah ah sen-TEER oon peh-KEN-yo pean-CHA-so.)
You can relax your fist.	*Usted puede relajar su puño.*	(oo-STED PWAY-day reh-la-HAR soo POON-yo.)
You can remove the bandage after about an hour or so.	*Usted podrá quitarse su vendaje en más o menos una hora.*	(oo-STED poe-DRAH key-TAR-say su ben-DA-hay en mas o MAY-nos oo-na OR-a.)
Do you need me to call an interpreter?	*¿Usted necesita que yo llame a un intérprete?*	(oo-STED nay-say-SEE-ta kay yo YA-meh a un in-TARE-pray-tay?)
You need to give us a urine sample for testing.	*Usted necesita darnos una muestra de su orina para el análisis.*	(oo-STED nay-say-SEE-tah DAR-nohs OO-nah MWAY-strah de soo oh-REEN-ah PAH-rah el ah-NAH-lee-sees.)
I will get the nurse.	*Voy a buscar a la enfermera.*	(Boy ah bus-CAHR ah lah an-fair-MAY-rah.)
Do you understand the instructions?	*¿Entiende usted estas instrucciones?*	(En-tee-EN-day oo-STED ES-tas in-strook-see-O-nays?)

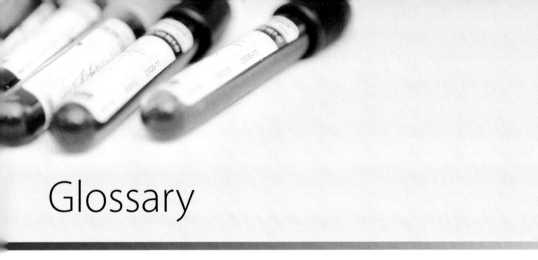

Glossary

Accreditation Process by which a program or institution documents meeting established guidelines

Accuracy Closeness of the measured result to the true value

Acid citrate dextrose (ACD) An additive that contains acid citrate to prevent clotting by binding calcium and dextrose to preserve red blood cells

Adipose (AD i pos) Pertaining to fat cells

Adrenocorticotropic hormone (a DRE no KOR ti ko TROP ik) Hormone produced by the anterior pituitary gland to stimulate secretion of adrenal cortex hormones

Aerosol (ER o SOL) Fine suspension of particles in air

Afferent neuron (AF er ent NU ron) Nerve cell carrying impulses to the brain and spinal cord (sensory neuron)

Airborne precautions (AR born pri KO shunz) Isolation practices associated with airborne diseases

Aldosterone (al DOS ter on) Hormone produced by the adrenal cortex to regulate electrolyte and water balance

Alimentary tract (AL i MEN tar e tract) Digestive tract

Aliquot (Al i kwot) Portion of a sample

Alternative medicine Medical procedures not generally considered to be proven by conventional scientific methods

Alveoli (al VE o li) Air sacs in the lungs where the exchange of O_2 and CO_2 occurs

Amino acids (a ME no AS ids) Building blocks for protein

Amniotic fluid (AM ne o tik FLOO id) Fluid surrounding the fetus in the uterus

Amphiarthrosis (AM fe ar THRO sis) Slightly movable joint

Amylase (AM i las) Pancreatic enzyme to digest starch

Anatomic position (AN a TOM ik po ZISH un) Body position used in anatomic descriptions (the body is erect and facing forward with the arms at the side and the palms facing forward)

Androgen (AN dro jen) Male hormone produced by the adrenal cortex to maintain secondary sex characteristics

Anemia (a NE me a) Deficiency of red blood cells

Antecubital (AN te KU bi tal) Area of the arm opposite the elbow (location of the large veins used in phlebotomy)

Antecubital fossa (AN te KU bi tal FOS a) Indentation of the midarm opposite the elbow (location of the large veins used in phlebotomy)

Anterior (ventral) Pertaining to the front of the body

Antibody (AN ti BOD e) Protein produced by exposure to antigen

Anticoagulant (AN ti ko AG u lant) Substance that prevents blood from clotting

Antidiuretic hormone (AN ti di u RET ik HOR mon) Hormone produced by the posterior pituitary gland to stimulate retention of water by the kidney

Antigen (AN ti jen) Substance that stimulates the formation of antibodies

Antiglycolytic agent (AN ti gli KOL i tik A jent) Substance that prevents the breakdown of glucose

Antiseptic (AN ti SEP tik) Substance that destroys or inhibits the growth of microorganisms

Aortic semilunar valve (a OR tik SEM e LU nar valv) Structure that prevents backflow of blood from the aorta to the left ventricle

Apheresis (a FER e sis) Removal of specific cellular components or plasma from a person's blood

Appendix (a PEN diks) Accessory organ of the digestive system that extends from the cecum

Arachnoid membrane (a RAK noyd MEM bran) Middle layer of the meninges

Arteriole (ar TE re ol) Small arterial branch leading into a capillary

Arteriospasm (ar TE re o spazm) Spontaneous constriction of an artery

Artery (AR ter e) Blood vessel carrying oxygenated blood from the heart to the tissues

Articulation (ar TIK u LA shun) A joint

Aseptic (a SEP tik) Free of contamination by microorganisms

Assault (a SAWLT) Attempt or threat to touch or injure another person

Atrioventricular valve (A tre o ven TRIK u lar valv) Structure that prevents backflow of blood from the right ventricle to the right atrium

Atrium (A tre um) One of two upper chambers of the heart

Autoimmunity (AW to im MU ni te) Condition in which a person produces antibodies that react with the person's own antigens

Autologous donation (aw TOL o gus do NA shun) Donation of a unit of blood designated to be available to the donor during surgery

Autologous transfusion (aw TOL o gus trans FU zhun) Transfusion of a person's own previously donated blood

Autonomic nervous system (aw to NOM ik NER ves SIS tem) System regulating the body's involuntary functions by carrying impulses from the brain and spinal cord to the muscles, glands, and internal organs

Autoverification (aw to VER i fi KA shun) An automated alert of nonmatching current and past patient results

Axon (AK son) Fiber of nerve cells that carries impulses away from the cell body of the neuron

B lymphocytes (LIM fo sits) Lymphocytes that transform into plasma cells to produce antibodies

Bacteria (bak TE re a) One-cell microorganisms

Bacteriology (bak TE re OL o je) The study of bacteria

Bacteriostatic (bak TE re o STAT ik) Capable of inhibiting the growth of bacteria

Bar code Computer identification system

Basal state (BA sal stat) Metabolic condition after 12 hours of fasting and lack of exercise

Basilic vein (ba SIL ik van) Vein located on the underside of the arm

Battery Unauthorized physical contact

Benign (be NIN) Noncancerous

Bevel Area of the needle point that has been cut on a slant

Bicuspid valve (bi KUS pid valv) Structure that prevents backflow of blood from the left ventricle to the left atrium

Bile (bil) Digestive juice to break up fat

Bilirubin (bil i ROO bin) Yellow-pigmented hemoglobin degradation product

Biohazardous (bi o HAZ ir dus) Pertaining to a hazard caused by infectious organisms

Biopsy (BI op se) Removal of a representative tissue for microscopic examination

Blood group Classification based on the presence or absence of A or B antigens on the red blood cells

Body substance isolation Guideline stating that all moist body substances are capable of transmitting disease

Bowman's capsule (BO mans CAP sel) Structure that encloses the glomerulus and collects filtered substances from the blood

Brainstem (BRAN stem) Portion of the brain that consists of the medulla, pons, and midbrain

Bronchioles (BRONG ke olz) Smallest air passageways within the lungs

Buccal (BUK al) Pertaining to the inside of the cheek

Bulbourethral glands (Bul bo u RE thral glanz) Glands on either side of the prostate gland that produce a mucous secretion before ejaculation

Bundle of His (BUN del ov his) Muscle fibers connecting the atria with the ventricles of the heart

Bursa (BUR sa) Sac of synovial fluid located between a tendon and a bone to decrease friction

Butterfly Winged blood collection set used for small veins

Calcaneus (kal KA ne us) Heel bone

Calcitonin (Kal si TO nin) Hormone produced by the thyroid gland to reduce calcium levels in the blood

Calibration (kal i BRA shun) Standardization of an instrument used to perform diagnostic tests

Cannula (Kan u la) Tube that can be inserted into a cavity

Capillary (KAP i LAR e) Small blood vessel connecting arteries and veins that allows the exchange of gases and nutrients between the cells and the blood

Carbaminohemoglobin (kar BAM i no HE mo GLO bin) Carbon dioxide combined with hemoglobin

Carcinogenic (KAR si no JEN ik) Capable of causing cancer

Cardiac muscle (KAR de ak MUS el) Striated muscle of the heart

Cardiologist (kar de OL o jist) Specialist in the study of the heart

Cardiovascular (KAR de o VAS ku lar) Pertaining to the heart and blood vessels

Carpals/metacarpals (KAR palz/ME ta CAR palz) Bones of the wrist and hands

Cartilage (KAR ti lij) Flexible connective tissue surrounded by gel (located where bones come together)

Cast Protein structure formed in the tubules of the kidney

Catheter (KATH e ter) Tube inserted into the body for injecting or withdrawing fluids

Cecum (SE kum) First part of the large intestine

Cell-mediated immunity (sel ME de a ted i MUN i te) Immune response by T lymphocytes to directly destroy foreign antigens

Central nervous system Brain and spinal cord

Central Venous Access Device (SEN tral VE nus AK ses di VIS) Catheter inserted into the superior vena cava

Centrifuge (SEN tri fuj) Instrument that spins test tubes at high speeds to separate the cellular and liquid portions of blood

Cephalic vein (sef a LEK van) Vein located on the thumb side of the arm

Cerebellum (ser e BEL um) Back part of the brain, responsible for voluntary muscle movements and balance

Cerebrospinal fluid (SER e BRO spi nal FLOO id) Fluid surrounding the brain and spinal cord

Cerebrum (SER e brum) Largest part of the brain, responsible for mental processes

Certification Documentation assuring that an individual has met certain professional standards

Chain of custody Documentation of the collection and handling of forensic specimens

Chain of infection Continuous link between six components that makes it possible for infections to occur

Civil lawsuit Court action between individuals, corporations, government bodies, or other organizations (compensation is monetary)

Clot Blood that has coagulated

Clot activator (klot AK ti VA tor) Clot-promoting substance such as glass particles, silica, and celite

Coccyx (KIK siks) Last four of five tiny vertebrae at the base of the spine (tailbone)

Code of Ethics The personal and professional rules of performance and moral behavior as set by members of a profession

Collecting duct Part of the renal tubule that extends from the distal convoluted tubule to the renal pelvis

Collateral circulation (ko LAT er al SER ku LA shun) Additional vessels supplying circulation to a particular area

Compatibility/crossmatch (kom PAT i BIL i ti/KROSS mach) Procedure that matches patient and donor blood before a transfusion

Confidentiality Maintaining the privacy of information

Congenital (kon JEN i tal) Existing at birth but not hereditary

Congenital hypothyroidism (kon JEN i tal HI po THI royd izm) Inadequate thyroid hormone production in newborn infants

Contact precautions Isolation practices to prevent the spread of disease caused by patient contact

Continuing education Maintenance of current knowledge and new additions to ones profession through journals, courses, and workshops

Continuous quality improvement Institutional program focusing on customer expectations

Control Substance of known concentration used to monitor the accuracy of test results

Cortisol (KOR ti sol) Hormone produced by the adrenal cortex to regulate the use of sugars, fats, and proteins by cells

Coumadin (KOO ma din) Anticoagulant monitored by the prothrombin time

Cranium (KRA ne um) Bones of the skull enclosing the brain

Criminal lawsuit Court action brought by the state for committing a crime against public welfare (punishment is imprisonment and/or a fine)

Critical value Laboratory test result critical to patient survival

Cross-training (kross TRA ning) Instruction to acquire additional patient care skills

Cryoprecipitate (KRI o pre SIP i tat) Component of fresh plasma that contains clotting factors

Cultural diversity The integration of language, customs, beliefs, religion, and values

Culture and sensitivity Microbiology test to identify microorganisms and determine antibiotic susceptibility

D-dimer (DI mer) Product of fibrinolysis

Decentralization Performance of procedures in various locations

Defamation Spoken or written words that can damage a person's reputation

Defendant Person against whom a law suit is filed

Delta check Comparison of a patient's current results with previous results

Dendrite (DEN drit) Fiber of nerve cells that carries impulses to the cell body of the neuron

Dermal (DER mal) Pertaining to the skin

Dermis (DER mis) Inner layer of the skin

Diagnosis-related group Government classification of a medical disorder for purposes of cost reimbursement

Diarrhea (di a RE a) Watery stools

Diarthrosis (di ar THRO sis) Freely movable joint

Diastole (di AS to le) Relaxation phase of the heartbeat

Diencephalon (DI en SEF a lon) Second portion of the brain, contains the thalamus and hypothalamus

Digestion (di JES chun) Breakdown of complex foods to simpler forms so that they can be used by cells

Disinfectant (dis in FEKT ant) Substance that destroys microorganisms (usually used on surfaces rather than on skin)

Distal convoluted tubule (DIS tal KON vo LOOT ed TU bul) Part of the renal tubule between the loop of Henle and the collecting duct

Diurnal variation (DI ur nal VAR i A shun) Normal changes in blood constituent levels at different times of the day

Documentation Recording of pertinent information such as test results, quality control, and observations

Droplet precautions Isolation practices to prevent the spread of microorganisms carried in fluid droplets

Duodenum (DU o DE num) First part of the small intestine

Dura mater (DU ra MA ter) Outermost layer of the meninges

Dysmenorrhea (DIS men o RE a) Painful menstruation

Ecchymoses (ek i MO sis) Hemorrhagic discoloration

Edema (e DE ma) Accumulation of fluid in the tissues

Efferent neuron (e FER ent NU ron) Nerve cell carrying impulses away from the brain and spinal cord (motor neuron)

Electrocardiography (e LEK tro KAR de o graf e) Recording of variations in the electrical activity of the heart muscle

Electroencephalography (e lek tro en SEF a lo graf e) Recording of electrical changes in various areas of the brain

Electrolytes (e LEK tro lits) Ions in the blood (primarily sodium, potassium, chloride, and carbon dioxide)

Electrophoresis (e LEK tro for E sis) Method of separation by electrical charge

Endocardium (En do KAR di um) Inner lining of the heart

Endocrine (EN do krin) Pertaining to ductless glands that secrete hormones directly into the bloodstream to affect other organs

Enzyme (EN zime) Protein capable of producing a chemical reaction with a specific substance (substrate)

Epicardium (EP i KAR di um) Outer layer of the heart

Epidermis (EP i DER mis) Outer layer of the skin

Epididymides (EP i DID i me des) Coiled organs of the testes where sperm mature

Epiglottis (EP i GLOT is) Leaf-shaped cartilage that covers the larynx during swallowing

Epinephrine (adrenalin) (EP i NEF rin) Hormone produced by the adrenal medulla to increase heart rate and blood pressure

Erythema (ER i THE ma) Redness from inflammation of the skin

Erythrocyte (e RITH ro sit) Red blood cell

Erythropoietin (e RITH ro POY e tin) Hormone produced by the kidney to increase red blood cell production

Estrogen (ES tro jen) Female hormone produced by the adrenal cortex and the ovaries to maintain secondary sex characteristics

Ethics Principles of personal and professional conduct

Ethylenediamine tetraacetic acid (EDTA) (ETH i len DI a men TET ra A se tic AS id) An anticoagulant that prevents clotting by binding or chelating calcium

Evacuated tubes (e VAK u at ed toobz) Blood collection tubes containing a premeasured amount of vacuum

Examination variables Processes that occur during testing of a sample

Exchange transfusion Removal of blood and replacement with an equal volume of donor blood

Exophthalmos (EKS of THAL mos) Abnormal protrusion of the eyeball

External respiration (EKS tern al res pir A shun) Exchange of O_2 and CO_2 at the lungs

Fallopian tubes (fa LO pe an toobz) Tubes connecting the ovaries and uterus

Fasting Abstinence from food and liquids (except water) for a specified period

Feathered edge Area of the blood smear where the microscopic examination is performed

Feces (FE sez) Waste product of digestion

Femur (FE mur) Long bone of the upper leg

Fertilization (fer TIL i za shun) Union of the sperm and ovum

Fibrin (FI brin) Protein substance produced in the coagulation process to form the foundation of a clot

Fibrinolysis (FI brin OL i sis) Breakdown of a fibrin clot

Fibula (FIB u la) Smaller long bone of the lower leg

First morning specimen The first voided urine specimen collected immediately upon arising; recommended screening specimen

Fistula (FIS tu la) Permanent surgical connection between an artery and a vein (used for dialysis)

Follicle-stimulating hormone (FOL i kel STIM yoo LAT ing HOR mon) Hormone produced by the anterior pituitary gland to stimulate estrogen secretion and egg production by the ovaries and sperm production by the testes

Forensic (for EN sik) Pertaining to legal proceedings

Fresh frozen plasma Plasma collected from a unit of blood and immediately frozen

Frontal (coronal) **plane** (FRUN tal plan) Vertical plane dividing the body into the anterior (front) and the posterior (back) portions

Galactosemia (ga LAK to SE me a) Genetic disorder in which the enzyme needed to metabolize galactose is absent

Gamete (GAM et) Male or female sex cell

Gastrin (GAS trin) Hormone produced by the gastric mucosa to stimulate gastric acid secretion

Gauge Unit of measure assigned to the diameter of a needle bore

Geriatric (JER e AT rik) Pertaining to old age

Gland (gland) Organ that secretes a substance

Glomerulus (glo MER u lus) Collection of capillaries enclosed by the Bowman's capsule where filtration occurs

Glucagon (GLOO ka gon) Hormone produced by the pancreas to stimulate conversion of glycogen to glucose

Glucosuria (GLOO ko SU re a) Glucose in the urine

Glycolysis (gli Kol i sis) Breakdown of glucose

Glycosuria (GLI ko SU re a) Glucose in the urine (glucosuria)

Gonads (GO nads) Ovaries and testes

Gram stain (gram stan) Stain used to classify bacteria

Growth hormone (groth HOR mon) Hormone produced by the anterior pituitary gland to stimulate growth of the bones and tissues

Health-care acquired infection Infection contact by a patient as the result of a hospital stay or an outpatient procedure

Health Insurance Portability and Accountability Act Legislation that guarantees the privacy if individual health information

Hematoma (HE ma TO ma) Discoloration produced by leakage of blood into the tissue

Hematopoiesis (HE ma to poy E sis) Formation of blood cells in the bone marrow

Hematuria/hemoglobinuria (HEM a TU re a/HE mo glo bin U re a) Blood or hemoglobin in the urine

Hemochromatosis (HE mo KRO ma TO sis) Excessive accumulation of iron in the body

Hemoconcentration (HE mo KON sin TRA shun) Increase in the ratio of formed elements to plasma

Hemoglobin (HE mo GLO bin) Red blood cell protein that transports O_2 and CO_2 in the bloodstream

Hemolysis (he MOL i sis) Destruction of red blood cells

Hemolytic disease of the newborn (HE mo LIT ik di ZEZ ov the NU born) Rh incompatibility between mother and fetus that can cause hemolysis of fetal red blood cells

Hemostasis (he MOS ta sis) Stoppage of blood flow from a damaged blood vessel

Hemostat (HE mo stat) Surgical clamp

Heparin (HEP a rin) An anticoagulant that prevents clotting by inhibiting thrombin

Heparin lock (HEP a rin lok) Device inserted into a vein for administering medications and collecting blood

Homeostasis (HO me o STA sis) State of equilibrium in the body

Hormone (HOR mon) Substance produced by a ductless gland and transported to parts of the body via the blood to control and regulate body functions

Hub The part of the needle that attaches to the syringe or blood collection holder

Human chorionic gonadotropin (HU man KO re on ic GON a do TRO pin) Hormone produced by the placenta during pregnancy to stimulate the ovaries to produce estrogen and progesterone

Humerus (HU mer us) Long bone of the upper arm

Humoral immunity (HU mor al i MU ni ti) Immune response that produces antibodies

Hyperbilirubinemia (HI per BIL i roo bin E me a) Increased serum bilirubin

Hyperglycemia (HI per gli SE me a) Elevated glucose levels in the blood

Hypodermic (HI po DER mik) Under the skin

Hypodermic needle (HI po DER mik NE del) Type of needle that attaches to a syringe

Hypotension (HI po TEN shun) Low blood pressure

Hypothalamus (HI po THAL a mus) Part of the brain that regulates body temperature and the secretions of the pituitary gland

Hypothyroidism (HI po THI royd izm) Reduced thyroid function

Iatrogenic (I at ro JEN ic) Pertaining to a condition caused by treatment, medications, or diagnostic procedures

Icteric (ik TER ik) Appearing yellow

Identification band Bracelet worn by patients that contains specific identification information

Ileum (IL e um) Last part of the small intestine

Immunochemistry (IM u no KEM is tre) Chemical analysis performed using antigens and antibodies

Immunoglobulin (IM u no GLOB u lin) Another name for antibody

Immunohematology (i mu no HEM TOL o je) The study of blood cell antigens and their antibodies

Immunology (IM u NOL o je) The study of the immune system

Incident report Detailed report of a condition that affected patient care or worker safety, documenting the incident and actions taken

Indwelling line Tube inserted into an artery or vein (primarily for administering fluids)

Infection (in FEK shun) Multiplication of microorganisms in body tissues

Infection control Procedures to control and monitor infections within an institution

Inferior Pertaining to a position below another structure

Inferior vena cava (in FE re or VE na CA va) Vein that transports blood from the lower body back to the heart

Informed consent Patient's right to know the method and risks before agreeing to treatment

Insertion (in SUR shun) Movable attachment point of a muscle to a bone

Insulin (IN su lin) Hormone produced by the pancreas to promote the use of glucose by the body

Internal respiration (in TUR nal res pir A shun) Exchange of O_2 and CO_2 between the blood and the cells of the body

International normalized ratio Standardized prothrombin time reporting system to equate results among reagent manufacturers

Interneuron (IN ter NU ron) Nerve cell entirely within the central nervous system

Interstitial fluid (IN ter STISH al FLOO id) Fluid located in the spaces between cells

Invasion of privacy Unauthorized release of information

Iontophoresis (i ON to fo RE sis) Electrical stimulation of soluble salt ions used in the collection of sweat electrolyte specimens

Isoenzyme (I so EN zim) Specific form of an enzyme

Jaundiced (JAWN dist) Appearing yellow

Jejunum (je JU num) Second part of the small intestine

Keratin (KER a tin) Tough protein found in the outer skin, hair, and nails

Ketonuria (ke to NU re a) Ketones in the urine

Labile (LA bil) Biologically or chemically unstable

Laboratory reference manual Document providing laboratory information to other areas of the hospital

Larynx (LAR inks) Organ between the pharynx and the trachea containing the vocal cords

Lean Management system focusing on elimination of waste

Leukemia (loo KEE me a) Malignant overproduction of white blood cells

Leukocyte (LOO ko sit) White blood cell

Libel Published writing that can damage a person's reputation

Ligament (LIG a ment) Fibrous connective tissue that binds bones together at the joint

Lipase (LI pas) Pancreatic enzyme that digests fats

Lipemia (li PE me a) Increased lipid content in the blood

Lipemic (li PE mic) Pertaining to turbidity (appears cloudy white) from lipids

Litigation Law suit

Local anesthetic (LO kal AN es THET ik) Substance that paralyzes nerve endings in the area of the injection

Loop of Henle (loop ov HEN le) Part of the renal tubule between the proximal convoluted tubule and the distal convoluted tubule

Lot Group of products manufactured at the same time under the same conditions

Lumbar puncture (LUM bar PUNK chur) Procedure used to remove cerebrospinal fluid from the lower spine

Luer tip (LU er tip) Part of a syringe that attaches to the needle

Lumen (LU men) Cavity of an organ or tube, such as a blood vessel or a needle

Luteinizing hormone (LU te in i zing HOR mon) Hormone produced by the anterior pituitary gland to stimulate ovulation

Lymph (limf) Fluid in the lymphatic vessels

Lymph node (limf nod) Lymph tissue that filters lymph as it passes to the circulatory system

Lymphedema (limf e DE ma) Retention of excess lymph fluid

Lymphokines (LIM fo kinz) Chemicals released by activated T cells that attract macrophages

Lymphostasis (LIM FOS ta sis) Stoppage of lymph flow

Macrophage (MAK ro faj) Cell derived from monocytes capable of phagocytosis of pathogens, damaged cells, and old red blood cells

Magnetic "flea" (mag NET ik flee) Small metal filing

Malignant (ma LIG nant) Cancerous

Malpractice Medical care that does not meet a reasonable standard and results in harm

Mastectomy (mas TEK to me) Excision of the breast

Median cubital vein (ME de an KU bi tal van) Vein located in the center of the antecubital area

Medulla oblongata (me DUL la OB long GA ta) Part of the brain that regulates heart rate, respiration, and blood pressure

Melanin (MEL a nin) Black pigment in the outer skin

Melanocyte-stimulating hormone (MEL an o sit STIM yoo LAT ing HOR mon) Hormone produced by the anterior pituitary gland to stimulate pigmentation of the skin

Melatonin (Mel a TO nin) Hormone produced by the pineal gland that influences circadian rhythms

Meninges (men IN jez) Protective membranes around the brain and spinal cord

Menopause (MEN o pawz) Permanent end of the monthly menstrual cycle

Menstruation (men stroo A shun) Monthly shedding of the uterine lining

Metabolic (MET a BOL ik) Pertaining to the chemical changes taking place in the body

Microbiology (MI kro bi OL o je) The study of microorganisms

Microorganism (mi kro OR gan izm) One-cell organism such as a bacterium or virus

Microsample A sample less than 1 mL in size

Midsagittal plane (mid SAJ i tal plan) Vertical plane dividing the body into equal right and left portions

Mitosis (mi TO sis) Cell division

Mitral valve (MI tral valv) Valve between the left atrium and left ventricle of the heart

Mnemonics (ne MON iks) Memory-aiding abbreviations

Multisample needle Type of needle that attaches to a holder to collect multiple blood collection tubes

Mycology (mi KOL o je) The study of fungi

Myelin sheath (MI el in) Tissue around the axon of the peripheral nerves

Myocardium (mi o KAR de um) Muscle layer of the heart

Necrosis (ne KRO sis) Death of cells

Negligence Failure to perform duties according to accepted standards

Neonatal (NE o NA tal) Pertaining to the first 4 weeks after birth

Nephron (NEF ron) Functional unit of the kidney that forms urine

Neuroglia (nu ROG le a) Connective tissue cells of the nervous system that do not carry impulses

Neuron (NU ron) Nerve cell

Norepinephrine (noradrenalin) (nor EP i nef rin) Hormone produced by the adrenal medulla to constrict blood vessels and increase blood pressure

Nosocomial infection (NOS o KO me al in FEK shun) Infection acquired in the hospital

Occluded (o KLUD ed) Obstructed

Olfactory receptors (ol FAK to re re SEP tors) Sensory receptors in the nasal cavity that provide the sense of smell

Opt-out-screening Patients have the right to refuse routine testing for HIV

Origin (or i JIN) Stationary attachment point of a muscle to a bone

Osteoblast (OS te o blast) Bone-producing cell

Osteochondritis (OS te o kon DRI tis) Inflammation of bone and cartilage

Osteoclast (OS te o klast) Bone-resorbing cell

Osteomyelitis (OS te o MI el i tis) Inflammation of the bone caused by infection

Ovaries (O va rez) Female gonads that produce ova

Ovulation (OV u LA shun) Release of the egg cell from the ovary

Ovum (pl. ova) (O vum) Female reproductive cell

Oxyhemoglobin (OK se HE mo GLO bin) Hemoglobin with O_2 attached

Oxytocin (OK se TO sin) Hormone produced by the posterior pituitary gland to stimulate contraction of the uterus at delivery and the release of milk into the breast ducts

Package insert Testing procedure information provided by the manufacturer of the testing materials

Packed cells Blood from which the plasma has been removed

Palmar (PAL mar) Pertaining to the palm of the hand

Palpation (pal pi TA shun) Examination by touch

Parasitology (PAR a si TOL o je) The study of parasites

Parathyroid hormone (par a THI royd HOR mon) Hormone produced by the parathyroid gland to regulate calcium levels in the blood

Partial pressure Amount of pressure exerted by an individual gas within a mixture of gases

Pathogen (PATH o jen) Microorganism capable of producing disease

Pathology (pa THOL o je) Branch of medicine specializing in the study of disease

Patient's Bill of Rights Document written by the American Hospital Association stating the patient's rights during treatment

Patient Care Partnership A revision of the Patient's Bill of rights

Patient-focused care Patient care that does not require transporting the patient to various locations

Patient Safety Goals Document published by the JC to better protect patients from medical errors

Peak level specimen Specimen collected when a serum drug level is highest

Pericardium (per i KAR de um) Membrane surrounding the heart

Peripheral nervous system (per IF er al NER ves SIS tem) All nerves outside the brain and spinal cord

Peristalsis (per i STAL sis) Wavelike muscular contractions to propel material through the digestive tract

Peritoneum (PER i to NE um) Membrane lining the abdominal cavity

Personal protective equipment Apparel worn to prevent contact with and transmission of pathogenic microorganisms

Petechiae (pe TE ke e) Small red spots appearing on the skin

Phagocytosis (FAG o si TO sis) Ingestion of bacteria or other foreign particles by a cell

Pharynx (FAR inks) Tubelike structure located behind the nose that is a passageway for air and food (throat)

Phenylalanine (Fen il AL a nin) Naturally occurring amino acid

Phenylketonuria (FEN il KE to NU re a) Presence of abnormal phenylalanine metabolites in the urine

Phlebotomy (fle BOT o me) Puncture or incision into a vein to obtain blood

Pia mater (PE a MA ter) Innermost layer of the meninges

Pilocarpine (PI lo KAR pin) Sweat-inducing chemical

Plaintiff Person who files a lawsuit

Plantar (PLAN tar) Pertaining to the sole of the foot

Plasma (PLAZ ma) Liquid portion of blood

Plasma cell (PLAZ ma cel) Cell derived from an activated B cell that produces antibodies to a specific antigen

Plasma separator tube (PST) Type of collection tube that contains a polymer gel that separates blood cells from the plasma when centrifuged

Platelet (PLAT let) Small, irregularly shaped disk formed from particles of a very large cell in the bone marrow called the megakaryocyte

Platelet plug (PLAT let plug) Initial blockage of a vascular puncture by platelets

Pleura (PLOO ra) Double-folded membrane surrounding each lung

Pneumatic tube system (nu MAT ik toob SIS tem) Air-driven transport system

Point-of-care testing Laboratory tests performed in the patient care area

Polycythemia (POL e si THE me a) Markedly increased numbers of red blood cells

Polydipsia (POL e DIP se a) Excessive thirst

Polymer gel (POL i mer jel) Substance that undergoes a temporary change in viscosity during centrifugation to create a barrier between cells and plasma or serum

Polyphagia (POL e FA je a) Excessive desire to eat

Polyuria (POL e U re a) Marked increase in the urine flow

Pons (ponz) Part of the brain stem that influences respiration

Postexaminational variables Processes that affect the reporting and interpretation of test results

Postexposure prophylaxis (post ik SPO zhur pro fi LAK sis) Preventive measures taken when a person is exposed to infectious disease

Posterior (dorsal) Pertaining to the back of the body

Postprandial (post PRAN de al) After eating

Potassium oxalate (po TAS e um OK sa lat) An anticoagulant that prevents clotting by binding calcium

Precision Reproducibility of a test result

Preexamination variables Processes that occur before collection of a sample

Procedure manual Detailed documentation of procedures and methods used in performing tests

Professionalism (pro FESH in a LIZ em) Conduct and qualities that typify a professional

Proficiency testing Performance of tests on specimens provided by an external monitoring agency

Progesterone (pro JES ter on) Female hormone produced by the adrenal cortex and the ovaries to promote conditions suitable for pregnancy

Prolactin (pro LAK tin) Hormone produced by the anterior pituitary gland to stimulate breast development and milk secretion

Prostate gland (PROS tat gland) Gland that surrounds the first inch of the male urethra and secretes an alkaline fluid to maintain sperm motility

Proteinuria (PRO te in U re a) Protein (albumin) in the urine

Prothrombin (pro THROM bin) Protein converted to thrombin in the coagulation process

Proximal convoluted tubule (PROK sim al KON vo LOOT ed TU bul) Part of the renal tubule between the Bowman's capsule and the loop of Henle

Pulmonary circulation (PUL mo ne re) Flow of blood from the heart to the lungs and back to the heart

Pulmonary semilunar valve (PUL mo ne re SEM e LU nar valv) Structure that prevents backflow of blood from the pulmonary arteries to the right ventricle

Pulse (puls) Measurement of the rhythm of ventricle contraction

Quality assessment Methods used to guarantee quality patient care

Quality control Methods used to monitor the accuracy of procedures

Quality Essentials A document containing information needed to perform quality laboratory work

Quality indicators Procedures to monitor each phase of testing

Quality Management System A plan to ensure quality results, staff competence, and organizational efficiency

Radioactivity (RA de o AK TIV i te) Emission of radiant energy

Radioisotope (RA de o I so top) Substance that emits radiant energy

Radius (RA de us) Shorter bone of the lower arm located on the lateral or thumb side

Reagent (re A jent) Substance used to produce a chemical reaction

Reagent strip/dipstick (re A jent strip/dip stik) Chemical- impregnated plastic strip used for analysis of urine

Rectum (REK tum) End part of the colon

Renal (RE nal) Pertaining to the kidney

Renal dialysis (RE nal di AL i sis) Procedure to remove waste products from the blood when the kidneys are not functioning

Renin (REN in) Hormone produced by the kidney to increase blood pressure

Requisition Form detailing orders for patient testing

Respiration rate (res pir A shun rat) Number of breaths per minute

Right lymphatic duct (rit lim FAT ik dukt) Duct that collects the lymph fluid from the upper right quadrant to return it to the blood

Risk Management A hospital department that develops policies to protect patients and workers

Root cause analysis Evaluation of the causative factors of variation in performance

Sacrum (SA krum) Five fused sacral vertebrae at the base of the spine

Sagittal plane (SAJ i tal plan) Vertical plane dividing the body into left and right portions

Sample One or more parts taken from a system

Sarcoma (sar KO ma) Malignant tumor containing embryonic connective tissue

Scapula (SKAP u la) Flat bone forming the back of the shoulder (shoulder blade)

Sclerosed (skle ROST) Hardened

Scrotum (SKRO tum) Sac that contains the male testes

Sebaceous gland (se BA shus) Oil-producing gland

Sebum (SE bum) Oily secretion of the sebaceous gland

Semen (SE men) Fluid containing spermatozoa

Seminal vesicles (SEM i nal VES i kalz) Glands that secrete alkaline fluid that becomes part of semen

Sentinel event An unanticipated death or permanent loss of function not related to a patient's illness or underlying condition

Septicemia (sep ti SE me a) Pathogenic microorganisms in the blood

Septum (SEP tum) Partition between the right and left sides of the heart

Serology (se ROL o je) The study of serum

Serum (SE rum) Clear yellow fluid that remains after clotted blood has been centrifuged and separated

Serum separator tube (SST) Type of collection tube that contains a polymer gel that separates the blood cells from the serum when centrifuged

Shaft The long portion of the needle

Shift Abrupt change in the mean of quality control results

Shock Sudden decrease in blood flow interfering with heart and tissue function

Sinoatrial node (SIN o A tre al nod) Mass of pacer cells considered the dominant pacemaker of the heart

Six Sigma A statistical method to reduce variables and decrease errors

Skeletal muscle (SKEL e tal MUS el) Striated voluntary muscle that moves bones

Slander False and malicious spoken words

Smooth muscle Unstriated involuntary muscle of the internal organs and blood vessels

Sodium citrate (SO de um SIT rate) An anticoagulant that prevents clotting by binding calcium

Sodium fluoride (SO de um FLOO rid) An additive that preserves glucose and inhibits microbial growth

Sodium polyanethol sulfonate (SPS) (SO de um POL e AN thol SUL fan at) An anticoagulant that prevents clotting by binding calcium and inhibits the actions of complement, phagocytosis, and certain antibiotics

Specimen Portion of a body fluid or tissue taken for examination such as an aliquot of plasma or serum

Spermatozoa (SPER mat o ZO a) Sperm cells/male gametes

Sphygmomanometer (SFIG mo man OM et er) Instrument that measures blood pressure

Standard precautions Guidelines describing personnel protective practices

Standard of Care Skill and knowledge requirements to perform patient care set up by regulatory and professional organizations

Steady state A 30-minute period of controlled stable oxygen consumption and no physical exercise

Sterile (STER il) Free of microorganisms

Sternum (STER num) Breastbone (alternate site for the collection of bone marrow specimens)

Stethoscope (STETH o skop) Instrument used for listening to sounds produced within the body

Stratum corneum (STRA tum KOR ne um) Outermost layer of the epidermis, consisting of dead cells filled with keratin

Stratum germinativum (STRA tum JER mi na tev um) Innermost layer of the epidermis in which cell division occurs

Streptokinase (STREP to KI nas) Clot lysis activator

Striated (STRI a ted) Marked with grooves or stripes

Subcutaneous layer (SUB ku TA ne us LA er) Innermost layer of skin, composed of connective tissue and fat

Sudoriferous gland (su dor IF er us gland) Sweat-producing gland

Superficial On the surface

Superior Pertaining to a position above another structure

Superior vena cava (soo PE re or VE na CA va) Vein that transports blood from the upper body back to the heart

Supine (su PIN) Lying on the back

Surfactant (sur FAK tant) Fluid that coats the walls of alveoli to reduce surface tension and allow inflation

Sweat electrolytes test (swet e LEK tro litz) Diagnostic test for the detection of cystic fibrosis

Synapse (SIN aps) Point at which an impulse is transmitted from one neuron to another

Synarthrosis (SIN ar THRO sis) Immovable joint

Syncope (SIN ko pe) Fainting

Synovial (sin O ve al) Pertaining to lubricating fluid secreted by membranes in joint capsules

Systemic circulation (sis TEM ik SER ku LA shun) Flow of blood between the heart and the tissues

Systole (SIS to le) Contraction phase of the heartbeat

T lymphocytes (LIM fo sits) Lymphocytes that act directly on an antigen to destroy it

Tachometer (tak O met er) Instrument for measuring speed

Tarsals/metatarsals (TAR salz/ ME ta TAR salz) Bones of the ankles and feet

Tendon (TEN dun) Connective tissue that binds muscles to bones

Testes (TES tes) Male gonads that produce sperm

Testosterone (tes TOS ter on) Hormone produced by the testes that is responsible for the development of male sexual characteristics

Thalamus (THAl a mus) Part of the brain that regulates subconscious sensations

Therapeutic phlebotomy Collection of a unit of blood performed as a patient treatment

Thoracic (tho RAS ik) Pertaining to the chest

Thoracic duct (tho RAS ik dukt) Duct that collects the lymph from the lower body and upper left quadrant to return it to the blood

Thrombin (THROM bin) Enzyme that converts fibrinogen to fibrin

Thrombocyte (THROM bo sit) Cell involved with clotting (platelet)

Thrombolytic therapy (throm bo LIT ik THER a pe) Administration of medication to enhance clot lysis

Thrombosis (throm BO sis) Formation of blood clots within the vascular system

Thrombus (THROM bus) Clot formed on the inner wall of a vein

Thymosin (THI mo sin) Hormone produced by the thymus gland for the maturation of T cells

Thyroid-stimulating hormone (THI royd STIM yoo LAT ing HOR mon) Hormone produced by the anterior pituitary gland to stimulate secretion of thyroid hormones

Thyroxine (thi ROKS in) Hormone produced by the thyroid gland to stimulate metabolism of cells

Tibia (TIB e a) Larger long bone of the lower leg

Tonicity (to NIS i te) Active resistance to stretching in muscles (maintains posture)

Tort Wrongful act committed by one person against another person or property

Total quality management Institutional policy to provide customer satisfaction

Toxicology (TOKS i KOL o je) Study of poisons

Trachea (TRA ke a) Organ that provides the opening between the larynx and the bronchi

Transmission-based precautions Isolation procedures based on airborne, droplet, and contact disease transmission

Transverse plane (trans VERS plan) Horizontal plane dividing the body into upper and lower portions

Trend (trend) Gradual change above or below the mean of quality control results

Tricuspid valve (tri KUS pid valv) Valve between the right atrium and right ventricle

Triiodothyronine (TRI i O do THI ro nen) Hormone produced by the thyroid gland to stimulate metabolism of cells

Trough level specimen Specimen collected when a serum drug level is lowest

Tunica adventitia (TU ni ka AD ven TISH e a) Outer layer of blood vessels, composed of connective tissue

Tunica intima (TU ni ka IN ti ma) Inner layer of blood vessels, composed of endothelial cells

Tunica media (TU ni ka ME de a) Middle layer of blood vessels, composed of smooth muscle tissue

Turn-around-time Amount of time between the request for a test and the reporting of results

Ulna (UL na) Larger long bone of the forearm opposite the thumb

Umbilicus (um bi LI kus) The navel

Unit of blood 405 to 495 mL of blood collected from a donor for a transfusion

Universal precautions Guideline stating that all patients are capable of transmitting bloodborne disease

Uremia (u RE me a) Increased urea in the blood

Ureters (U re terz) Tubes that carry urine from the kidney to the bladder

Urethra (u RE thra) Organ that carries urine from the bladder to the outside of the body

Urinalysis (U ri NAL i sis) Physical, chemical, and microscopic analysis of urine

Urokinase (u ro KI nas) Clot lysis activator

Uterus (U ter us) Female organ that forms a placenta to nourish a developing embryo

Valve Structure in veins and the heart that closes an opening so blood will flow in only one direction

Variable Measurable condition used to evaluate the quality of patient care or laboratory specimens

Vas deferens (vas DEF er enz) Tube that carries sperm from the epididymides to the ejaculatory duct

Vascular (VAS ku lar) Pertaining to blood vessels

Vasovagal reaction (VAS o VA gal re AK shun) Stimulation of the blood vessels by the vagus nerve

Vector (VEK tor) Carrier that transfers an infective agent from one host to another

Vein (van) Blood vessel carrying deoxygenated blood from the tissues to the heart

Ventilation device (VEN ti LA shun di VIS) Apparatus to control the amount of oxygen inhaled

Ventricle (Ven trik l) One of two lower chambers of the heart

Venule (VEN ul) Small vein leading from a capillary to a vein

Virology (vi ROL o je) The study of viruses

Visceral (VIS er al) Pertaining to organs within a body cavity

Volar (VO lar) Pertaining to the palm side of the forearm

Waived test Laboratory test requiring no special training

Winged blood collection set A stainless steel needle and tubing apparatus attached to plastic wings

Zone of Comfort The amount of distance between two people when communicating

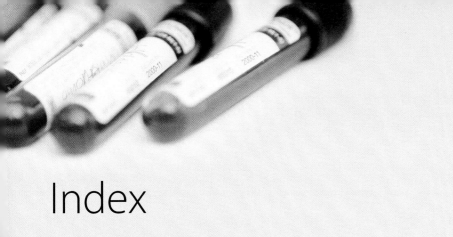

Index